Hemodialysis
High-Efficiency Treatments

CONTEMPORARY ISSUES IN NEPHROLOGY

VOLUME 27

Series Editor
Jay H. Stein, M.D.

Series Editors, Vols. 1-21
Barry M. Brenner, M.D.
Jay H. Stein, M.D.

Volumes Already Published

VOLUME 3
Immunologic Mechanisms of Renal Disease
Curtis B. Wilson, M.D., Guest Editor

VOLUME 4
Hormonal Function and the Kidney

VOLUME 7
Chronic Renal Failure

VOLUME 9
Nephrotic Syndrome

VOLUME 11
Divalent Ion Homeostasis

VOLUME 12
Pediatric Nephrology
Bruce M. Tune, M.D., and Stanley A. Mendoza, M.D., Guest Editors

VOLUME 13
The Heart and Renal Disease
Robert A. O'Rourke, M.D., Guest Editor

VOLUME 14
The Progressive Nature of Renal Disease
William E. Mitch, M.D., Guest Editor

VOLUME 15
Modern Techniques of Ion Transport

VOLUME 16
Body Fluid Homeostasis

VOLUME 17
Pharmacotherapy of Renal Disease and Hypertension
William M. Bennett, M.D., and David A. McCarron, M.D., Guest Editors

VOLUME 18
Immunopathology of Renal Disease
Curtis B. Wilson, M.D., Guest Editor

VOLUME 19
Renal Transplantation
Edgar L. Milford, M.D., Guest Editor

VOLUME 20
The Kidney in Diabetes Mellitus

VOLUME 21
Atrial Natriuretic Peptides

VOLUME 22
Peritoneal Dialysis
Zbylut J. Twardowski, M.D., Karl D. Nolph, M.D., F.R.C.P.S. (Glasgow), and Ramesh Khanna, M.D., Guest Editors

VOLUME 23
Hormones, Autacoids, and the Kidney
Stanley Goldfarb, M.D., and Fuad N. Ziyadeh, M.D., Guest Editors

VOLUME 24
Lipids and Renal Disease
William F. Keane, M.D., Guest Editor

VOLUME 25
Diagnostic Techniques in Renal Disease
Robert G. Narins, M.D., Guest Editor

VOLUME 26
The Progressive Nature of Renal Disease, 2nd Ed.
William E. Mitch, M.D., Guest Editor

Hemodialysis
High-Efficiency Treatments

Guest Editor
JUAN P. BOSCH, M.D., F.A.C.P., F.A.C.N.
Professor
Division of Renal Diseases and Hypertension
Department of Medicine
The George Washington University School of Medicine
and Health Sciences
Director
Division of Renal Diseases and Hypertension
Department of Medicine
The George Washington University Medical Center
Washington, DC

Series Editor
JAY H. STEIN, M.D.
Professor and Chairman
Department of Medicine
Dan F. Parman Chair in Medicine
University of Texas Medical School at San Antonio
San Antonio, Texas

CHURCHILL LIVINGSTONE
New York, Edinburgh, London, Madrid, Melbourne, Tokyo

Library of Congress Cataloging-in-Publication Data

Hemodialysis : high-efficiency treatments / guest editor, Juan P. Bosch.
p. cm. — (Contemporary issues in nephrology ; v. 27)
Includes bibliographical references and index.
ISBN 0-443-08848-9
1. Hemodialysis. I. Bosch, Juan P. II. Series: Contemporary issues in nephrology ; vol. 27.
[DNLM: 1. Hemodialysis. 2. Kidney Diseases—complications. 3. Kidney Diseases—therapy. W1 C0769MR v. 27]
RC901.7.H45H45 1993
617.4'61059—dc20
DNLM/DLC
for Library of Congress 92-48307
CIP

Distributed in the United Kingdom by Churchill Livingstone, Robert Stevenson House, 1–3 Baxter's Place, Leith Walk, Edinburgh EH1 3AF, and by associated companies, branches, and representatives throughout the world.

Accurate indications, adverse reactions, and dosage schedules for drugs are provided in this book, but it is possible that they may change. The reader is urged to review the package information data of the manufacturers of the medications mentioned.

The Publishers have made every effort to trace the copyright holders for borrowed material. If they have inadvertently overlooked any, they will be pleased to make the necessary arrangements at the first opportunity.

Acquisitions Editor: *Robert A. Hurley*
Copy Editor: *Lorene Johnson*
Production Designer: *Maryann King*
Production Supervisor: *Jeanine Furino*

Printed in the United States of America

First published in 1993 7 6 5 4 3 2

A Mis Padres

J.P.B.

Contributors

Sergio R. Acchiardo, M.D.
Professor and Medical Director, Division of Nephrology, Department of Medicine, Artificial Kidney Medical Center, University of Tennessee, Memphis, College of Medicine, Memphis, Tennessee

Juan P. Bosch, M.D., F.A.C.P., F.A.C.N.
Professor, Division of Renal Diseases and Hypertension, Department of Medicine, The George Washington University School of Medicine and Health Sciences; Director, Division of Renal Diseases and Hypertension, Department of Medicine, The George Washington University Medical Center, Washington, D.C.

Alessandra Brendolan, M.D.
Assistant Clinical Nephrologist, Department of Nephrology, St. Bortolo Hospital, Vicenza, Italy

George W. Buffaloe, Ph.D.
Senior Scientist, Renal Care Division, Department of Research and Development, COBE Laboratories Incorporated, Lakewood, Colorado

Allan J. Collins, M.D.
Assistant Professor, Department of Medicine, University of Minnesota Medical School—Minneapolis; Executive Director, Metropolitan Dialysis Division, The Regional Kidney Disease Program, Minneapolis, Minnesota

Carlo Crepaldi, M.D.
Assistant Clinical Nephrologist, Department of Nephrology, St. Bortolo Hospital, Vicenza, Italy

Pang-Yen Fan, M.D.
Fellow, Division of Nephrology, Department of Medicine, Duke University School of Medicine, Durham, North Carolina

Babatunde Fariyike, M.D.
Fellow, Division of Nephrology and Hypertension, Department of Medicine, Beth Israel Medical Center, New York, New York

John R. Gleason, M.D.
Fellow, Division of Nephrology, Department of Medicine, and Fellow, Kidney Disease Program, University of Louisville School of Medicine; Louisville, Kentucky

Thomas A. Golper, M.D.
Professor, Department of Medicine, and Director, Dialysis Related Services, Kidney Disease Program, University of Louisville School of Medicine, Louisville, Kentucky

Lee W. Henderson, M.D.
Vice President, Renal Division, Department of Scientific Affairs, Baxter Healthcare Corporation, Round Lake, Illinois

Paul L. Kimmel. M.D.
Professor, Division of Renal Diseases and Hypertension, Department of Medicine, The George Washington University School of Medicine and Health Sciences; Attending Physician, Division of Renal Diseases and Hypertension, Department of Medicine, The George Washington University Medical Center, Washington, D.C.

Peter Konstantin, Ph.D.
Vice President, Department of Research and Development, Fresenius AG, St. Wendel, Germany

Ingrid Ledebo, Ph.D.
Manager, International Scientific Support, Gambro Renal Division, Lund, Sweden

Nathan W. Levin, M.D.
Professor, Department of Medicine, Mount Sinai School of Medicine of the City University of New York; Chief, Division of Nephrology and Hypertension, Department of Medicine, Beth Israel Medical Center, New York, New York

Susie Q. Lew, M.D.
Assistant Professor, Division of Renal Diseases and Hypertension, Department of Medicine, The George Washington University School of Medicine and Health Sciences, Washington, D.C.

Atef Wadie B. Morcos, M.D.
Postgraduate Researcher, Division of Nephrology, Department of Medicine, University of California, Los Angeles, UCLA School of Medicine, Los Angeles, California

Allen R. Nissenson, M.D.
Professor, Department of Medicine, and Director, Dialysis Program, University of California, Los Angeles, UCLA School of Medicine, Los Angeles, California

Terry M. Phillips, Ph.D., D.Sc.
Professor, Division of Renal Diseases and Hypertension, Department of Medicine, The George Washington University School of Medicine and Health Sciences; Director, Immunochemistry Laboratory, The George Washington University Medical Center, Washington, D.C.

Claudio Ronco, M.D.
Associate Clinical Nephrologist, Department of Nephrology, St. Bortolo Hospital, Vicenza, Italy

Steve J. Schwab, M.D.
Associate Professor, Department of Medicine, Duke University School of Medicine; Associate Director and Clinical Director, Division of Nephrology, Department of Medicine, Duke University Medical Center, Durham, North Carolina

Manuel T. Velasquez, M.D.
Associate Professor, Division of Renal Diseases and Hypertension, Department of Medicine, The George Washington University School of Medicine and Health Sciences; Attending Physician, Division of Renal Diseases and Hypertension, Department of Medicine, The George Washington University Medical Center, Washington, DC

Hieronymus H. Vincent
Department of Internal Medicine and Nephrology, St. Anthony's Hospital, Mieuwegein, The Netherlands

Margreet C. Vos
Department of Microbiology, St. Elizabeth's Hospital, Tilburg, The Netherlands

Preface

When I was asked to be the guest editor on a volume dedicated to hemodialysis in this prestigious series, *Contemporary Issues in Nephrology*, I was very pleased. Finally, hemodialysis, an important area of nephrology, was going to be represented in the series. The original idea was to have this volume dedicated to *advances in hemodialysis*. Ultimately, the emphasis of the monograph changed to reflect the global rapid diffusion of high-efficiency treatments. The volume is now divided into two sections: "High-Efficiency Treatments: A Guide for the Practitioner," and "Advances in Hemodialysis."

In the first section, all aspects of high-efficiency treatments are covered with an emphasis on the how to approach. First, the technical advances that made high-efficiency treatments possible are described: bicarbonate dialysate, high blood flows during the treatment, and the new equipment available to perform these therapies. These topics are followed by a description of each of the high-efficiency treatments currently available: high-efficiency hemodialysis, high-flux hemodialysis, and hemodiafiltration. In each of these treatments the dialyzer and equipment specifications are included. The issues related to prescription of high-efficiency treatments as well as the issues of treatment actually delivered to the patient are also emphasized. The section ends with a variety of issues, such as water quality, drug clearances, treatment of anemia, and biocompatibility which are of critical importance for a successful program of high-efficiency treatments.

In the second section, several practical issues are covered by well-known experts: the treatment of hypertension in dialysis patients, the complication of metabolic alkalosis in hemodialysis patients, sleep apnea, and the relevance of cytokines for extracorporeal therapy.

As you can see the essential bricks to build your knowledge in the area of high-efficiency treatments are included. I hope that the efforts of my collaborators will help you deliver the best treatment for your patients.

Juan P. Bosch, M.D., F.A.C.P., F.A.C.N.

Contents

1

The Evolution of High-Efficiency Treatments from Conventional Hemodialysis

Juan P. Bosch

INTRODUCTION

The decade since the early 1980s has seen the culmination of a series of technical developments in the field of hemodialysis. The result of these innovations has been the clinical introduction of the so-called high-efficiency hemodialysis treatments (the term *high-efficiency* refers to solute [urea] clearances in excess of 170 to 180 ml/min. These hemodialysis techniques have become rapidly accepted and widely used throughout the United States and the world.

There are powerful reasons why this expansion has taken place. First and foremost, patients have always wanted a shorter treatment time since the time spent on therapy is an important factor in their rehabilitation. A treatment time of 3 hours or less would significantly add to their quality of life. Second, a reduction in treatment time has an important impact on the cost of the procedure, especially in industrialized countries, where the personnel expense exceeds the cost of materials and overhead. Third—and this is perhaps the most understated advantage of these therapies—high-efficiency treatments may provide the same amount of therapy as conventional treatments in a shorter time. In addition, by increasing the range (i.e., molecular size) of solutes removed, these treatments may approximate the function of the human kidney. Thus, for the first time nephrologists may prescribe and administer a "greater dose of a more physiologic hemodialysis" in an acceptable period of time and examine the outcome of such a strategy. It is likely therefore, that use of these high-efficiency treatments will continue to expand throughout the world, and in the future these new techniques will probably replace conventional hemodialysis as the main form of treatment for patients with chronic renal failure.

BACKGROUND

In the 1970s it was clearly demonstrated that in acetate hemodialysis the dialysance of total carbon dioxide (bicarbonate) was identical to that of urea nitrogen[1] (Fig. 1-1). The amount of a given solute removed during dialysis is proportional to its dialysance or clearance

(solute removal rate (mg/min) = solute clearance (ml/min) × Plasma solute concentration (mg/ml).

Thus, the greater the clearance of urea, the greater will be the quantity of bicarbonate removed per unit time. In the 1970s it was also known that the rate of metabolism of sodium acetate to bicarbonate was limited,[2] and therefore, that there was an upper limit of 2.5 to 3.5 mEq/kg/h to the quantity of bicarbonate that could be removed during the treatment without the development of metabolic acidosis.[3] Therefore, the maximal dialysance of total carbon dioxide that could be achieved without untoward effects was 175 ml/min.[4] The maximal urea nitrogen dialysance that can be achieved in acetate hemodialysis is also approximately 170 to 180 ml/min. These are the limitations to what is now called *conventional hemodialysis*. A greater urea nitrogen dialysance can be achieved only with bicarbonate dialysate if the tolerance of the treatment is to be maintained.

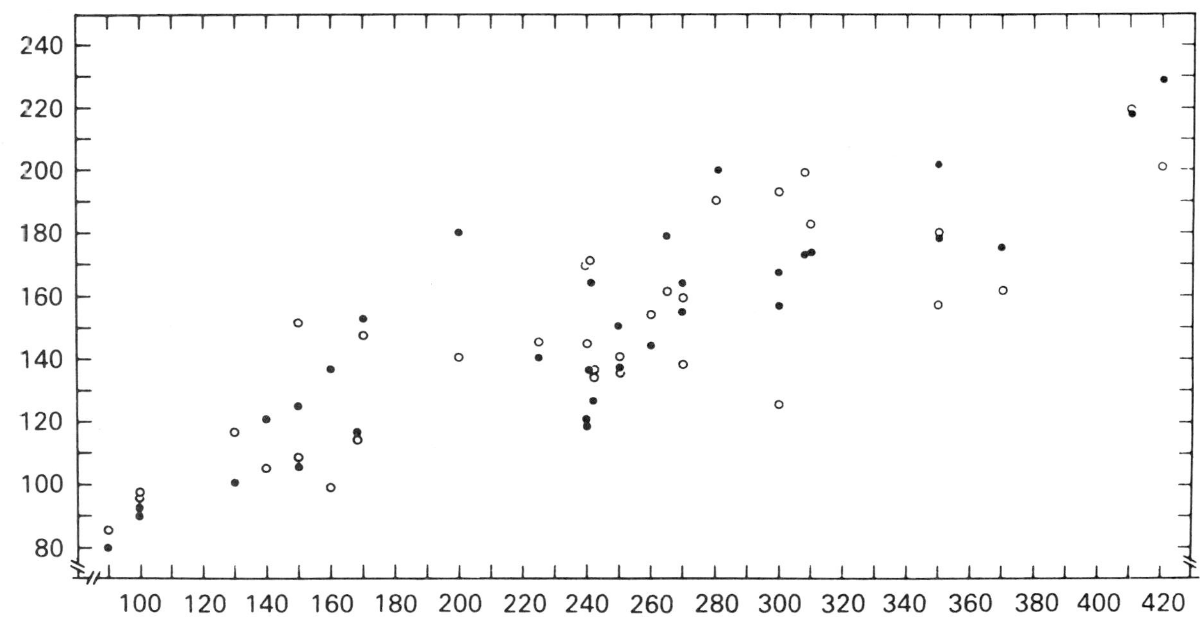

Fig. 1-1. Effects of blood flow on urea and carbon dioxide dialysance in acetate hemodialysis. Open circles indicate dialysance and dark circles indicate urea nitrogen dialysance.

DEVELOPMENTS

High-efficiency treatments are possible owing to the clinical introduction of a series of technical advances namely, bicarbonate dialysate, high blood flows, and special equipment.

Bicarbonate dialysate is required to increase the efficiency (clearance) of hemodialysis to provide urea clearances above 170 to 180 ml/min. The technical and clinical aspects of bicarbonate dialysate are covered in Chapter 2 of this volume.

In the late 1970s, when investigators were exploring alternatives to hemodialysis, such as hemofiltration, for the treatment of chronic renal failure, it was recognized that *high blood flows* (>250 to 300 ml/min) were possible in patients on maintenance extracorporeal therapy.[5] This *reserve for efficiency* can now be easily tapped, since it has been recognized that vascular access via grafts or fistulas generally provides blood flows in excess of 400 ml/min and that most modern hemodialysis facilities include blood pumps that can deliver blood flows in excess of 300 ml/min. It has also been demonstrated that high blood flows per se do not produce any systemic hemodynamic changes, which is as expected since the volume of blood in the extracorporeal circuit is independent of the flow rate.[6]

Special equipment made available by industry in a relatively short time period provides the technical features required for high-efficiency treatments. The alarm and monitoring functions of the extracorporeal circuit must be able to handle the higher pressures resulting from the high blood flow rates. A prerequisite for the use of membranes with greater hydraulic permeability is automated ultrafiltration control that provides for positive dialysate pressure and precise programmable weight loss rates throughout the treatment. This is achieved either by direct volumetric control with self-adjusting dialysate pressures or by automated continuous adjustments of transmembrane pressure by direct measurements of differential dialysate flow rates.

Dialyzers with increased surface area (at least 1.5 to 2.0 m^2) are used to optimally exploit the higher blood flow rates. The dialyzer membranes range in composition from conventional cellulosic membranes to synthetic ones with enhanced diffusivity and convective permeability, such as polysulfone, polyacrylonitrile, and polymethylmethacrylate membranes. The other components of the extracorporeal circuit, such as blood lines, must be able to withstand the higher pressures and should have fail-safe connectors. Large-diameter pump segments are necessary to deliver high flow rates with available occlusive blood pumps. A unique and important component of high-efficiency treatments is the needle used to cannulate the vascular access. Depending on the viscosity and hematocrit of the blood, the needle lumen should have an internal diameter of 1.8 to 2.0 mm to avoid pressure differentials across the needle at high blood flow rates.[7]

BASIC ASSUMPTIONS

In a very general sense, the objective of a dialysis session is to remove a certain quantity of solutes and water. No definite agreement exists as to the nature (i.e., molecular size) of the solutes that must be removed. There is a clinically accepted view that urea is a good marker to use in guiding the prescription of a dialysis treatment. It is also agreed that the minimal quantity of urea to be removed during hemodialysis is at least 60 to 65 percent of the pretreatment total body urea or expressed in a different way, Kt/V must equal 1 (where V is the urea distribution volume removed during dialysis, K is the dialyzer clearance, and t is the treatment time).[8] Therefore, to remove a given amount of urea in a given patient, a dialyzer with a low urea clearance will require a longer treatment time than a dialyzer with a high urea clearance.

Long treatment time × low clearance = short treatment time × high clearance

The quality of the dialysis treatment will depend on the presence or absence of symptoms during the treatment. The majority of the symptoms experienced by patients during hemodialysis are related to their tolerance of fluid removal. The shortest treatment time cannot be reduced below the point which removal of the weight gain is associated with a minimum of symptoms. The appearance of symptoms in a given patient during removal of the interdialytic weight gain rather than not the efficiency of the dialyzer may be the limiting factor in reducing treatment. The ability to increase solute removal rate has created a conceptual difference between treatment time and "dose" or extent of treatment. In the past, when efficiency was low and varied little among patients, the amount of treatment was satisfactorily defined by time which averaged 4 hours. Today, treatment time is meaningless as a definition of treatment extent, since efficiency can vary greatly from center to center. A short treatment time is no longer synonymous with less therapy. Conversely, long treatment periods do not necessarily imply greater solute removal during treatment.

PITFALLS IN CLINICAL PRACTICE

The successful application of high-efficiency treatments in clinical practice requires a comprehensive approach, with recognition of the underlying clinical principles and technical aspects. The dialysis team (nephrologist, nurses, dieticians) must be aware of these principles and have a clear understanding of possible pitfalls in their implementation. Compliance with treatment time by patients and staff is more important in high-efficiency treatments than in conventional dialysis: 15 minutes lost in a 240-minute treatment is only 6 percent of total treatment time, but 15 minutes lost in a 120-minute treatment represents 12.5 percent. The impact of time lost and of other possible pitfalls in carrying out these treatments warrants mandatory implementation of strict quality assuarance programs. It is imperative that the treatment be assessed on a routine basis as to whether it is being delivered as prescribed.

REUSE

High-efficiency treatments, with the exception of high-efficiency hemodialysis, may necessitate reprocessing the dialyzer. This is especially the case in hemodiafiltration which requires two high-flux dialyzers. My experience has been that patients are willing to accept reuse in order to improve the quality of their treatment. Reuse should also be considered imperative from an ecologic point of view. Disposition of medical waste in our society is expensive and technically difficult. In high-efficiency treatment the choice is between high-efficiency hemodialysis, with no dialyzer reuse, and high-flux hemodialysis or hemodiafiltration both of which provide additional clearance of intermediate-size solutes with dialyzer reuse.

DEFINITIONS

High-Efficiency Hemodialysis

High-efficiency hemodialysis[9] is a further development of conventional hemodialysis and depends primarily on enhanced diffusive transport of solute. It is preformed with equipment that provides with bicarbonate capability and, preferably ultrafiltration control. The dialyzers used contain conventional membranes with low hydraulic permeability and large surface area. Enhanced clearance of small solutes results from the greater flow rates and larger membrane surface area, and ultrafiltration is equal to the weight loss during the treatment. Several cuprophane dialyzers are available that are suited for use in this treatment. They provide, at blood flows of 300 to 400 ml/min and in the absence of recirculation, a urea clearance of approximately 200 to 225 ml/min. It is apparent that these devices can provide adequate hemodialysis (Kt/V = 1.0) in less than 180 minutes for patients with low, lean body mass. High-efficiency hemodialysis is ideal for elderly and small patients. In larger patients (weighing over >70 kg) treatments shorter than 210 minutes may not provide adequate therapy.

High-Flux Hemodialysis

High-flux hemodialysis[10] was developed to provide simultaneous diffusive and convective transport in a single device. Its essential feature is the use of synthetic "open" membranes with high diffusive and hydraulic permeability.

These membranes must be used with equipment that provides volumetric ultrafiltration control. Simultaneous ultrafiltration of blood and backfiltration of dialysate occur in response to oppositely directed pressure gradients within the dialyzer, thereby augmenting convective transport. When used in conjunction with high blood and dialysate flow rates, high-flux dialysis offers both greater efficiency and transport of a wider size range of solutes than conventional or even high-efficiency hemodialysis. In this modality total ultrafiltration during treatment far exceeds the weight gain between treatments.

Hemodiafiltration

The concept of simultaneous diffusive and convective transport is further extended in hemodiafiltration.[11] This technique attempts to approximate the function of the human glomerulus over the size range of filtered solutes. It can be performed with the same type of dialyzer membranes and dialysis equipment used in high-flux hemodialysis. Ultrafiltration exceeds by far the weight gained between treatments and volume losses are replaced by either substitution fluid or prefiltered dialysate.

High-Flux Hemodiafiltration

High-flux hemodiafiltration, described in detail elsewhere[12] is performed with two highly permeable dialyzers in series. It provides both a large membrane surface area for diffusion and high rates of simultaneous ultrafiltration and replacement by backfiltration of prefiltered dialysate. Because of its unsurpassed high diffusive and convective solute transport rates, this treatment offers both the greatest efficiency and widest range of solute size removal of all therapies for end-stage renal disease.

REFERENCES

1. Bosch, JP, Glabman, S, Moutoussis, G et al: Carbon dioxide removal in acetate hemodialysis: effects on acid base balance. Kidney Int 25:830, 1984
2. Lunquist F: Production and utilization of free acetate in man. Nature 193:579, 1962
3. Kveim M, Nebaskkew R: Utilization of exogenous acetate during hemodialysis. Trans Am Soc Artif Intern Organs 21:138, 1975
4. Groefe U, Milutinovich J, Follette WC et al: Less dialysis-induced morbidity and vascular instability with bicarbonate in dialysate. Ann Intern Med 88:332, 1978
5. Kubota K, Kawauchi A, Nakajima M et al: Arteriovenous shunt flow measurement by ultrasonic duplex system. Trans Am Soc Artif Intern Organs 33:144, 1987

6. Ronco C, Brendolan A, Bragantini L et al: Technical and clinical evaluation of different short, highly efficient dialysis techniques. Contrib Nephrol 61:46, 1988
7. Von Albertini B, Bosch JP: Short hemodialysis. Am J Nephrol 11:169, 1991
8. Daurgidas JT: The pre:post dialysis plasma urea nitrogen ratio of estimate Kt/V and NPCR: validation. Int J Artif Organs 12:420, 1989
9. Keshaviah P, Collins A: Rapid high-efficiency bicarbonate hemodialysis. Trans Am Soc Artif Intern Organs 32:17, 1986
10. Streicher E, Schneider H: The next generation of dialysis membranes: barriers or pathways. Contrib Nephrol 44:125, 1985
11. Shinaberger JH, Miller JH, Gardner PW: Short treatment. p. 360. In Maher JF (ed): Replacement of Renal Function by Dialysis. 3rd Ed. Kluwer, Boston, 1989
12. Miller JH, von Albertini B, Gardner PW, Shinaberger JH: Technical aspects of high-flux hemodiafiltration for adequate short (under 2 hours) treatment. Trans Am Soc Artif Intern Organs 30:377, 1984

2

Bicarbonate in High-Efficiency Hemodialysis

Ingrid Ledebo

FROM BICARBONATE TO ACETATE

Since the composition of dialysis fluid should mirror that of normal plasma water, the choice of bicarbonate as buffer is so self-evident that it hardly deserves a chapter of its own. Krebs and Henseleit in 1932 were the first to report the preparation of a parenteral solution with the same pH, buffering capacity, and composition of inorganic ions as human plasma. Their solution contained bicarbonate and carbon dioxide as buffering agent. Kolff used bicarbonate in his first clinical hemodialysis on March 17, 1943 but later had to omit it several times because of problems with calcium precipitation.[1] The closed dialysis system described by Alwall in 1946 was designed for carbon dioxide bubbling into the bicarbonate-containing fluid.[2] This was the method adopted by others in the 1950s to keep the calcium and the bicarbonate ions in solution.

The expansion of the dialysis program during the early 1960s necessitated simplified preparation of the dialysis fluid. An automatic system, which mixed water with a concentrated electrolyte solution in the right proportions, was developed by Grimsrud et al. in Seattle.[3] Since bicarbonate could not be kept in a concentrated solution with the other electrolytes, a separate proportioning pump and a separate bicarbonate solution had to be used. Since this procedure was still complicated, a search for a more convenient buffering agent was initiated. In 1964 the Seattle group proposed that sodium acetate be substituted for sodium bicarbonate in the dialysis fluid in view of the fact that each mole of acetate metabolized yields one mole of bicarbonate.[4] Under the dialysis conditions used in those days, with urea clearance below 100 ml/min and treatment times of 15 to 17 hours, it was found that acetate concentrations of 35 to 40 mmol/L could restore the plasma bicarbonate level to normal values during dialysis without problems. The acetate influx during this form of dialysis was far below the normal metabolic utilization rate in humans of 300 mmol/h.[5] The practical advantages of using acetate rather than bicarbonate were so convincing that it became generally accepted within only a few years.

CONSEQUENCES OF USING ACETATE

The other side of the coin became evident when dialysis efficiency was increased. With a higher mass transfer rate of small solutes, the acetate influx exceeded the maximum metabolic acetate utilization rate.[6,7] At the same time the removal of bicarbonate and carbon dioxide was accelerated. The result was acetate accumulation, bicarbonate depletion, and aggravation of acidosis. Vascular instability and consequently reduced ultrafiltration rates and general morbidity were also reported under these conditions.[8] In these early studies the increased dialysis efficiency was achieved with large-surface-area dialyzers (2.5 m^2 cellulose acetate), while the flow rates for blood and dialysis fluid were still maintained in the standard range. This gave urea clearances of approximately 200 ml/min. The dialysance of acetate into the blood under these conditions was around 150 ml/min. The peak acetate level in plasma and the final acid-base status were shown to depend directly on the metabolic capacity of the patient and on the efficiency of solute transport.[7]

METABOLISM OF ACETATE

The acetate metabolism in connection with dialysis takes place mainly in the mitochondria of muscle cells.[9] The metabolic capacity is reduced in uremic patients, and utilization rates of 2.5 to 3.5 mmol/h/kg have been measured.[6] Thus, the body weight and, more specifically, muscle mass are important. Patients with small muscle mass (e.g., older patients, inactive patients, and women) have been identified as poor metabolizers of acetate.[10] Proper circulation and oxygenation are also prerequisites for optimal acetate metabolism, since all muscle cells must be provided with fuel.

Normal metabolism of acetate starts with its conversion to the corresponding acid, in which process bicarbonate is formed from carbon dioxide. The acetic acid is then activated by coenzyme A in an energy-consuming reaction, and the active acetate proceeds through the Krebs cycle, yielding carbon dioxide and water. Since each molecule of acetate metabolized requires one molecule of carbon dioxide to form bicarbonate, the respiratory drive is reduced and hypoxemia occurs.

When large amounts of acetate are metabolized, the main route through the Krebs cycle becomes overloaded, and intermediates such as citrate and β-hydroxybutyrate, along with breakdown products such as adenosine monophosphate (AMP), phosphates, and adenosine, may accumulate. Acetate may also be channeled into other pathways for synthesis of fatty acids, cholesterol, and keto acids or may be reduced to acetaldehyde.[9,11] During acetate dialysis the influx of acetate is so large that its utilization becomes the major metabolic activity in the body. This may affect the metabolism of other substrates such as glucose.[12] Diabetic patients, who have a disturbed carbohydrate metabolism, also have problems with acetate.[13]

ACID-BASE CORRECTION WITH ACETATE

When the influx of acetate exceeds its metabolic utilization, acetate will accumulate in plasma, and the reduced concentration gradient will slow down its diffusion into the blood. A steady state will develop in which acetate influx equals acetate utilization. In a similar way the bicarbonate efflux will adjust itself to the metabolic production of bicarbonate. Assuming a constant acetate metabolism, the steady-state plasma bicarbonate level during dialysis will be inversely proportional to the efficiency of solute transport[14] (Fig. 2-1); the more efficient the treatment, the lower the bicarbonate level. Only at the end of dialysis, when the accumulated acetate has been metabolized and no more bicarbonate is being lost, will the plasma bicarbonate levels increase.

The final degree of acid-base correction is determined by the difference between the total influx of acetate and efflux of bicarbonate (i.e., the buffer balance). In all situations in which the acetate load exceeds the metabolic

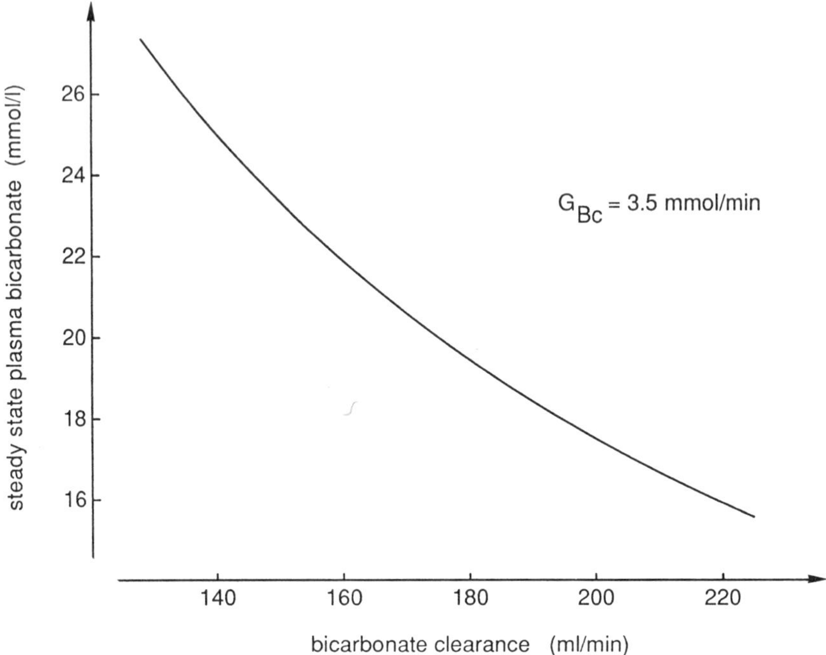

Fig. 2-1. The relationship between the steady-state plasma bicarbonate concentration and the clearance of bicarbonate during acetate hemodialysis. A bicarbonate metabolic generation rate (G_{Bc}) of 3.5 mmol/min was used. (From Ledebo,[14] with permission).

capacity, it is the metabolic rate that controls the process of acid-base correction. Only when acetate is supplied at rates below the maximum metabolic rate will the actual acetate load affect the final acid-base balance. Dialysis conditions since the early 1980s and persisting today have been such that the majority of all patients treated by acetate dialysis are in a state of chronic acidosis, since the amount of bicarbonate generated from acetate is not sufficient to compensate both for the bicarbonate losses during dialysis and for the intradialytic generation of acid.

CLINICAL SYMPTOMS WITH ACETATE

Most of the clinical symptoms associated with the use of acetate in dialysis are a direct consequence of the metabolic activities induced by the large acetate load. The hemodynamic instability, manifested as reduced peripheral resistance and falling blood pressure, could come from acetate accumulation as the acetate ion itself is a potent vasodilator.[15] Adenosine release and tissue hypoxia from the metabolism of large amounts of acetate would enhance the vasodilation.[9] All this impairs the vascular refilling, which is vital during conditions of fluid removal, and the result is hypovolemia.[16] It is also accompanied by all the clinical symptoms associated with symptomatic hypotension.

Many symptoms associated with acetate dialysis (e.g., headache, nausea, and fatigue) could be caused by formation of acetaldehyde.[11] It is tempting to compare an acetate dialysis to a large intake of alcohol, both giving a typical hangover.

The severity of the acetate-induced symptoms depends mainly on the acetate load, on the fluid removal rate, and on the cardiovascular status of the patient. Metabolic capacity seems to have less of an impact, since adverse conditions could be generated by acetate metabolism as well as by acetate accumulation. Therefore, attempts to correlate plasma acetate levels with symptoms have not always been successful.[17]

THE IMPACT OF INCREASED DIALYSIS EFFICIENCY

At urea clearances of about 170 ml/min, the influx of acetate corresponds to the normal metabolic utilization rate in uremic patients. At higher dialysis efficiency the increased acetate load will cause metabolic stress and more clinical problems. The higher ultrafiltration rates usually accompanying high-efficiency treatments will be poorly tolerated. This was illustrated by Keshaviah and Collins of the Minneapolis group in their pilot study of increased efficiency and reduced treatment time[18] (Table 2-1). The symptoms were frequent even on standard hemodialysis with acetate. An increase in efficiency aggravated the situation when acetate was used but was well tolerated when a switch was made to bicarbonate.

Higher efficiency also increases loss of bicarbonate, leading to more severe acidosis during the treatment. When the accumulated acetate is finally metabolized after the treatment, this causes a rebound of bicarbonate concentration, which is uncontrolled and is often not sufficient to achieve physiologic acid-base correction.[7]

Table 2-1. Effects of Changing Buffer and Treatment Efficiency

	Standard HD Ac	Rapid HD Ac	Rapid HD Bc
Urea clearance (ml/min)	187	266	266
Hypotension (%)	17	21	12
Nausea (%)	16	20	5
Vomiting (%)	8	10	1
Weight loss achieved (kg)	2.1	1.6	2.2

Abbreviations: HD, hemodialysis; Ac, acetate; Bc, bicarbonate. (Data from Keshaviah and Collins.[18])

FROM ACETATE TO BICARBONATE

The consequences of using acetate as a buffer source in the dialysis fluid were well described as early as the late 1970s, but the use of acetate persisted except in a few pioneering centers. One reason for this was probably that treatment efficiency was maintained at urea clearances about 150 to 175 ml/min, which gave an acceptable treatment quality for most patients. Bicarbonate was prescribed mainly for patients who were critically ill or especially unstable during acetate dialysis. The added cost of bicarbonate and the need for special equipment were also important factors. A third reason for the delay in conversion to bicarbonate was the ongoing debate about its benefits in relation to elevated sodium levels in the dialysis fluid. Since sodium was both simpler and less expensive to administer, it was often preferred.[19] It was finally the trend toward higher-efficiency treatments that convinced dialysis practitioners of the benefits of bicarbonate, not only for these treatments but for all forms of dialysis. Today the majority of all hemodialysis patients in North America, western Europe, and Japan, together representing almost 90 percent of the world population treated by hemodialysis, are using bicarbonate in both standard and high-efficiency treatments. The actual percentage of patients receiving bicarbonate treatment is difficult to predict since it is increasing every month. At the end of 1990 it was calculated to be 70 percent in the above-mentioned regions.

Since most of the symptoms associated with acetate dialysis are directly caused by acetate or its metabolism, they do not appear during bicarbonate dialysis. The bicarbonate ion as such has no direct pharmacologic effect on the cardiovascular system, but also it does not interfere with the physiologic compensation of fluid removal. Bicarbonate dialysis therefore results in a slight nonsympathetic vasoconstriction,[15] which, together with the better tissue oxygenation and normal carbon dioxide pressure (PCO_2) values, better preserves the plasma volume.[16]

Since bicarbonate does not need to be metabolized, its use in dialysis increases the plasma bicarbonate levels directly, and the degree of acid-base correction depends on the amount of bicarbonate gained during the treatment.

HOW MUCH BICARBONATE IS NEEDED?

To maintain a patient in acid-base balance, the dialysis treatment should provide an amount of buffer corresponding to the endogenous generation of acid occurring in the interdialytic period, but it must also compensate for the losses of buffer during the treatment. The metabolic production of hydrogen ions is a consequence of the protein intake and can be estimated from the protein catabolic rate[20]; it corresponds approximately to 1 mmol per kilogram of body weight per day. The buffer losses consist mainly of organic anions with a buffer potential and bicarbonate that are convectively lost in the ultrafiltrate.[7,21] The impact on the acid-base status of the bicarbonate loss during dialysis was shown by Fabris et al., who found that reducing the interdialytic weight gain by fluid restriction significantly improved predialysis plasma bicarbonate values.[22]

When careful buffer balance studies are made, it becomes evident that compensation for the acid production and the buffer loss may not be sufficient to bring a patient's plasma bicarbonate values into the physiologic range of 24 to 27 mmol/L. In some cases up to 60 to 70 percent of the buffer supplied may be used by the body to restore nonbicarbonate buffers rather than to increase the plasma bicarbonate level.[20,23] Patients with depleted buffer stores can be identified by their enlarged apparent bicarbonate distribution space, normally corresponding to 40 to 50 percent of total body weight.[24] The buffer deficit can be seen as the accumulated positive hydrogen balance and usually has little correlation with the plasma bicarbonate level, since it is compensated by nonbicarbonate buffers, mainly bone. The nonbicarbonate buffering in the body is believed to be regulated both by hormones and by the metabolism. Bone buffering has been shown to depend on the availability of active vitamin D metabolites and parathyroid hormone (PTH) since vitamin D administration alone increased the plasma bicarbonate levels in a group of dialysis patients.[25] Acetazolamide, an inhibitor of carbonic anhydrase, causes severe metabolic acidosis in uremic patients, probably by interfering with bone buffering; this has been attenuated by vitamin D administration.[26]

A certain amount of the bicarbonate provided during dialysis is used to restore the nonextracellular buffering capacity, and the rest remains in the extracellular space and raises the plasma bicarbonate level. The equilibrium plasma bicarbonate concentration, sometimes referred to as the *setpoint,* is an individual parameter affected by the acid-base status, the buffering capacity, the hormonal regulation, and the uremic state. It has been claimed that this set-point represents a normalized acid-base correction in uremic patients and that it can not be raised even by increased bicarbonate administration.[27] However, evidence based on the experience of many years with bicarbonate dialysis indicates that long periods of positive buffer balance seem to gradually restore the nonbicarbonate buffers, raising the setpoint into the physiologic range. When the acid-base status becomes normalized, the fluctuations of the plasma bicarbonate level, both pre- and postdialysis, seem to be smaller, indicating that the total buffering capacity of the body is greater in this range.[28]

SELECTING THE DIALYSATE BICARBONATE CONCENTRATION

When estimating the buffer concentration needed in the dialysis fluid, all the parameters discussed above and all the buffer-related treatment variables listed in Table 2-2 should be considered.

Table 2-2. Buffer Related Treatment Variables

Factors affecting the buffer need during dialysis	
Protein intake → generation of acid	
Loss of organic anions	
Ultrafiltrate volume → loss of bicarbonate	
Predialysis plasma bicarbonate level	
Nonbicarbonate buffer depletion	
Body weight	
Factors affecting the buffer gain during bicarbonate dialysis	
Bicarbonate concentration in dialysis fluid	} Total buffer concentration
Acetate concentration in dialysis fluid	
Acid concentration in dialysis fluid	
Dialysis efficiency	
Predialysis plasma bicarbonate level	
Treatment time	

On the basis of the varying degrees of acid-base correction achieved in 35 patients who underwent dialysis with five different buffer compositions during 3 months (Fig. 2-2), Mioni et al.[23] proposed a formula for the concentration of total buffer in the dialysis fluid needed to obtain a certain postdialysis plasma bicarbonate level.

$$\text{Total buffer conc} = (\text{postBc conc} - 1.7 - 0.30 \text{ preBc conc}) / 0.42$$

where conc = concentration and Bc = bicarbonate. Since this formula considers neither patient-specific factors such as body size and degree of buffer depletion nor treatment-dependent factors, it is not widely applicable but

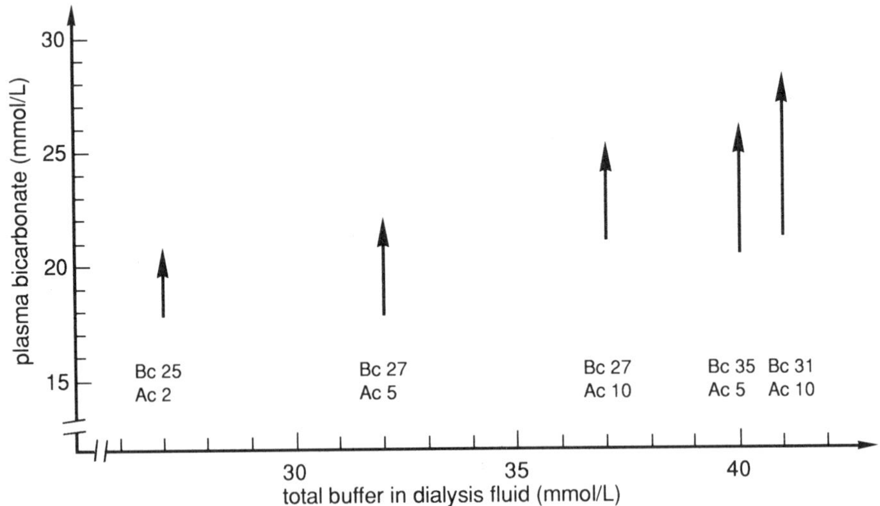

Fig. 2-2. Change of plasma bicarbonate level during dialysis in relation to the total buffer concentration in the dialysis fluid. The exact buffers used are indicated below the respective sums. Bc, bicarbonate; Ac, acetate. (Data from Mioni et al.[23])

may serve as a guide when starting bicarbonate dialysis. Whichever buffer concentration is used initially, the general advice is to regularly follow the patient's plasma bicarbonate values pre- and postdialysis. If the patient is in the acidotic range, the buffer dose should be increased, which is most easily done by raising the bicarbonate concentration in the dialysis fluid. As long as the postdialysis values do not extend into the alkalotic region, the buffer dose can be safely augmented, but a certain period of equilibration at each level is advisable. Postdialysis plasma levels of 29 to 30 mmol/L have been widely reported without accompanying clinical problems, but allowable levels must be carefully judged on an individual basis. Assuming that the nonbicarbonate buffers become gradually regenerated under conditions of positive buffer balance, a state of complete buffer replenishment may eventually be reached. This will be characterized by a normalized apparent bicarbonate space and by plasma bicarbonate values both before and after dialysis that are within or close to the physiologic range. In this condition it may be necessary to adjust the bicarbonate dose by reducing its concentration in the dialysis fluid.

For some patients the buffer dose during dialysis may need to be supplemented with an oral agent, such as bicarbonate or citrate. If a patient's protein intake is large, which is today encouraged, the endogenous generation of acid may be so high that it cannot be adequately compensated with an intermittent treatment.

HIGH-EFFICIENCY BICARBONATE DIALYSIS

When patients are switched from standard dialysis to high-efficiency dialysis, an accompanying change from acetate to bicarbonate may be made. Even if the use of bicarbonate does not by itself lead to normalized acid-base values, it generally results in a positive buffer balance, which should be manifested by increasing plasma bicarbonate levels, at least in the initial postdialysis period. The optimal dialysate bicarbonate concentration must then be empirically selected, as outlined above.

If the patient has already undergone dialysis with bicarbonate before the transfer to a high-efficiency procedure and the total treatment dose expressed as Kt/V for urea (where K is dialyzer clearance, V is urea distribution volume, and t is treatment time) is maintained together with the bicarbonate concentration in the dialysis fluid, there should be no immediate effect on the acid-base balance. It is still important to monitor the plasma bicarbonate levels regularly, since they may be indirectly affected by the new therapy (e.g., as a consequence of changed diet or phosphate accumulation).

CONSEQUENCES OF METABOLIC ACIDOSIS

Normalization of the plasma bicarbonate levels for the complete interdialytic period may not be possible to achieve with intermittent dialysis therapy, but keeping the fluctuations within the physiologic range of 24 to

27 mmol/L should be the goal. The majority of all hemodialysis patients, even those treated with bicarbonate, are still exposed to some degree of acidosis most of the time. The main reason for this is probably that the beneficial effect of bicarbonate on the treatment symptomatology has overshadowed its potential for acid-base correction at the time that the value of a fully corrected acid-base balance has been discussed.

Today many benefits of a normalized acid-base balance are gradually being revealed. The catabolic effect of acidosis has been shown by several groups in animals, in uremic patients, and in dialysis patients and is believed to contribute to the abnormal protein metabolism and malnutrition often found in dialysis patients.[29–31] Acidosis has also been identified as one of the risk factors for increased mortality among dialysis patients.[32]

The role of acidosis in uremic bone disease is controversial, but recent studies are strengthening the belief that the extensive bone buffering associated with chronic acidosis aggravates osteodystrophy.[33] Lefebvre et al.[34] have reported that the progression of uremic osteodystrophy was halted by optimal correction of acidosis in a group of patients observed for 18 months. De Marchi and Cecchin[35] have proposed that the acidosis-induced bone buffering is a PTH-controlled and vitamin D-mediated process and that the degree of metabolic acidosis may influence the level of secondary hyperparathyroidism. If these observations are further confirmed, the optimal correction of metabolic acidosis during dialysis will become a central issue in preventing uremic osteodystrophy.

CHEMICAL AND TECHNICAL ASPECTS IN BICARBONATE DIALYSIS

The chemical problems associated with using bicarbonate in dialysis are still the same as when Kolff mixed his dialysis fluid in 1943. To maintain calcium and bicarbonate ions in solution at the concentrations required for dialysis, the pH should be 7.3 or lower. In more concentrated solutions the ions have to be completely separated. Methods for achieving this pH at the moment of mixing the dialysis fluid should be simple and practical. Originally carbon dioxide was bubbled into the mixing tank, and this was a cumbersome procedure. Today an acid is included in the calcium-containing concentrate, the A component, which is diluted with water in a first mixing step. This solution is then mixed with bicarbonate, the B component, and in this process carbon dioxide is formed (Fig. 2-3). As long as the gas is kept in solution, the pH is maintained in the desired range, and precipitation of calcium carbonate is prevented.

The above basic principle for preparing dialysis fluid with bicarbonate is used by all manufacturers of dialysis machines. Older machines usually have an extra module for bicarbonate proportioning, whereas this function is integrated in all modern equipment. Most machines can be operated in

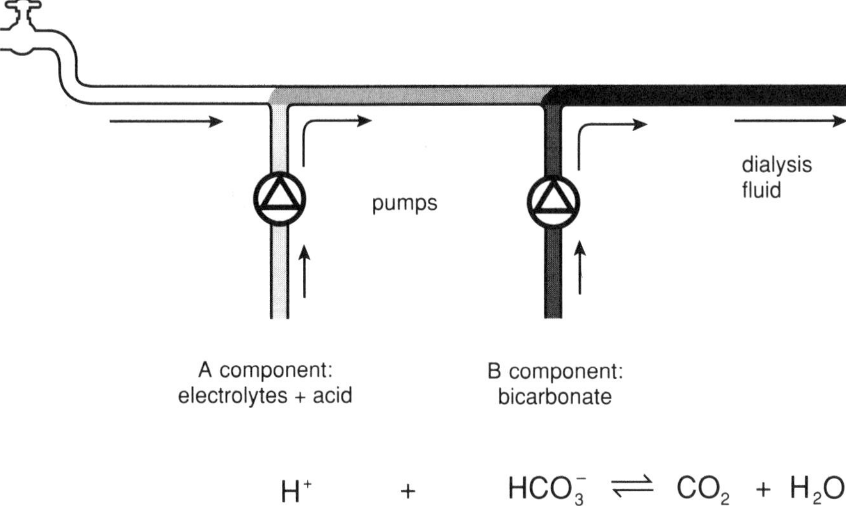

Fig. 2-3. Two-step proportioning of dialysis fluid with bicarbonate. The production of carbon dioxide in the second step creates the chemical conditions required to maintain the calcium and bicarbonate ions in solution during passage through the dialyzer.

either acetate or bicarbonate mode. The two-step proportioning is controlled by fixed volume or by conductivity. Separate control systems are needed for the two pumps, since high accuracy is essential in each mixing step. Some form of safety system, such as a pH electrode or a pump speed check, ensures that the correct concentrate is used with the respective pump; use of the wrong concentrate would be dangerous, since the machines measure the ionic rather than the overall chemical composition of the final fluid. Modern machines should permit adjustment of the bicarbonate concentration in the final fluid independently of the sodium concentration. This gives proportional change in concentration of other ions, but since their concentrations are low, this can generally be disregarded. Thus the same concentrates could be used to prepare dialysis fluids with varying bicarbonate and sodium content.

Central delivery systems for bicarbonate dialysis are generally designed on the basis of the same mixing principle, and the final fluid is distributed to the bedside monitors. In a special hybrid system the bicarbonate component is first mixed with water and then distributed to the individual dialysis machines of the acetate type, in which a one-step mixing with the A component produces the final dialysis fluid.[36] This has been described as an economical system, since conventional machines can be used, but a great deal of maintenance and microbiologic know-how are required to operate it safely.

The amount of acid in the A component mainly influences the final pH of the dialysis solution and thus determines the safety margin for calcium carbonate precipitation. Today most units have switched from 2 to

3 mmol/L of acetic acid to avoid some calcification problems. However, even with this acid concentration the result is a supersaturated solution, which remains stable only during the passage through the machine and the dialyzer. Using freshly prepared bicarbonate fluid, such as that produced online from a powder cartridge, and a machine with a short uncomplicated flow path gives the best result.[37] Aged bicarbonate concentrate, a higher bicarbonate concentration, and a longer flow path as in central delivery systems will predispose to a more rapid precipitation and thus require increased levels of acid. The acid level should be increased to 4 mmol/L when the bicarbonate concentration exceeds 35 mmol/L and standard liquid B concentrate is used. However, when the on-line produced B component from powder is used, this higher acid level is needed at bicarbonate concentrations above 38 mmol/L. For central delivery of bicarbonate fluids an even higher acid concentration is generally recommended. In Japan where central delivery systems are frequently used, pH values around 7.0 are often found in the final dialysis solution.

In spite of the chemical benefits there seems to be a certain reluctance in using acid levels above 2 to 3 mmol/L. This may be due to a concern about the higher PCO_2 levels and acetate levels. Using more acid gives a lower pH and as a direct consequence a higher PCO_2 in the fluid, according to the classic Henderson-Hasselbalch equation. The PCO_2 values in bicarbonate fluid may be about twice as high as in normal blood. The clinical result of this is hyperventilation and unloading of carbon dioxide, and the PCO_2 level in the arterial blood remains unchanged[38] (Fig. 2-4). Increasing the acid concentration also means including more anions, usually acetate. The possible adverse effect of this acetate has been discussed, and use of other acids with less harmful anions has been suggested.[39] However, no practical solutions for this problem exist today. For most dialysis patients the acetate influx during bicarbonate dialysis is far below the metabolic utilization rate.[11,17]

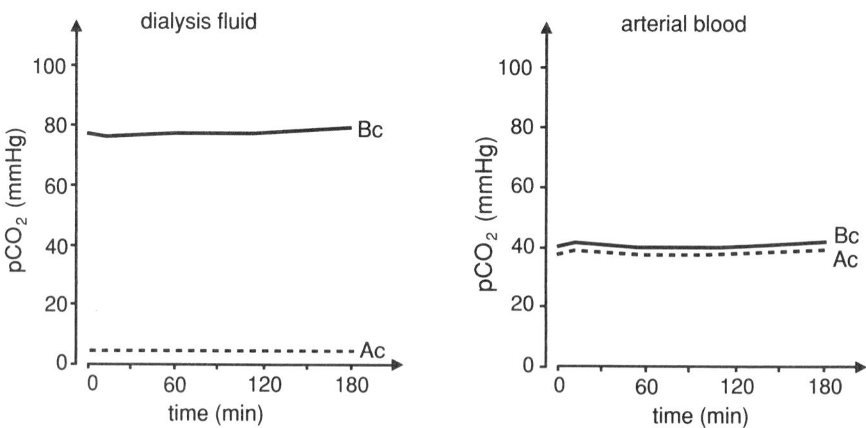

Fig. 2-4. The PCO_2 in dialysis fluid and in arterial blood during hemodialysis with acetate or bicarbonate. Ac, acetate; Bc, bicarbonate. (Data from De Broe et al.[38])

MICROBIOLOGIC ASPECTS OF BICARBONATE DIALYSIS

Bicarbonate concentrates have a salt content of approximately 1 mmol/L and could sustain the growth of bacteria. They should therefore never be produced under unsterile conditions and stored.[40] Manual preparation of bicarbonate solutions should always follow the quality assurance guidelines from the Food and Drug Administration and the manufacturers.[41] Most brands of commercially produced bicarbonate concentrate are not registered as a sterile product; thus there is a risk of contamination even before the container is opened. Once it has been opened, the contents should be used the same day or discarded. Many incidents with grossly contaminated bicarbonate concentrate have been reported, and the frequency of pyrogenic reactions in dialysis has increased with the widespread use of bicarbonate.[42] The best safeguard against microbiologically contaminated concentrate is use of a dry powder cartridge (BiCart), from which a fresh bicarbonate concentrate is automatically produced by the dialysis machine.[43]

However, the concentrate is not the only source of microbiologic contamination in dialysis. The water quality and the design and maintenance of the water treatment and distribution equipment are equally important for the final microbiologic quality of the dialysis fluid (see Ch. 6). Use of ultrapure fluid for all dialysis treatments is today strongly advocated.[44] Central delivery systems for bicarbonate-containing fluid involve a great risk, even if the whole system is frequently sterilized, and ultraviolet disinfection of the fluid can not be considered adequate.[45]

The final link in this hygienic chain is the dialysis machine. Again, both design and maintenance are vital issues. Dead ends, complicated valve systems, and other potential areas of stagnation should be avoided. In addition to regular disinfection, decalcification of the machine is necessary when bicarbonate is used, since calcium carbonate deposits promote bacterial growth and may disturb the accuracy of the control systems. Any acid may be used to dissolve the calcium carbonate, but the stronger it is, the more effective it will be. If consideration is also given to the aggressive action on the machine and the practical handling, citric acid appears to be the best choice. It owes its effectiveness to both its acidity and its chelating power. The recommendations of the respective machine manufacturers should be followed regarding both the frequency and the duration of decalcification and disinfection, since differences in material resistance may be a restriction. All the factors that increase the risk of calcium carbonate precipitation, discussed above, may lead to a greater need for decalcification.

PRACTICAL ASPECTS IN BICARBONATE DIALYSIS

When comparing the practical routines surrounding a dialysis treatment with bicarbonate or acetate, there is often more work and worry connected with the former. In some units the procedure starts with mixing the bicarbonate concentrate. Before the treatment the two different concentrate containers, weighing about 25 lb each, should be carried to the machine and properly connected. After the treatment, time is required for extra rinsing, disinfection, and decalcification of the machine. Reports of pyrogenic reactions during the treatment have caused concern among staff personnel.

All these aspects make it understandable that the use of bicarbonate has met with some resistance, delaying its general acceptance. For the acceptance and correct use of bicarbonate by the staff it is important to facilitate its handling and to institute logical routines. The modern equipment available today is useful in this respect.

BENEFITS OF BICARBONATE

From a physiologic point of view, bicarbonate has always been the first choice for a dialysis buffer, but in reality it was not widely accepted until it proved to be a vital component of high-efficiency treatments. The high fluid removal rates and the rapid mass transfer of solutes across the membrane would have been poorly tolerated by the patients if superimposed on acetate-induced symptoms. With use of bicarbonate instead, the treatment comfort in high-efficiency dialysis can usually be maintained at a level comparable with that of standard dialysis. The greatest benefit of bicarbonate with respect to symptomatology during treatment is achieved when it is used for unstable patients without increasing dialysis efficiency. To generalize, one could say that bicarbonate is used in dialysis either to increase efficiency with maintained hemodynamic stability or to improve hemodynamic stability with maintained efficiency (Fig. 2-5).

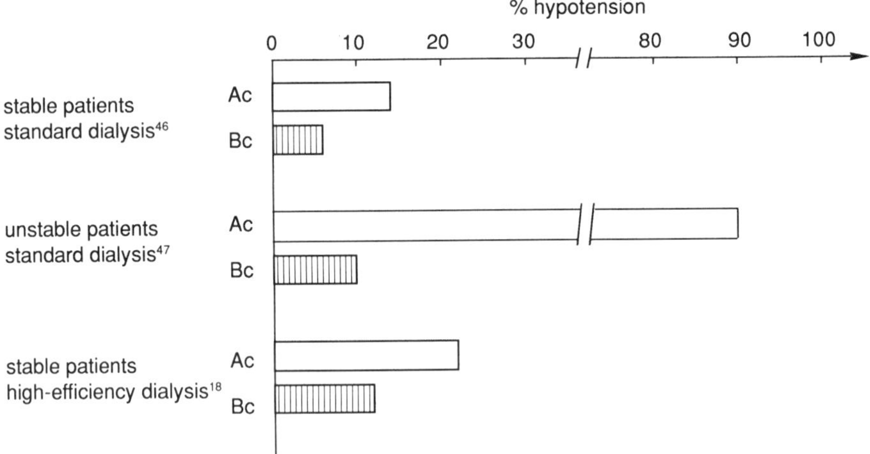

Fig. 2-5. Incidence of hypotension during hemodialysis in stable and unstable patients receiving standard and high-efficiency treatment. The effect of using acetate or bicarbonate was studied for each set of conditions. (Data from Keshaviah and Collins,[18] Oettinger and Oliver,[46] and Mastrangelo et al.[47])

With the widespread use of bicarbonate in dialysis today, the potential for a physiologic correction of the acid-base balance is becoming evident. Future benefits of bicarbonate dialysis may therefore be related to a normalized acid-base status and could include improved nutritional status and better management of uremic osteodystrophy.

REFERENCES

1. Kolff WJ: De Kunstmatige Nier (The artificial kidney). MD Thesis, University of Groningen, JH Kok NV, Kampen, the Netherlands, 1946 (in Dutch)
2. Alwall N: Recent technical modifications of the author's artificial kidney (dialyser, ultrafilter) in clinical use since 1946. p. 2. In: Therapeutic and Diagnostic Problems in Severe Renal Failure. Svenska Bokförlaget, Stockholm, 1963
3. Grimsrud R, Cole JJ, Lehman GA et al: A central system for the continuous preparation and distribution of hemodialysis fluid. Trans Am Soc Artif Intern Organs 10:107, 1964
4. Mion CM, Hegstrom RM, Boen ST, Scribner BH: Substitution of sodium acetate for sodium bicarbonate in the bath fluid for hemodialysis. Trans Am Soc Artif Intern Organs 10:110, 1964
5. Lundquist F: Production and utilization of free acetate in man. Nature 193:579, 1962
6. Tolchin N, Roberts JL, Hayashi J, Lewis EJ: Metabolic consequences of high mass-transfer hemodialysis. Kidney Int 11:366, 1977
7. Vreman HJ, Assomull VM, Kaiser BA et al: Acetate metabolism and acid-base homeostasis during hemodialysis: influence of dialyzer efficiency and rate of acetate metabolism. Kidney Int, suppl. 10:S62, 1980
8. Graefe U, Milutinovich J, Follette WC et al: Less dialysis-induced morbidity and vascular instability with bicarbonate in dialysate. Ann Intern Med 88:332, 1978
9. Vinay P, Cardoso M, Tejedor A et al: Acetate metabolism during hemodialysis: metabolic considerations. Am J Nephrol 7:337, 1987
10. Danielsson A, Gutierrez A, Hultman E, Bergström J: Patient-related factors influencing the plasma acetate concentration during haemodialysis. Nephrol Dial Transplant 2:526, 1987
11. Cairns HS, Rediout JM, Peters TJ et al: Changes in blood acetaldehyde concentrations during acetate hemodialysis. Nephrol Dial Transplant 3:637, 1988
12. Panzetta G, Tessitore N, Schiavon R et al: Effects of acetate on glucose metabolism and cellular ATP content during hemodialysis. Clin Nephrol 29:179, 1988
13. Knowles SE, Jarrett IG, Filsell OH, Ballard FJ: Production and utilization of acetate in mammals. Biochem J 142:401, 1974
14. Ledebo I: Correction of acid-base balance in dialysis. p. 74. In: Acetate vs Bicarbonate in Everyday Dialysis. Gambro AB, Lund, Sweden, 1990
15. Baldamus CA, Ernst W, Freu U, Koch KM: Sympathetic and hemodynamic response to volume removal during different forms of renal replacement therapy. Nephron 31:324, 1982
16. Leunissen KML, Cheriex EC, Janssen J et al: Influence of left ventricular function on changes in plasma volume during acetate and bicarbonate dialysis. Nephrol Dial Transplant 2:99, 1987

17. Mansell MA, Morgan SH, Moore R et al: Cardiovascular and acid-base effects of acetate and bicarbonate haemodialysis. Nephrol Dial Transplant 1:229, 1987
18. Keshaviah, P, Collins A: Rapid high-efficiency bicarbonate hemodialysis. Trans Am Soc Artif Intern Organs 32:17, 1986
19. Keshaviah PR: The role of acetate in the etiology of symptomatic hypotension. Artif Organs 6:378, 1982
20. Gotch FA, Sargent JA, Keen ML: Hydrogen ion balance in dialysis therapy. Artif Organs 6:388, 1982
21. Bosch JP, Glabman S, Moutoussis G et al: Carbon dioxide removal in acetate hemodialysis: effects on acid base balance. Kidney Int 25:830, 1984
22. Fabris A, La Greca G, Chiaramonte S et al: The importance of ultrafiltration on acid-base status in a dialysis population ASAIO Trans 34:200, 1988
23. Mioni G, Favazza A, Messa P: Acid-base metabolism in short dialysis. p. 197. In Cambi V (ed): Short Dialysis. Martinus Niijhoff, Boston, 1987
24. Fernandez PC, Cohen RM, Feldman GM: The concept of bicarbonate distribution space: the crucial role of body buffers. Kidney Int 36:747, 1989
25. Mioni G, Messa P, Favazza A et al: Bone tissue metabolism and acid-base status in uraemic patients. Miner Metab Res Ital 4:69, 1983
26. De Marchi S, Cecchin E: Severe metabolic acidosis and disturbances of calcium metabolism induced by acetazolamide in patients on haemodialysis. Clin Sci 78:295, 1990
27. Gennari FJ: Acid-base balance in dialysis patients. Kidney Int 28:678, 1985
28. Ahmad S, Pagel M, Vizzo J, Scribner BH: Effect of the normalization of acid-base balance on postdialysis plasma bicarbonate. Trans Am Soc Artif Intern Organs 26:318, 1980
29. May RC, Kelly RA, Mitch WE: Mechanisms for defects in muscle protein metabolism in rats with chronic uremia. J Clin Invest 79:1099, 1987
30. Jenkins D, Burton PR, Bennett SE et al: The metabolic consequences of the correction of acidosis in uraemia. Nephrol Dial Transplant 4:92, 1989
31. Bergström J, Alvestrand A, Fürst P: Plasma and muscle free amino acids in maintenance hemodialysis patients without protein malnutrition. Kidney Int 38:108, 1990
32. Lowrie EG, Lew NL: Death risk in hemodialysis patients: the predictive value of commonly measured variables and an evaluation of death rate differences between facilities. Am J Kidney Dis 15:458, 1990
33. Green J, Kleeman CR: Role of bone regulation of systemic acid-base balance. Kidney Int 39:9, 1991
34. Lefebvre A, de Vernejoul MC, Gueris J et al: Optimal correction of acidosis changes progression of dialysis osteodystrophy. Kidney Int 36:1112, 1989
35. De Marchi S, Cecchin E: Bone buffering and acidosis in end-stage renal disease. Semin Dial 4:148, 1991
36. Luehmann D, Hirsch D, Ebben J et al: Hybrid hardware scheme for bicarbonate dialysis. p. 188. In Nosé Y, Kjellstrand C, Ivanovich P (eds): Progress in Artificial Organs—1985. Int Soc Artif Organs Press No. 205, Cleveland, 1986
37. Delin K, Attman PO, Dahlberg M, Aurell M: A clinical test of a new device for on-line preparation of dialysis fluid from bicarbonate powder: the Gambro BiCart. Dial Transplant 17:468, 1988
38. De Broe ME, Van Waeleghem JP, Boberg U et al: Effect of CO_2 loading on ventilation and acid-base during bicarbonate dialysis, abstracted. Blood Purif 8:92, 1990

39. Veech RL: The untoward effects of the anions of dialysis fluids. Kidney Int 34:587, 1988
40. Ebben JP, Hirsch DN, Luehmann DA et al: Microbiological contamination of liquid bicarbonate concentrate for hemodialysis. ASAIO Trans 33:269, 1987
41. Quality Assurance Guidelines for Hemodialysis Devices. U.S. Food and Drug Administration, Center for Devices and Radiological Health, Washington, D.C., Feb 1991
42. Alter MJ, Favero MS, Moyer LA, Bland LE: National surveillance of dialysis-associated diseases in the United States, 1989. ASAIO Trans 37:97, 1991
43. Leunissen KML, Claessens PJM, Movy JMV et al: Chronic haemodialysis with bicarbonate dialysate. Technical and clinical aspects. Blood Purif 8:347, 1990
44. Mion C, Canaud B, Garred LJ et al: Sterile and pyrogen-free bicarbonate dialysate: a necessity for hemodialysis today. Adv Nephrol 19:275, 1990
45. Klein E, Pass T, Harding GB et al: Microbiological and endotoxin contamination in water and dialysate in the central United States. Artif Organs 14:85, 1990
46. Oettinger CW, Oliver JC: An economical new process for incenter bicarbonate dialysate production: comparison with acetate in a large dialysis population. Artif Organs 13:432, 1989
47. Mastrangelo F, Rizzelli S, Corliano C: Benefits of bicarbonate dialysis. Kidney Int 28 (suppl 17):S188, 1985

3

Vascular Access and Rapid Hemodialysis

Pang-Yen Fan
Steve J. Schwab

INTRODUCTION

As the population of patients with end-stage renal disease continues to grow, vascular access for hemodialysis is becoming an increasingly important concern. Burgeoning numbers of elderly or seriously ill patients on maintenance hemodialysis pose a challenging problem for the establishment and maintenance of adequate vascular access. Indeed, vascular access-related problems account for approximately one-quarter of all admissions and hospitalization days for hemodialysis patients.[1,2] In addition, technical advances such as high-efficiency dialysis have placed new demands for higher blood flows than previously required. Finally, longer survival of patients on maintenance hemodialysis has made vascular access one of the major limitations on survival.

TYPES OF VASCULAR ACCESS

Arteriovenous (AV) fistulas constructed from native vessels remain the first choice for vascular access (Fig. 3-1). These fistulas have the advantages of long survival and low incidence of infection. However, native AV fistulas are difficult, if not impossible, to establish in many patients, particularly the elderly or those with peripheral vascular disease. Even with careful selection of patients for native fistula placement, as many as 30 to 40 percent of these fistulas fail to develop adequately.[3] Owing to these limitations, less than 30 percent of dialysis patients in most centers have native AV fistulas.

AV fistulas constructed with synthetic vessels, most commonly composed of polytetrafluoroethylene (PTFE), provide excellent vascular access in most patients who fail primary AV fistula placement (Fig. 3-2). These grafts have the advantage of relatively short maturation time but are more likely to be lost to thrombosis or infection than native fistulas.[4] In addition, synthetic grafts have a limited life since the graft material eventually wears out from repeated needle sticks.

Double-lumen cuffed Silastic catheters (Permcath and others) provide acceptable access in patients in whom native or synthetic fistulas can not be placed (Fig. 3-3). These catheters can be used for several months before replacement. With careful attention to sterile technique and placement of a Dacron cuff, infectious complications can be minimized. Catheter thrombosis can be treated by instillation of thrombolytic agents.

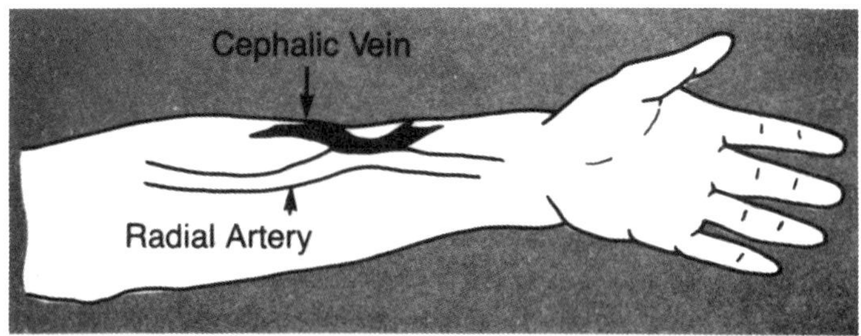

Fig. 3-1. Native AV fistula in the forearm position. (From Schwab,[3] with permission.)

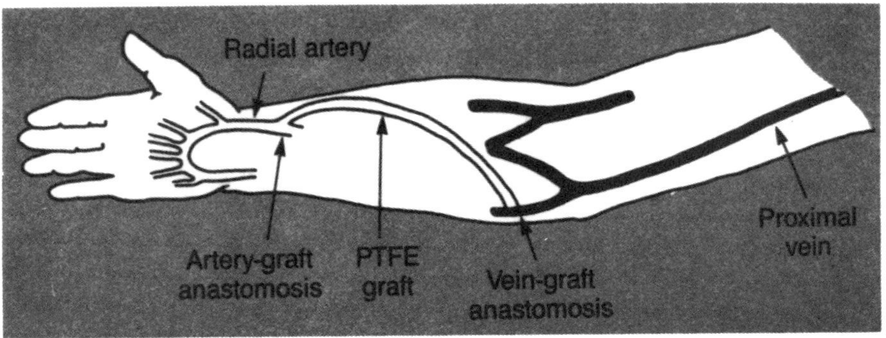

Fig. 3-2. PTFE vascular access in the forearm position. (From Schwab et al.,[19] with permission.)

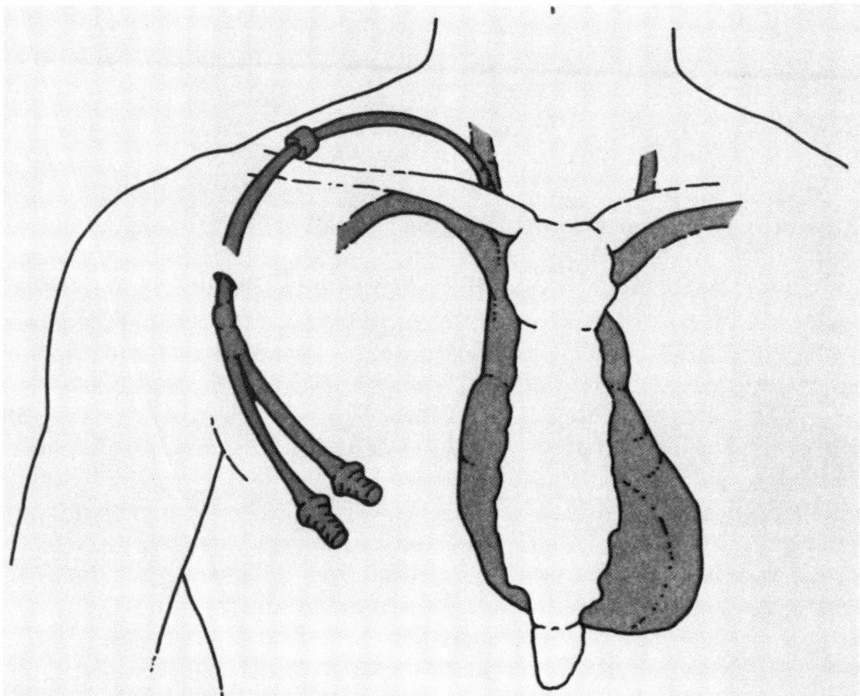

Fig. 3-3. Cuffed hemodialysis catheter inserted in the right interval jugular position. (From Schwab et al.,[23] with permission.)

ADEQUACY OF BLOOD FLOWS FOR HIGH-EFFICIENCY HEMODIALYSIS

Vascular access must provide adequate blood flow, since insufficient flow leads to increased recirculation of blood through the dialyzer as dialyzed blood reenters the dialysis circuit rather than the systemic circulation. The higher dialyzer flows necessitated by high-efficiency hemodialysis exacerbate this problem, since recirculation increases as dialyzer blood flow increases. In severe cases the increase in recirculation may reduce urea clearance enough to offset the benefit of the increased dialyzer flow rates.

Unfortunately, fistula blood flow remains difficult to directly measure. Fistulograms can define fistula anatomy but not function. Electromagnetic flow probes can provide direct measurements for research purposes but are not practical for routine clinical use. Duplex Doppler ultrasound color flow studies may be useful but have not been validated by concomitant flow probe measurements. In addition, they are limited by the technical difficulties posed by the turbulent blood flow in fistulas and are extremely operator-dependent. Other techniques such as thermodilution, dye dilution or isotope dilution are also poorly validated or technically impractical for routine clinical use.

Studies employing flow probes and Doppler ultrasonography have demonstrated that many new native and synthetic fistulas achieve mean blood flows of 800 ml/min, with some reaching flows in excess of 1,000 ml/min.[5,6] The location of the fistula may affect blood flow, more proximal arterial anastamoses appearing to yield higher flows.[6,7] Although only limited data are available, in general radial fistulas appear to yield lower blood flow rates than brachial or upper arm fistulas. The role of the venous anastamotic site in fistula flow remains unknown. In addition, the natural history of fistula blood flow remains to be determined, as flow rates may change over time. Flow in PTFE fistulas probably decreases progressively as intimal hyperplasia and subsequent venous stenoses develop. However, flow may actually increase in native AV fistulas as the venous anastamosis matures.

In general, double-lumen cuffed Silastic catheters can not provide flow rates as high as native or synthetic AV fistulas. While no studies on the adequacy of these catheters for high-efficiency hemodialysis have yet been published, we have usually obtained blood flows of 300 ml/min, with approximately 50 percent attaining 400 to 450 ml/min, while maintaining recirculation ratios of less than 20 percent.

COMPLICATIONS OF VASCULAR ACCESS

Infection

Infection is a serious cause of vascular access loss and accounts for 15 to 20 percent of vascular access complications.[4] While sometimes related to systemic infection from other sites, vascular access infection most commonly results from improper needle insertion technique. Although infection rates are low in relation to the great number of venipunctures performed, vascular access infection remains an important quality assurance issue for dialysis units. In our studies infection rates have correlated with the experience of the dialysis unit staff performing the venipunctures. This association is most striking for new hemodialysis units, with which infection rates are higher initially but improve rapidly as the staff gains expertise. Other predisposing factors for infection include intravenous drug use, dermatitis overlying the fistula, and excessive scratching of needle insertion sites.

While native fistulas can frequently be salvaged, synthetic fistulas or Silastic catheters must generally be removed. No studies have directly addressed the possibility that the incidence of vascular access infection may differ between high-efficiency and conventional hemodialysis units. However, in our dialysis units the rate of access infections has remained stable even though the great majority of patients have been switched from conventional to high-efficiency hemodialysis.

Thrombosis

Thrombosis is the most common cause of vascular access loss and is presumably associated with decreased fistula flow. Fistula thrombosis can result from hypotension, decreased cardiac output, hypovolemia, or prolonged external pressure on the fistula site. However, repeated thrombosis is most commonly due to stenosis at the venous anastomosis or more proximally in the venous system. In addition, the rate of thrombosis appears to be higher with synthetic fistulas.

We have recently examined rates of fistula thrombosis with high-efficiency hemodialysis. In our initial studies thrombosis rates in our units have remained stable even though the majority of our dialysis population has been converted to high-efficiency regimens. With our vascular access monitoring techniques (discussed below) and prompt correction of all venous stenoses, our patients average 0.26 thrombosis and require 0.09 fistula replacement per patient-year of dialysis.[5] These results compare favorably with fistula thrombosis and replacement rates that we observed in our studies using conventional hemodialysis.

Arterial and Venous Stenoses

Arterial stenoses are relatively uncommon complications of vascular access. However, venous stenoses occur frequently and are associated with up to 80 percent of episodes of thrombosis. Approximately 50 percent of venous stenoses result from intimal hyperplasia at the venous anastomosis of the fistula while the rest occur more proximally in the venous circulation. The pathogenesis of these proximal lesions remains unknown but may involve calcification or fibrosis of venous valves or endothelial trauma at certain anatomic pressure points such as the elbow or axilla. Up to 20 percent of venous stenoses involve central veins. These central stenoses may be associated with prior central venous cannulation but can also occur without it.

Endothelial injury from chronic turbulent blood flow may be a factor in the development of venous stenoses. In such cases high blood flows necessary for high-efficiency hemodialysis could potentially worsen intravascular turbulence and hasten the formation of stenotic sites. No studies have addressed this question. Indeed, longer follow-up will likely be needed to determine the role, if any, that high-efficiency dialysis regimens play in the pathogenesis of venous stenoses.

Cardiac Complications

Vascular access-related cardiac decompensation occurs occasionally in patients with underlying cardiac dysfunction, particularly those with severe cardiomyopathies. Such patients can develop high-output cardiac failure after access placement if fistula flow exceeds 20 percent of the cardiac output. Limiting fistula flow by shunt ligation or banding usually corrects the problem.

Available data, though limited, suggest that high-efficiency hemodialysis itself has relatively minor effects on cardiac physiology. Doppler ultrasonographic measurements of fistula flow show no change from baseline flow with high-efficiency hemodialysis.[8] In studies with small groups of patients, mean arterial pressures have remained stable and noninvasive assessment of cardiac output and peripheral resistance has demonstrated only minimal changes with high-efficiency dialysis relative to predialysis baselines.[9] In addition, echocardiographic data demonstrate that cardiac chamber size remains unaffected.[8] Therefore, high-efficiency hemodialysis does not appear to significantly alter cardiac physiology in patients who can hemodynamically tolerate a fistula with adequate blood flow.

However, high-efficiency treatments may have adverse cardiac effects in patients with large interdialytic weight gain, since the excess volume must be removed more rapidly. Patients with large interdialytic weight gains may suffer more frequent episodes of hypotension during high-efficiency dialysis, as the rate of volume removal overwhelms the compensatory mechanisms for maintenance of intravascular volume.

Steal Syndrome

In patients with severe peripheral vascular disease, placement of AV fistulas can result in distal hypoperfusion from significant shunting of arterial blood (the steal syndrome). In severe cases patients can develop digital ischemia and require fistula takedown. However, these complications are solely dependent on fistula flow and are unrelated to the extracorporeal blood flow rate.

Aneurysms and Pseudoaneurysms

Aneurysms and pseudoaneurysms are relatively infrequent complications of vascular access. They usually result from repeated needle sticks the same location and can be avoided by rotation of insertion sites. They can generally be easily managed by surgical fistula revision, with removal or ligation of the involved area. At present there is no evidence to suggest any difference in the incidence of these complications with conventional versus high-efficiency hemodialysis.

EVALUATION OF ACCESS PATENCY

Maintenance of access patency is one of the principal challenges facing nephrologists. With improved patient survival, preservation of the limited available vascular access sites becomes of paramount importance.

Access patency rates vary widely. For conventional hemodialysis, fistula patency rates are approximately 60 percent at 1 year and 50 percent at 2 years.[3] On the average, 0.5 to 0.8 episode of fistula thrombosis occurs per patient-year of dialysis.[3] Access patency for patients undergoing high-efficiency hemodialysis appears to be similar to that for patients undergoing conventional hemodialysis but has not yet been rigorously reviewed.

Venous Dialysis Pressures

Venous dialysis pressures are useful in monitoring access patency for patients undergoing conventional hemodialysis. Persistently elevated venous pressures (when measured at blood flows of 225 ml/min or less) that occur during at least three consecutive treatments can reliably identify patients at high risk for fistula thrombosis from venous stenosis.[10] Early correction of venous stenosis with angioplasty or fistula revision can prolong access viability.

Unfortunately, venous dialysis pressures have less predictive value at higher blood flows because the distinction between patients with patent fistulas and those with venous stenosis becomes blurred under these conditions. The increase in venous dialysis pressures at higher extracorporeal blood flow rates appears to be due to increasing intravascular turbulence. Therefore, venous dialysis pressures are currently of limited usefulness for predicting venous stenosis in patients undergoing high-efficiency dialysis. However, pressure and resistance measurement at multiple sites along the fistula appears to hold promise as a diagnostic tool, but current studies are still in early investigational stages.

Urea Recirculation

Recirculation involves the reentry of dialyzed blood into the dialyzer without passing through the systemic circulation. Elevated recirculation levels reduce effective urea clearance. Increased recirculation is frequently caused by improper placement of the dialysis needles, resulting in inadequate distance between the arterial inflow and venous outflow sites. However, recirculation levels also increase when fistula flow is insufficient to meet dialyzer blood requirements.

Increasing dialyzer blood flow increases recirculation, but the relationship is not necessarily linear.[11] Indeed, recirculation increases most dramatically in patients with limited fistula flow due to reduction in either arterial inflow or venous outflow. These patients may have moderate or even low recirculation rates at conventional dialyzer blood flows but develop extremely high recirculation rates when blood flows are increased beyond the capacity of the fistula, since all additional blood flow must come from recirculated blood. Therefore, elevated urea recirculation should be useful for prospectively detecting venous stenoses. In fact, recirculation studies have been used successfully to predict stenosis in selected patients undergoing high-efficiency hemodialysis.[12]

Urea recirculation is calculated from blood urea nitrogen (BUN) by the formula

(Systemic BUN − dialyzer arterial BUN)/
(systemic BUN − dialyzer venous BUN)

as shown in Figure 3-4. In determinations based on three samples, systemic BUN is usually measured as peripheral venous BUN, with blood samples drawn from the dialyzer lines and the contralateral arm. Unlike the three-sample techniques, which necessitates peripheral venipuncture or stop-flow, two-sample techniques require only blood from the dialyzer lines. Urea recirculation values are obtained by substituting the arterial line BUN from samples drawn before or after the dialysis session for the system BUN,[13-14] although ratios calculated in this fashion may be less accurate. In the stop-flow technique, dialyzer arterial and venous line samples are drawn, and dialyzer flow is then halted briefly to allow fistula blood BUN to equilibrate with peripheral venous blood.[15] A sample is then drawn from the dialyzer arterial line; this should closely approximate the systemic BUN. Recirculation measurements by this method correlate with values determined by the standard three-needle technique.[15,16]

Urea recirculation ratios may vary with a number of factors that can affect fistula blood flow (Table 3-1). While venous stenosis may be the primary concern of the nephrologist, decreased cardiac output, hypotension, or reduced intravascular volume status can also potentially increase recircula-

$$\frac{P - A}{P - V} = \% \text{ RECIRCULATION}$$

P = PERIPHERAL UREA
A = ARTERIAL (DIALYZER INFLOW) UREA
V = VENOUS (DIALYZER OUTFLOW) UREA

Fig. 3-4. Formula for calculation of recirculation.

Table 3-1. Factors Affecting Urea Recirculation

Needle placement
Extracorporeal blood flow
Hypotension
Decreased cardiac output
Intravascular volume depletion
Venous stenosis
Arterial stenosis

tion. Measurements should be performed at uniform times, preferably during the first hour of dialysis, and close attention should be paid to intravascular volume to avoid these potentially confounding variables.

To investigate the usefulness of urea recirculation ratios for detecting fistula stenosis in patients undergoing high-efficiency hemodialysis, we prospectively followed monthly recirculation ratios for 52 such patients over 6 months.[17] The study group consisted of the entire patient population of one dialysis center. Recirculation was measured at blood flows of 300 and 400 ml/min, and the results were compared by fistula location as well. In patients with recirculation in excess of 15 percent at a 400-ml/min flow rate, measurements were repeated and a fistulogram was obtained if recirculation remained elevated. To compare the recirculation ratios obtained by the stop-flow method with those calculated from contralateral arm peripheral venous samples, the measurements were determined by both techniques at 30, 60, and 120 minutes into the dialysis treatment.

We and other investigators have shown that urea recirculation increases as extracorporeal blood flow rate increases. Our overall mean urea recirculation was 8 percent at 300 ml/min but increased to 17 percent at 400 ml/min. Although recirculation did not correlate with fistula location at blood flows of 300 ml/min or less, we observed a statistically significant correlation at higher flows, radial fistulas having the greatest increase in recirculation. Brachial fistulas also had statistically significant increases at higher dialyzer blood flows, but upper arm fistula ratios, although slightly increased, were not significantly affected.

Recirculation ratios proved useful in identifying patients with significant venous stenoses. Increasing levels of recirculation correlated with increasing likelihood of stenosis, as we identified venous stenoses in 79 percent of patients with ratios higher than 20 percent. Since recirculation ratios for upper arm fistulas do not increase significantly, even at a flow of 400 ml/min, a lower threshold ratio may be necessary for detection of stenoses in patients with this type of access. In our study we identified stenotic lesions in 80 percent of patients with upper arm fistulas and urea recirculation ratios greater than 15 percent. Our results agree with those previously reported in a more highly selected patient population.[12]

In comparing the stop-flow and contralateral arm peripheral venous sample methods of measuring urea recirculation ratios (Table 3-2), we obtained similar recirculation ratios by both techniques at both 30 and 60 minutes

Table 3-2. Urea Recirculation Analysis at a Blood Flow of 400 ml/min

Dialysis Duration	Stop-Flow Technique	Contralateral Arm Technique
30 minutes	16 ± 3	17 ± 3
60 minutes	17 ± 2	17 ± 3
120 minutes	19 ± 3	24 ± 4[a]

[a] $P < .05$.

into the dialysis treatment. In fact, ratios calculated by the stop-flow method were similar at 30, 60, and 120 minutes, but at 120 minutes the peripheral venous sample technique yielded statistically significantly higher recirculation ratios. Our study does not address the validity of either technique but does demonstrate the importance of consistency in the technique and timing of recirculation measurements.

Duplex Doppler Color Flow Studies

Duplex Doppler color flow studies may accurately measure fistula flow and may ultimately prove useful in monitoring vascular access patency for patients undergoing high-efficiency hemodialysis. Serial measurements of fistula flow may provide an additional means of prospectively identifying venous stenoses. However, the usefulness of this technique is presently limited by cost and operator dependence.

Intravascular Ultrasonography

Intravascular ultrasonography may provide a useful adjunct for evaluation of fistula patency (Fig. 3-5.) This technique is particularly useful for determining the characteristics of a stenotic lesion, thereby yielding valuable information regarding the degree and nature of the stenosis.[18] Such information is frequently helpful in consideration of therapeutic options such as angioplasty. In addition, since intravascular ultrasonography can measure internal fistula dimensions, it has substantial potential as a research tool when used in conjunction with a electromagnetic flow velocity probe to provide accurate measurements of fistula blood flow.

Fistulography

Fistulography remains the gold standard for assessment of vascular access patency. By providing detailed visualization of the fistula lumen, venous anastomosis, and proximal venous system, this technique allows the clinician to identify any anatomic lesion. However, the fistulogram provides no information on fistula blood flow and furthermore, it is of limited utililty as a screening test since the overall prevalence of venous stenoses in the dialysis population is relatively low.

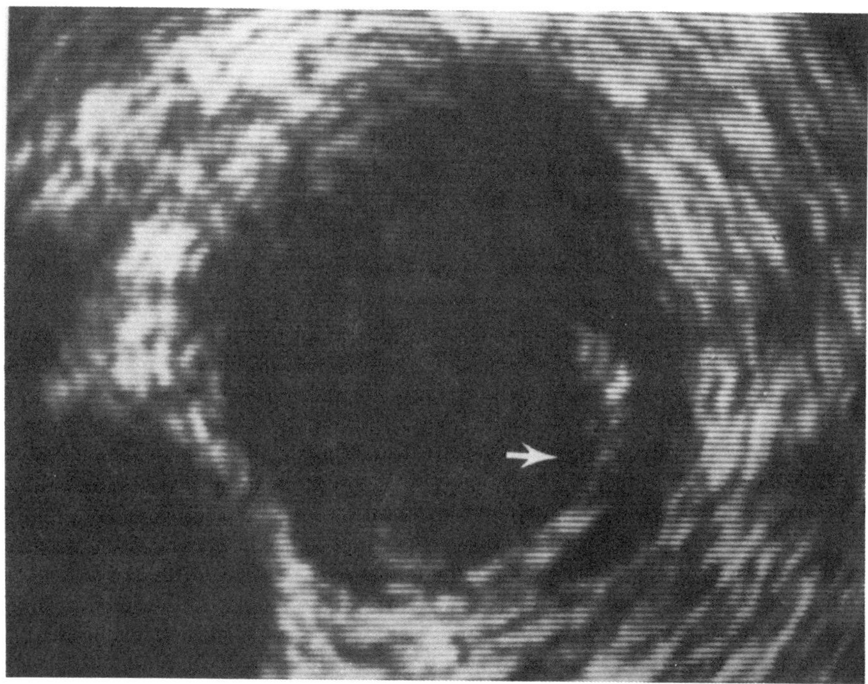

Fig. 3-5. Intravascular ultrasonogram of a brachial venous dissection (arrow) noted after percutaneous transluminal angioplasty. (From Davidson et al.,[18] with permission.)

THERAPEUTIC INTERVENTIONS

Angioplasty

Percutaneous transluminal angioplasty is an excellent means of correcting venous stenoses in both native and synthetic fistulas (Fig. 3-6). Successful angioplasty improves fistula function and prolongs access survival.[19] In addition, angioplasty can be performed as an outpatient procedure. However, stenosis recurs more frequently after angioplasty than after surgical fistula revision.[20]

Angioplasty can also correct proximal stenoses. In fact, this intervention is the preferred procedure for central vein stenoses, surgical correction of which is impractical because of their intrathoracic location. Even total central vein stenoses can sometimes be opened by angioplasty, either alone or with adjunctive thrombolytic infusion to the affected area.[21]

At our institution we obtain initial technical success with angioplasty in 85 percent of stenoses involving the fistulovenous anastomosis or proximal peripheral veins. For central vein stenoses, we achieve initial success with angioplasty in 95 percent of cases. Our restenosis rates at 1 year are 20 percent for lesions at the fistula anastomosis, 33 percent for proximal veins,

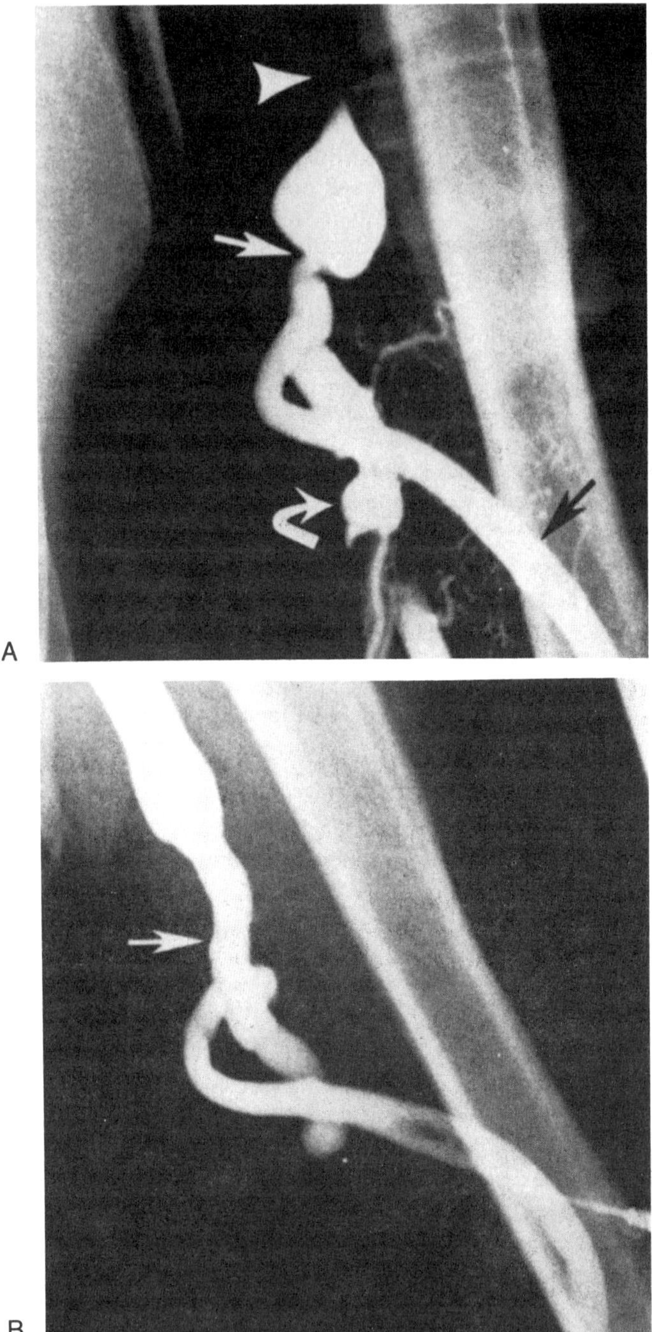

Fig. 3-6. (A) Diagnostic fistulogram showing a stenosis at the Gore-Tex graft-vein anastomosis (straight white arrow). The proximal vein is occluded by a pressure cuff (arrowhead). Black arrow shows distal vein. The arterial limb is not shown. (B) Fistulogram after percutaneous transluminal angioplasty shows adequate dilation of the stenosis (arrow), with good proximal venous runoff. (From Schwab et al.,[19] with permission.)

and 50 percent for central veins.[22] However, 75 percent of the restenoses are successfully treated by repeat angioplasty.[22]

Intravascular ultrasonography may help to identify atheromatous lesions that would be amenable to atherectomy via a Simpson catheter. Such intervention may reduce recurrence of stenosis in certain cases. However, relatively few lesions are suitable for atherectomy since the great majority of venous stenoses are thin-walled.

Surgical Fistula Revision

Surgical fistula revision remains the most definitive intervention for venous stenosis. This procedure results in the lowest stenosis recurrence rates but has the disadvantages of necessitating hospitalization and also extension of the fistula, thereby reducing the number of sites available for later vascular access placement.

SUMMARY AND CONCLUSIONS

Establishment and maintenance of vascular access have become increasingly important and are now significant factors in patient survival. High-efficiency hemodialysis places new demands on vascular access. Both native and synthetic fistulas, and sometimes even double-lumen Silastic catheters, can provide adequate blood flows for high-efficiency hemodialysis in the majority of patients. The vascular access complication rate for high-efficiency regimens appears similar to that for conventional hemodialysis, although differences may become apparent with further follow-up. Vascular access patency and function can be preserved by careful monitoring and prospective detection of venous stenoses. Recirculation ratios provide valuable information for identifying patients with significant stenoses. Other modalities such as Doppler flow studies and intravascular ultrasonography may also prove useful in evaluating fistula function. Aggressive correction of venous stenoses with percutaneous transluminal angioplasty improves fistula function and prolongs access patency, although surgical fistula revision remains the definitive intervention.

REFERENCES

1. Besarab A, Dorrell S, Moritz M et al: What can be done to preserve vascular access for dialysis? Semin Dial 4:155, 1991
2. Carlson DM, Duncan DA, Naessens JM, Johnson WJ: Hospitalization in dialysis patients. Mayo Clin Proc 59:769, 1984
3. Schwab SJ: Hemodialysis vascular access. p. 769. In Jacobson H, Striker G, Klahr S (eds): The Principles and Practice of Nephrology. 1st Ed. BC Decker, Philadelphia, 1991

4. Munda R, First MR, Alexander JW et al: Polytetrafluoroethylene graft survival in hemodialysis. JAMA 249:219, 1983
5. Burdick JF, Scott W, Cosimi AB: Experience with Dacron graft arteriovenous fistulas for dialysis access. Ann Surg 187:262, 1978
6. Rittgers SE, Garcia-Valdez C, McCormick JT, Posner MP: Noninvasive blood flow measurement in expanded polytetrafluoroethylene grafts for hemodialysis access. J Vasc Surg 3:635, 1986
7. Anderson CB, Etheredge EE, Harter HR et al: Blood flow measurements in arteriovenous dialysis fistulas. Surgery 81:459, 1977
8. Ronco C, Brendolan A, Bragantini L et al: Technical and clinical evaluation of different short, highly efficient dialysis techniques. Contrib Nephrol 61:46, 1988
9. Dalal S, Yu AW, Gupta DK et al: L-Lactate high efficiency hemodialysis: hemodynamics, blood gas changes, potassium/phosphorous, and symptoms. Kidney Int 38:896, 1990
10. Schwab SJ, Raymond JR, Saeed M et al: Prevention of hemodialysis fistula thrombosis: early detection of venous stenosis. Kidney Int 36:707, 1989
11. Sherman RA, Levy SS: Rate-related recirculation: the effect of altering blood flow on dialyzer recirculation. Am J Kidney Dis 17:170, 1991
12. Windus DW, Audrain J, Vanderson R et al: Optimization of high-efficiency hemodialysis by detection and correction of fistula dysfunction. Kidney Int 38:337, 1990
13. Pederson JA, Dunlay R, Williams C, Llach F: Two-needle calculation of recirculation compared with standard three needle method. Clin Nephrol 33:203, 1990
14. Kobrin SM, Kriger FL, Raja RM: Measurement of hemodialysis access recirculation: a two-needle method at the start of dialysis. ASAIO Trans 35:508, 1989
15. Gibson SM, von Albertini B, Bosch JP: Reproducible measurement of recirculation without peripheral venipuncture, abstracted. Kidney Int 37:297, 1990
16. Sherman RA, Levy SS: Assessment of a two-needle technique for measurement of recirculation during hemodialysis, abstracted. J Am Soc Nephrol 1:377, 1990
17. Schwab S, Lambert M, Collins D et al: Fistula dysfunction: effect on rapid hemodialysis, abstracted. J. Am Soc Nephrol 2:350, 1991
18. Davidson CJ, Newman GE, Sheikh KH et al: Mechanisms of angioplasty in hemodialysis fistula stenoses evaluated by intravascular ultrasound. Kidney Int 40:91, 1991
19. Schwab SJ, Saeed M, Sussman SK et al: Transluminal angioplasty of venous stenoses in polytetrafluoroethylene vascular access grafts. Kidney Int 32:395, 1987
20. Brooks JL, Sigley RD, May KJ, Mack RM: Transluminal angioplasty versus surgical repair for stenosis of hemodialysis grafts. Am J Surg 153:530, 1987
21. Newman GE, Saeed M, Himmelstein S et al: Total central vein obstruction: resolution with angioplasty and fibrinolysis. Kidney Int 39:761, 1991
22. Newman GE, Davidson CJ, McCann RL, Schwab SJ: Functional restenosis rate after hemodialysis graft angioplasty, abstracted. J Am Soc Nephrol 2:341, 1991
23. Schwab SJ, Buller G, McCann R et al: Prospective evaluation of a Dacron-cuffed hemodialysis catheter for prolonged use. Am J Kidney Dis 11:166, 1988

4

Water and Dialysate Treatment for Hemodialysis

Claudio Ronco
Alessandra Brendolan
Carlo Crepaldi

INTRODUCTION

The problem of water and dialysate quality in hemodialysis has been underestimated or neglected over the past several years.[1] New interest in this field has been spurred by the wide use of highly permeable membranes in clinical practice and by the increased number of pyrogenic reactions reported in the literature.[2–4] In addition, an increased number of possible contaminants have been found, both in tap water and in the dialysate, thanks to new and more sophisticated analytic methods.[2,5–7] Therefore water treatment for hemodialysis must efficiently remove all different types of contaminants in order to make extremely pure and refined water available at the individual dialysis bed station.

The same level of care must be given to the final preparation of dialysate. Dialysate quality must be checked and defined in terms of chemical, physical, and microbiologic characteristics. The choice of concentrates and the disinfection of the dialysis machine as well as the microbiologic control of the final dialysate are crucial points in the achievement of a "pure" dialysate. The requirement for such a dialysate has become particularly important in recent years, concurrently with the wide use of highly permeable membranes.[7] Therefore the use of such membranes in different treatments will be discussed in order to define the optimal dialysate preparation for each specific operative condition.

WATER TREATMENT MODALITIES

Several factors contribute to the increasing contamination of tap water. Increased water consumption, large urban areas, high population density, industrial waste products, and use of fertilizers in agriculture account for the most common sources of contamination. All these factors may contribute significant degrees of physical, chemical, and microbiologic pollution[8–10] (Fig. 4-1). Figure 4-2, shows some of these contaminants and methods of detecting and separating them according to their molecular size and weight. All these substances must be removed to achieve high-quality water. The standards for dialysis water recommended by the American Association for the Advancement of Medical Instrumentation (AAMI) and the Canadian Science Association (CSA)[7–12] are outlined in Table 4-1. The use of high-flux dialysis may sometimes require larger dialysate flow rates and, as a consequence, larger amounts of treated water per unit of time. Under such conditions, the equipment originally installed in one center may not be capable of maintaining effective and efficient water treatment meeting recommended AAMI standards, and improvements or equipment modification may be required. When such modifications are planned, they must involve the entire system, since the final water quality is a function of the accurate and optimal performance of each individual component. Therefore the water refining system must be considered as a complex apparatus in which water treatment equipment—circuits, tanks, and distribution pipes—are crucial parts of a whole.

Different substances can be removed with various modalities applied in series. Filtration of particles such as coal dust, beach sand, vegetable particles is achieved by sediment or media filters (Fig. 4-3). These filters are also used to protect other water treatment equipment downstream from clogging and damage. Sediment filters do not remove organic contaminants such as chloramine derivatives or compounds that can liberate free chlorine. These substances must be absorbed by carbon filters[8] (Fig. 4-4).

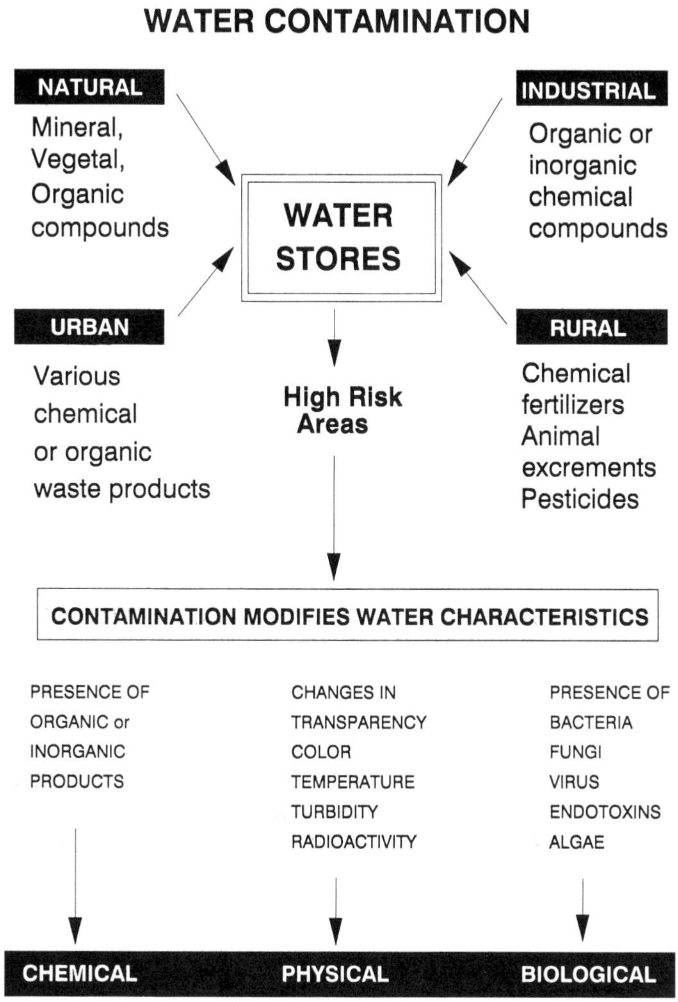

WATER CONTAMINATION

NATURAL
Mineral, Vegetal, Organic compounds

INDUSTRIAL
Organic or inorganic chemical compounds

WATER STORES

URBAN
Various chemical or organic waste products

RURAL
Chemical fertilizers
Animal excrements
Pesticides

High Risk Areas

CONTAMINATION MODIFIES WATER CHARACTERISTICS

PRESENCE OF ORGANIC or INORGANIC PRODUCTS

CHANGES IN TRANSPARENCY
COLOR
TEMPERATURE
TURBIDITY
RADIOACTIVITY

PRESENCE OF BACTERIA
FUNGI
VIRUS
ENDOTOXINS
ALGAE

CHEMICAL PHYSICAL BIOLOGICAL

Fig. 4-1. Sources and effects of water contaminants.

The European Economic Community has defined a maximal content of chlorinated solvents (30 ppb) after a series of reports concerning clinical problems related to contamination of dialysis water. For the same reason, the World Health Organization has defined a maximum of 30 pCi/L as the standard for radioactive substances in tap water.

According to these suggestions and AAMI-recommended standards, additional controls and procedures must be used for efficient water treatment.

Inorganic chemical contaminants such as aluminum, fluoride, sodium, magnesium, iron, copper, and manganese generally originate from substances in the ground or from industrial waste. These and other chemical contaminants must be removed by further water treatments, the most com-

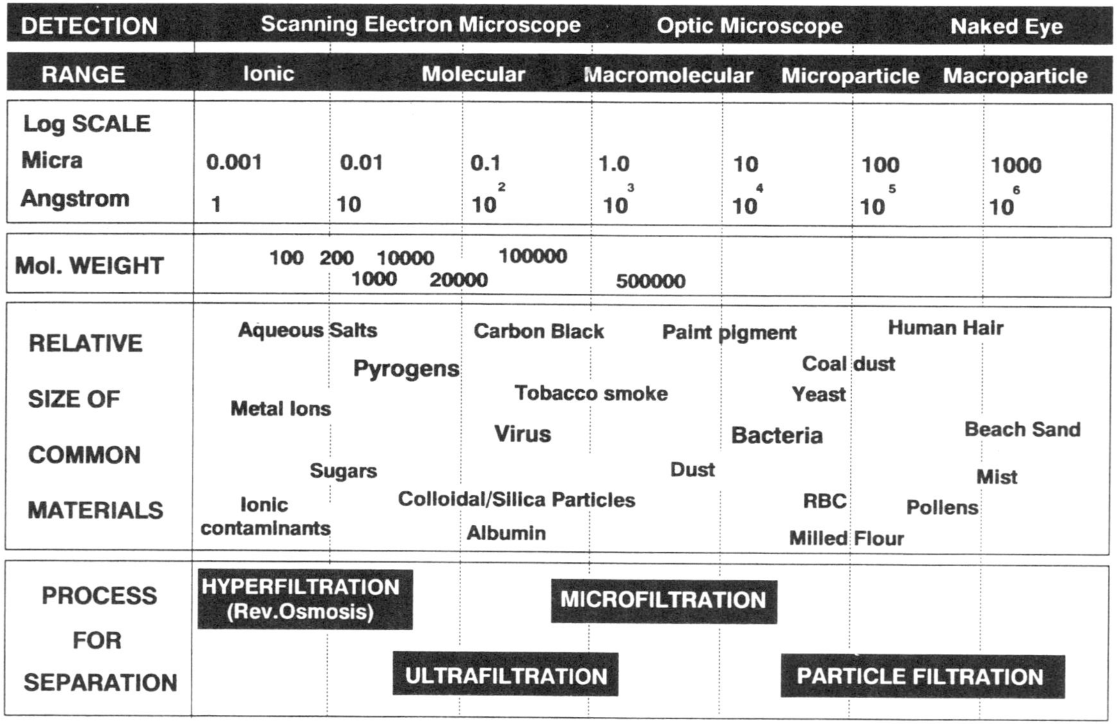

DETECTION	Scanning Electron Microscope			Optic Microscope			Naked Eye
RANGE	Ionic	Molecular		Macromolecular	Microparticle		Macroparticle
Log SCALE							
Micra	0.001	0.01	0.1	1.0	10	100	1000
Angstrom	1	10	10^2	10^3	10^4	10^5	10^6
Mol. WEIGHT	100 200	10000 1000	20000 100000	500000			
RELATIVE SIZE OF COMMON MATERIALS	Aqueous Salts Metal Ions Ionic contaminants	Pyrogens Sugars Colloidal/Silica Particles	Carbon Black Tobacco smoke Virus Albumin	Paint pigment Dust	Bacteria Yeast RBC Milled Flour	Coal dust Human Hair Pollens	Beach Sand Mist
PROCESS FOR SEPARATION	HYPERFILTRATION (Rev.Osmosis)	ULTRAFILTRATION		MICROFILTRATION	PARTICLE FILTRATION		

Fig. 4-2. Various contaminants present in tap water, methods of detection, and processes for separation according to their molecular size. (Modified from Osmonics).

Table 4-1. Proposed Dialysis Water Standards

Maximum Allowable Level mg/L	AAMI	CSA
Sodium	70	70
Potassium	8	8
Calcium	10	10
Magnesium	4	4
Fluoride	0.2	0.2
Chloride	0.5	0.5
Chloramines	0.1	0.1
Nitrate	2	2
Sulfate	100	100
Copper, barium, zinc (each)	0.1	0.1
Arsenic, chromium, lead, silver (each)	0.05	0.05
Cadmium, selenium, aluminum (each)	0.01	0.01
Mercury	0.002	0.0002
Colony count	<200/ml	<200/ml

Abbreviations: AAMI, American Association for the Advancement of Medical Instrumentation; CSA, Canadian Science Association.

monly used of which methods employ softeners, deionizers, and reverse osmosis equipment.

Softeners are employed primarily to reduce the calcium, and magnesium concentration of tap water and to protect other equipment. Calcium and magnesium ions are trapped inside columns packed with cationic resins, where they are exchanged for sodium ions. This is a partial water treatment, which cannot be safely used alone.

Deionizers use cationic and anionic resins to exchange various ions for hydrogen and hydroxyl ions, which combine to form water. Such systems must be periodically regenerated and disinfected to avoid major complications due to bacterial infestation as well as to avoid production of poor water quality[13–16] (Fig. 4-5).

Reverse osmosis, also called hyperfiltration, consists of the application of high hydrostatic pressures to membranes that reject 98 to 100 percent of chemical contaminants with production of ultrapure water. Water produced with this equipment is characterized by a resistivity higher than 1 megohm/cm. Although reverse osmosis has been widely used for industrial purposes and presently represents the best water treatment for hemodialysis, it may not be entirely free of complications (Fig. 4-6).

All these systems can be used in series. Additional filters with 0.5 and 0.2 μm resolution can be used to ensure better functioning of the whole apparatus. Water quality is continuously ensured by resistivity monitors. Water that does not meet the required standards is generally recirculated and reprocessed in the reverse osmosis system. A 0.2-mμ filter is generally included in this loop to avoid bacterial contamination of the reverse osmosis membranes by the recirculating water[14–18] (Fig. 4-7).

Various contaminants and the relative removal capacities of different equipment are schematically outlined in Table 4-2. As previously noted, all these systems can become potential sources of contamination because of

SEDIMENT OR MEDIA FILTERS

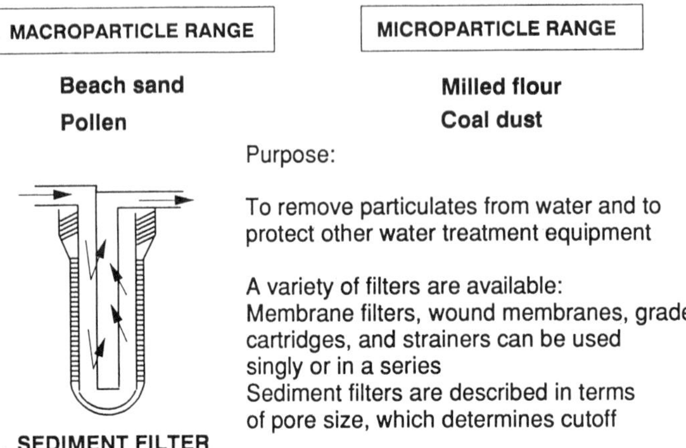

POSSIBLE PROBLEMS WITH SEDIMENT FILTERS

EVENT	CAUSE	CONSEQUENCE
Bacterial Growth inside the filter	Inadequate disinfection	Pyrogenic reactions, sepsis, bacteremia
Contaminants in treated water	Elution of substances from the resins	Hemolytic Anemia
Seal leaks or particle breakthrough	Poor quality of treated water	Damage of equipment for water treatment
Sloughing of filter media	Improper design Poor mechanical integrity	Damage to other equipment from clogging
Transluscent materials of filter housing	Algae growth in the filter	Pyrogenic reactions

Fig. 4-3. Function and possible problems with sediment or media filters.

bacterial infestation or system failure and exhaustion. In these circumstances, despite the remarkable quality of treated water, chemical and microbiologic contaminants can be found in significant amounts in the final dialysate. Figures 4-3 to 4-6 schematically describe the possible complications related to malfunction of the various systems or their inappropriate utilization. It appears evident that several clinical symptoms may be related to these problems and that the final composition of dialysis fluid may strongly affect the patient's clinical tolerance of dialysis therapy.[17,18]

CARBON FILTERS

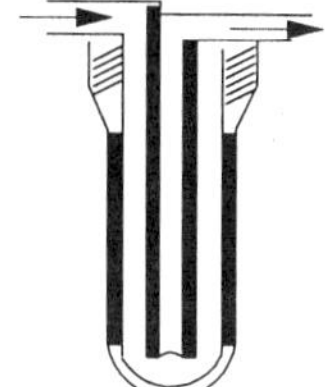

Carbon filters are adsorptive filters used to remove molecules with molecular weights in the range of 60–300 (free chlorine, chloramines, pyrogens etc.)

They can be used as pretreatment for certain types of R.O. equipment

They can contain different types of carbon: this causes different effectiveness in removing chloramines. Carbon filter cartridges can be disposable or reusable. In the latter case, a regeneration process is required (backwashing with sodium hydroxide and rinsing)

POSSIBLE PROBLEMS WITH CARBON FILTERS

EVENT	CAUSE	CONSEQUENCE
Bacterial growth inside the filter	Inadequate disinfection	Pyrogenic reactions, antibody production
Inadequate removal of chloramines	Type or source of carbon used	Chills, Hemolysis Shock, Sudden death.
High pH and [Na] in water supply	Inadequate rinse out of sodium hydroxide	Damage to water treatment equipment
Release of carbon particles	Manufacturing process/quality control	Damage to other equipment downstream from the filter
Release of adsorbed substances	Use beyond point of filter exhaustion	Toxicity depends on the substance released

Fig. 4-4. R.O., reverse osmosis. Function and possible problems with carbon filters.

DIALYSATE CONTAMINATION

The above-mentioned procedures render the treated water almost 100 percent free of contaminants. Analysis of final dialysate, however, demonstrates a significant presence of trace elements and bacterial contamination. Trace elements are contained in the salts used for preparation of the concentrate. Despite innovative procedures such as complexation with macromolecules (e.g., transferrin), significant improvement in dialysate quality from this point of view cannot be anticipated at present.

DEIONIZERS

DEIONIZERS WORK ON ION-EXCHANGE PRINCIPLE

Remove all types of cations and anions and replace them with hydrogen and hydroxide ions, which combine to form water.

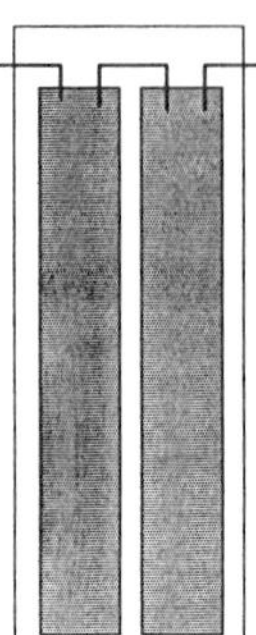

Dual-bed or mixed bed configurations produce water with a resistivity greater than 1 MOhm/cm, neutral pH, and a residual ionic concentration lower than 1 mg/L.

The system must be regenerated periodically with hydrochloric acid and sodium hydroxide.

Use beyond resins exhaustion may result in clinical risks and hazards

Bacterial contamination occurs easily because of the porous structure of the resins.

POSSIBLE PROBLEMS WITH DEIONIZERS

EVENT	CAUSE	CONSEQUENCE
Bacterial contamination	Inherent to design Poor disinfection	Pyrogenic reactions, chills, sepsis
Elution of Fluoride or Copper	DI near exhaustion Acidic effluent water	Nausea, vomiting, pain, chills, pyrogenic reactions
Undetected DI exhaustion	Monitoring system malfunction	Toxicity from poor water quality
Continued use of DI beyond point of exhaustion	Monitoring system malfunction	All risks associated with poor water quality and toxic substances
Acidic effluent water	Use beyond point of DI exhaustion	Headaches, tachycardia, clotting of dialyzers

Fig. 4-5. DI, deionizer. Function and possible problems with deionizers.

Exposure of patients undergoing dialysis to these contaminants is much greater than that observed in normal subjects drinking the same water. The patient's blood is directly exposed to an average volume of 450 L/wk of contaminated fluid, and the membranes employed are not able to prevent diffusion of trace elements.[18–28]

On the other hand, it is well known that piping, storage, and delivery systems after water treatment, as well as dialysis machines, can be sites of bacterial contamination. Inadequate piping layout, water stagnation, and inaccurate disinfection may be the most common causes of the presence of

REVERSE OSMOSIS SYSTEMS

R.O. is often used as a primary method of water treatment for HD

Hydrostatic pressures greater than the osmotic pressure of the solution are applied. This produces pure water from an aqueous solution with different ionic concentration.

R.O. membranes operate on the basis of molecular weight sieving, but also involve ionic exclusion (Cellulose Acetate Membranes).

Rejection Coefficients	System Configurations
NaCl = 0.95	Plate and Frame
Divalent Ions = 0.98	Tubular
Bacteria = 1.00	Helical
Viruses = 1.00	Spiral wound
Pyrogens = 1.00 (in absence of leaks)	Hollow fiber

POSSIBLE PROBLEMS WITH R.O. SYSTEMS

EVENT	CAUSE	CONSEQUENCE
Premature failure of R.O. Membrane	Inadequate pretreatment of water	Poor water quality
Ruptures	Improper operation of equipment such as excessive positive pressure	No consequences if readily detected by resistivity monitors
Bacterial Contamination	Inadequate disinfection Leaks not detected by resistivity monitors	Pyrogenic reactions Chills Sepsis Bacteremia

Fig. 4-6. R.O., reverse osmosis; HD, hemodialysis. Function and possible problems with reverse osmosis.

bacteria in treated water. Furthermore, dialysate contamination may depend on the quality and age of the concentrate. While acid concentrates preclude bacterial growth because of their high osmolality, a high risk of bacterial contamination and growth has been demonstrated for liquid bicarbonate concentrate. Several authors have reported the presence of bacterial contamination and remarkable concentrations of bacterial degradation products in LBC.[14,15]

Since the most common species found in treated water and liquid bicarbonate concentrate are gram-negative organisms, the formation of endotoxins

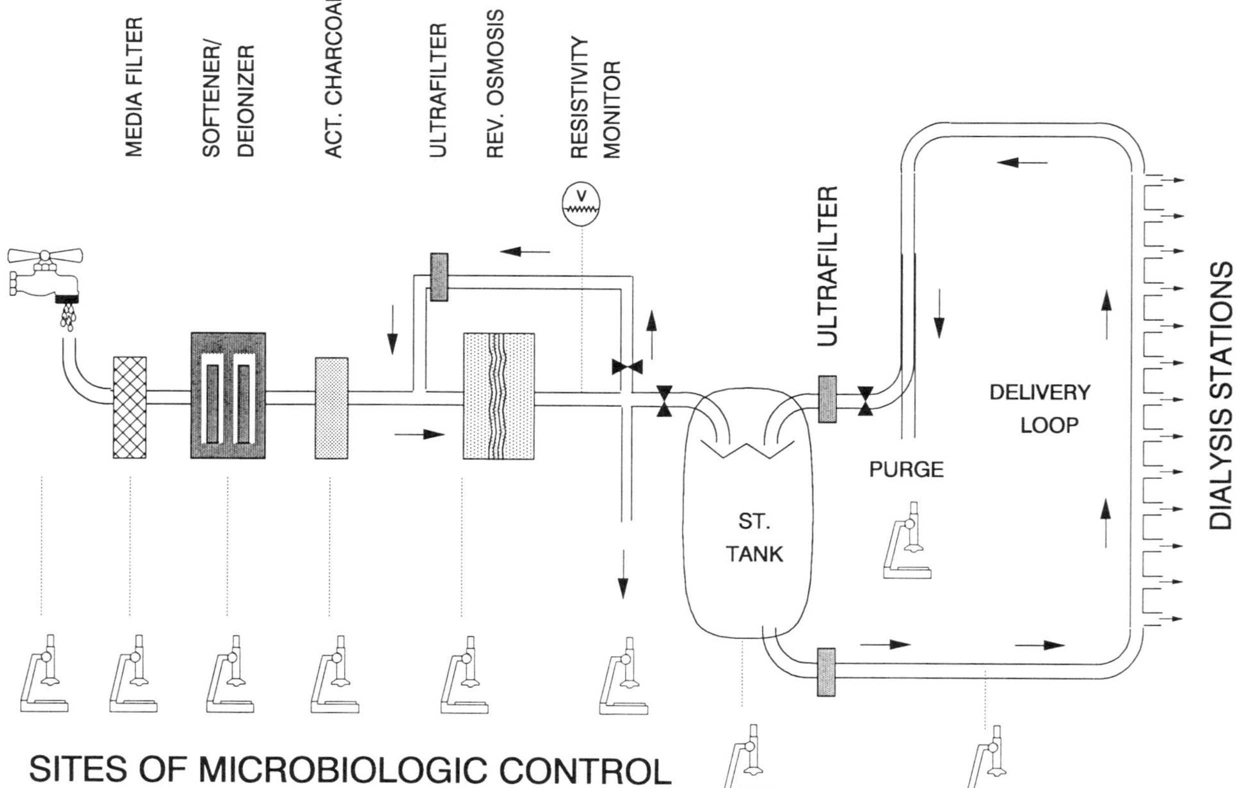

Fig. 4-7. Schematic representation of a possible circuit for water treatment and delivery. All components of the system may become a hidden source of contamination. They must be disinfected, controlled, and eventually replaced when damaged. The piping layout must ensure continuous water flow and avoid stagnation or dead spaces in the circuit.

Table 4-2. Effectiveness of Commonly Used Water Treatment Equipment

	Sediment Filters	Carbon Filters	Softeners	Deionizers	Reverse Osmosis
Aluminum				X	X
Arsenic				X	X
Barium				X	X
Cadmium				X	X
Calcium			X	X	X
Chloramine		X		X	X
Chlorine		X			
Chromium				X	X
Copper				X	X
Fluoride				X	X
Lead				X	X
Magnesium			X	X	X
Mercury				X	X
Nitrate				X	X
Potassium				X	X
Selenium				X	X
Silver				X	X
Sodium				X	X
Sulfate				X	X
Zinc				X	X
Viruses		X		X	X
Organic material		X		X	X
Endotoxins		X		X	X
Particles	X	X		X	X
Bacteria	X	X		X	X

Abbreviation: X, effective.

and their products is likely to occur. Such contaminants can be found in various concentrations in the final dialysate and include the complex lipopolysaccharide, with a molecular weight of 100,000 which represents the "intact" endotoxin. The lipopolysaccharide, which is detected by a positive reaction in the limulus amebocyte lysate (LAL) test and causes a pyrogenic reaction in the rabbit, can generate various LAL-positive fragments with molecular weights ranging between 1,000 to 20,000. Enzymatic degradation of gram-positive bacteria may also release peptidoglycans such as LAL-negative muramylpeptides, with molecular weights ranging between 400 to 1,000, which may cause monocyte activation and immunostimulation, resulting in the production of cytokines such as interleukin-1.

Minimal doses of these substances (1 to 2 ng/kg) may produce a significant pyrogenic reaction in humans.[17] On the other hand, it has been shown that concentrations of endotoxins ranging from 0.1 to 200 ng/ml can be commonly observed in standard dialysate. Furthermore, a series of pyrogenic reactions, including fever and discomfort, has been described in relation to the use of contaminated dialysate.[14,16,20,29,30]

The crux of the issue centers upon whether endotoxins are capable of crossing specific dialysis membranes. This aspect is still a matter of controversy. Different supporting and opposing data regarding this question may be found in the literature.[14,19–21] Apparently, small fragments can cross intact cellulosic membranes by backdiffusion, while larger fragments can be transported across synthetic membranes by both backdiffusion and backfiltration. However, while cellulosic membranes display very low sieving coefficients for such molecules, thus retaining these substances in the dialysate compartment, synthetic membranes seem to have specific adsorptive capacities that greatly reduce the probability of endotoxin transfer across their intact structures.

According to Mion et al.,[14] the contradictory results of various experimental studies investigating endotoxin transfer across intact dialysis membranes are probably due to problems in methodology. Several factors must be considered. Results can be different depending on whether saline solution or blood is used in the experimental circuit. When thermostated blood is used, plasma proteins seem to be the critical factor in permitting transfer of endotoxin fragments across dialysis membranes. This is further confirmed by the observation that endotoxin fragments do not cross the membrane when protein-free saline solution is used in the dialyzer blood compartment.[14] Different endotoxins may cause opposing clinical responses and cause variable interactions with dialysis membranes. This could explain, at least in part, the clinical observation of febrile reactions occurring with negative blood cultures when dialysate contamination is present. On the other hand, endotoxin antibodies found in the blood of patients treated with contaminated dialysate may be related not to the dialytic treatment but to other, pre-existing pathologic events. The characteristics of the membrane may not only play a role in terms of permeability but may also affect the biologic interaction of the membrane with endotoxins.

Adsorption and trapping of endotoxins in the membrane structure might lead to their possible contact with pseudopods of human monocytes. Under such conditions the release of cytokines from monocytes can be expected even in the absence of detectable endotoxin levels in the blood. In addition, the behavior of the membrane after reuse may not be comparable with its behavior during the first dialysis treatment. Despite the observation of a few clinically evident pyrogenic reactions in dialysis practice, even with highly permeable membranes, we do not know what results subclinical stimulation produced by endotoxins might produce in the long run. Therefore, a cautious approach is advisable.

Theoretically speaking, cellulosic and synthetic membranes show different diffusivity coefficients for various endotoxin fragments with molecular weights ranging from 1,000 to 20,000. For small molecules, diffusivity is relatively high in both cuprophane and polysulfone membranes. However, although the diffusion coefficient for small molecules is slightly higher in synthetic membranes, this represents only one of the factors affecting overall diffusive flux. Temperature, surface of the membrane, concentration gradient, and membrane thickness all influence net diffusive flux. The last parameter, in fact, plays a pivotal role in determining the final diffusive flux. The lower thickness of cuprophane permits better diffusion of small molecules as compared with polysulfone. For this reason, Colton has suggested that small endotoxin fragments with molecular weights in the range of 400 to 2,000 may be transferred easily from dialysate into the blood by backdiffusion.[6]

Different behavior is shown by larger molecules (10,000 to 20,000) which have very low free diffusion coefficients, not only in dialysis membranes but also in aqueous solutions. In this case the molecules tend to be restrained more by their low diffusivity than by the membrane itself. It is evident, however, that since the permeability of synthetic membranes is higher for these molecules than that of cuprophane, different behavior may be expected when convective flux is an important component of the dialytic treatment. When high ultrafiltration rates are used with polysulfone membranes, the possibility of backdiffusion of these molecules is partially reduced. On the other hand, when backfiltration is present, backdiffusion of small molecules may be enhanced and larger endotoxin fragments may be transported back into the blood by convection (backfiltration flux). According to this view, use of ultrapure dialysate is strongly advisable in order to avoid the risks associated with backdiffusion in cellulosic membranes and backfiltration in synthetic membranes.[22–24]

DIALYSATE CONTAMINATION AND HIGH-FLUX MEMBRANES

Since a large number of adverse reactions have apparently been related to the use of highly permeable membranes, we will discuss some possible approaches to the clinical use of these membranes. Several solutions have been proposed to reduce the negative effects of microbiologic contamination of dialysate. These possible approaches may be divided into two categories: strategies aimed at avoiding backfiltration and strategies that permit backfiltration but include specific dialysate treatments.[23,24] These approaches are shown schematically in Figure 4-8.

Hemodiafiltration, which is commonly used in Europe, consists of mixed diffusive-convective therapy, with the ultrafiltration rate always maintained in a high range to avoid backfiltration. Large amounts of fluids are removed during treatment, and use of a commercially prepared, sterile replacement solution is mandatory. A 9- to 15-L portion of this solution is reinfused in a postdilutional mode; specific dialysate purification is not used. In all cases the ultrafiltration rate is higher than the critical filtration rate, and backfiltration is thus avoided (Fig. 4-8).

A different situation is encountered in high-flux dialysis. In this treatment convection is also largely used, but it is less evident since significant amounts of backfiltration reduce the absolute value of net filtration. Use of both extremely high quality water and carefully controlled dialysate is both strongly recommended.

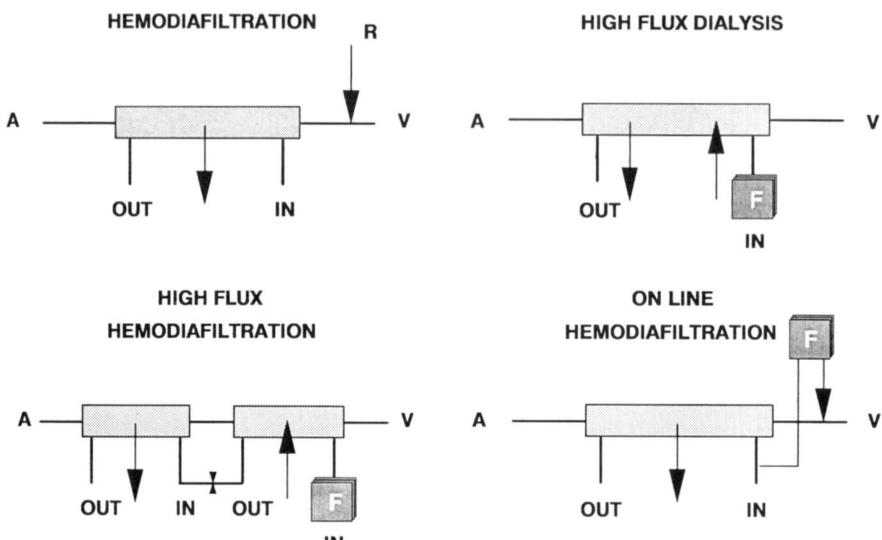

Fig. 4-8. Different methods of using highly permeable membranes. (**A**) Hemodiafiltration maintains a high convective flux and avoids backfiltration but requires the reinfusion of substitution fluid. (**B**) High-flux dialysis operates with low net ultrafiltration, achieved because of high filtration and backfiltration flows. Treatment of dialysate is recommended. (**C**) High-flux hemodiafiltration uses two dialyzers in series. In the first ultrafiltration occurs, while in the second backfiltration takes place. Since the filtration and backfiltration fluxes are greater than in high-flux dialysis, dialysate treatment is even more important. (**D**) On-line hemodiafiltration is a compromise that maintains ultrafiltration sufficiently high to avoid backfiltration. The replacement solution is prepared on line from fresh inlet dialysate.

Despite the fact that treatment of dialysate is not a standard procedure in most centers using high-flux dialysis, we would like to emphasize the importance of such a procedure in view of the following considerations. All water treatment systems may be hidden sources of contamination when disinfection procedures are inadequate. Even in the case of a properly operating water treatment, several possible contamination sites may be present in the circuit; these include the piping system, the liquid bicarbonate concentrate, and the dialysis machine itself. Therefore, not only is stringent disinfection of the whole system required, but final dialysate treatment just before the dialyzer is also recommended. Most dialysis companies presently supply a built-in system for ultrafiltration of the dialysate, which includes a large surface area hollow-fiber ultrafilter equipped with different synthetic membranes. Such a system guarantees the high quality and purity of the dialysate during treatment. Table 4-3 outlines the main characteristics of three filters commonly used for this purpose.

Two specific aspects of these filters must be considered. The first concerns the ability of the membrane to retain endotoxins and endotoxin fragments. This is expressed as the ratio of the logarithm of the concentration in a

Table 4-3. Characteristics of Three Different Filters for Dialysate Treatment

Company	Amicon	Fresenius	Gambro
Name	Diaclean	Diasafe	UV 7000
Membrane	PSF 75 μ	PSF 30 μ	Polyamide
Surface area	2.4 m^2	1.8 m^2	2.0 m^2
Pressure drop (Qd 500)	40 mmHg	135 mmHg	75 mmHg
Bacterial retention	100%	100%	100%
Endotoxin reduction factor[a]	5	7.5	4

[a] Native endotoxin reduction factor is calculated from the ratio log endotoxin units in challenge suspension/log endotoxin units in the filtrate. Experimental conditions: log bacterial challenge, 7; log endotoxin challenge, 4.

challenge suspension to the logarithm of the concentration in the filtrate. The reduction factor for these filters is found to be between 4 and 7.5, which demonstrates that a significant effect of these devices on the final endotoxin concentration in dialysate can be expected. Considering an average concentration of endotoxins between 0.1 and 200 endotoxin units per milliliter (E.U./ml), the use of these filters should provide an LAL-negative, "ultrapure" dialysate. Most of this characteristic is probably due to adsorption of endotoxins and their fragments on the inner structure of the membrane. The filters therefore must be changed periodically in order to avoid using them beyond the point of exhaustion of their adsorptive capacity.

The second aspect concerns the hydraulics of the dialysate circuit. All these filters are characterized by a transmembrane pressure drop that is proportional to the dialysate flow crossing the membrane. This creates a positive pressure before the filter, which must be considered when using standard dialysis machines. Some older dialysis machines may not be able to compensate for the higher pressure in the dialysate circuit, and dialysate delivery may become inaccurate. When the filter is a built-in component of the machine, the circuit automatically adjusts to different pressure levels, and the prescribed dialysate flow is accurately delivered. Periodic air purging of the filter is also suggested in order to avoid surface loss due to air trapping in the filter. Dialysis machines with built-in filters are equipped with an automatic system for filter purging.

Dialysate ultrafiltration, in our view, is strongly recommended when using treatments that involve higher surface areas and backfiltration flows, such as high-flux hemodiafiltration.[19] In this treatment filtration takes place in the first filter, and backfiltration occurs in the second filter (Fig. 4-8C). Filtration and backfiltration fluxes up to 150 ml/min have been reported, and high transmembrane pressures are commonly used.

A possible compromise between the above-described approaches is offered by hemodiafiltration, with on-line production of the replacement solution. This method, still under investigation, does not provide full dialysate treatment; instead, part of the fresh incoming dialysate is ultrafiltered with a 0.7 m^2 polysulfone membrane and a 0.2 μm filter in series and is then reinfused into the venous line of the circuit. This permits blood ultrafiltration to be maintained at a level up to 4 to 6 L/h thus avoiding backfiltration during treatment (Fig. 4-8D). The system requires an efficient ultrafiltration control apparatus, which serves as a dialysate inlet and outlet flux equalizer. In other words, the amount of fresh dialysate used for reinfusion is replaced in the exhausted dialysate by the amount of ultrafiltrate. The system permits the treatment of only part of the dialysate and does not require commercially prepared solutions for reinfusion. This system is still being clinically evaluated but may represent an interesting approach for the future.

PRACTICAL RECOMMENDATIONS

Continuous and effective surveillance of water and dialysate characteristics is an important aspect of the quality of hemodialysis treatment. Several problems may be caused by inadequate water treatment or inaccurate microbiologic dialysate control, and physicians and technicians may not have been specifically trained to avoid such complications.[31] For this reason we consider it appropriate to add some practical guidelines to supplement the theoretical approach described in the previous sections of this chapter.

Monitoring Procedures

Special sampling points are generally provided at the sites of microbiologic control throughout the entire system of water treatment and delivery (Fig. 4-7). Water samples should be collected from each sampling port after a flushing period of 30 seconds. Samples of water to be used for dialysate preparation must be collected immediately prior to mixing with dialysate concentrate. Dialysate samples should be collected at least weekly immediately ahead of the dialyzer any time during the dialysis treatment. Samples from internal fluid pathways within the dialysis machine should also be collected before and after disinfection procedures. Samples should be subjected to microbiologic assays by the spread plate technique or membrane filtration. The culture medium should be tryptic soy agar, and cultures should be incubated at 37°C for 48 hours. Endotoxin concentrations should be measured by LAL assay. Table 4-4 outlines the standards recommended for microbial and endotoxin contamination in dialysis fluids.[32]

Table 4-4. Microbiologic and Endotoxin Standards for Dialysis Fluids

Type of Fluid	Microbial Count (cfu/ml)	Endotoxin Concentration (ng/ml)
Treated water to prepare dialysate	<200	No standard
Dialysate	<2,000	No standard
Treated water to reprocess dialyzers	<200	<1
Treated water for dialyzer disinfectant	<200	<1

[a] *Abbreviation:* cfu, colony-forming unit.

The quality of treated water must also be checked with resistivity monitors and possibly by a continuous graphic recording of the resistivity value. When the treated water does not meet the required values of resistivity (Fig. 4-7), specific alarms activate a recirculation loop, and water is thereby reprocessed. It is also helpful, however, to maintain the graphic recording during the entire period of water treatment since daily variations related to temperature, flow rates, and pressures may interfere with system performance and with the final quality of the delivered water.

Bacterial Growth Prevention

Normally tap water contains less than 100 bacterial colonies per milliliter. The quality of the hydraulic installation and the water treatment chain used to prepare pure water for hemodialysis may be important factors affecting bacterial growth. As far as the hydraulic installation is concerned, three criteria should be considered for optimal performance:

1. A design of the hydraulic circuit should ensures linear circulation of water, with elimination of any valve or lateral arm that may create stagnation zones.
2. Bacterial adhesion to the inner surfaces of the piping should be prevented (a small diameter of the conduit yields high water velocity and shear rate). Despite the use polyvinylchloride in several older systems, use of stainless steel in newer systems is strongly recommended.
3. Water circulation should be continuous, since any stagnation is inevitably accompanied by bacterial proliferation.

As far as the water treatment chain is considered, media filters, ion-exchange resins (water softeners or deionizers), and activated carbon filters are potential sites of bacterial growth. Cartridge filters are made of felt, cotton cloth, or fiberglass. These porous materials are easily penetrated by waterborne bacteria, which can proliferate in situ. Resins are also excellent materials for bacterial proliferation, and the backwashing procedure during regeneration may not completely remove bacteria. Activated carbon is an excellent site for bacterial growth. Its high affinity for organic substances facilitates bacterial fixation and proliferation.

To reduce bacterial contamination, media filters, carbon cartridges, and ion-exchange resins must be periodically changed or regenerated and disinfected (if possible every week but at least on a monthly basis). The disinfection procedures must be accurate and performed by professionally trained personnel. Manufacturers generally provide a specific instruction manual for each piece of water treatment equipment, and the advised procedures for disinfection, regeneration, or substitution should be accurately followed.

A special comment about activated carbon filters is in order. These filters are used to remove chloramines and other organic products. Chloramines found in dialysis equipment have molecular weights of 51.5 to 120.4 and easily cross filtration membranes. A concentration of 0.25 mg/L is sufficient to cause hemolysis and metahemoglobinemia.[33] They originate from water containing ammonia or to which ammonia is added to stabilize chlorine (to avoid formation of chloroform) that has been added for disinfection procedures. Carbon filters can efficiently remove chloramines, but the activated carbon must be periodically regenerated or changed. It is critical to perform a periodic test for chloramines and to maintain optimal efficiency of the activated carbon, since minimal concentrations of these substances may cause life-threatening hemolytic syndromes.

Special care should also be used in the monitoring and disinfection of the internal fluid pathways of the dialysis machine. Even when very highly purified water is delivered at the bed station, the dialysis machine may in fact represent a site of contamination and bacterial growth. The final quality of dialysate will therefore depend on the accuracy of all sterilization procedures.

System Disinfection

A real understanding of the functions and interactions of individual components of the water treatment for hemodialysis is required to achieve an effective performance of the system. For this reason we strongly suggest specific training of the personnel involved in the system maintenance and strict adherence to the procedures recommended by the manufacturers of the different components.

Disinfection procedures for hemodialysis systems are mostly directed toward gram-negative bacteria that can survive and multiply in water. Routine disinfection of only isolated components of the water treatment chain can frequently produce inadequate results. When disinfection procedures are considered, they must be applied to the entire system. Aqueous formaldehyde solutions (1 to 2 percent) generally produce consistent results. Formaldehyde has good vapor-phase germicidal activity and penetrating characteristics. Sometimes irritating fumes can be observed in the ambient air; staff members may be exposed to health hazards if the concentration in the air exceeds the safety standards.

Once disinfection has been completed, several commercial test kits can be used for determining residual formaldehyde levels in water and for ensuring a complete rinse-out of the germicide prior to resumption of dialysis treatment. Chlorine-based disinfectants, such as sodium hypochlorite solutions, are convenient and effective when used at a concentration of about 500 ppm. Because of the corrosive nature of chlorine, the disinfectant is usually rinsed out from the system with treated water after 30 minutes. Then, if the system is not immediately used, bacterial growth from the stagnant water can be expected even after disinfection. Therefore chlorine-based disinfection should be carried out during the morning hours just before the beginning of dialysis center activity, instead of in the late evening.

Complete disinfection of the system is generally planned on a weekly basis, but more frequent disinfection procedures can be scheduled when microbiologic or clinical evidence of bacterial colonization is observed. As far as the dialysis machine is concerned, complete disinfection of the external surfaces of the machine as well as of the inner fluid pathways is recommended. The external surface can be disinfected on a daily basis with chemical detergents and disinfectants to avoid transmission of bloodborne viruses such as hepatitis B. Internal fluid pathways in each dialysis machine must be disinfected at the end of its continuous use. Bacteria do not colonize or adhere to inner surfaces during dialysis flow; therefore if the machine is kept running, disinfection between each treatment is unnecessary.

Despite the fact that in most dialysis machines dialysate does not recirculate, possible patient to patient contamination with viruses has been suggested, and various policies of isolation have been proposed for infected patients. Use of a complete disposable dialysate circuit in our center has made it possible to limit spread of hepatitis C infection (Chiaramonte S, Ronco C, LaGreca G: Center policy for infected patients. Unpublished data presented at internal meetings, St. Bortolo Hospital, Vicenza, Italy). Chemical germicides containing glutaraldehyde or hydrogen peroxide/peroxyacetic acid (or citric acid) are commercially available and specifically designed for hemodialysis machines. These products offer the combined advantage of disinfection and removal of encrusted calcium carbonate crystals from the inner fluid pathways of the dialysis machine. All these germicides must be used in strict accordance with the instructions on the manufacturer's label. Germicides containing 4 percent formaldehyde or hydrogen peroxide/peroxyacetic acid have also been used for dialyzer reprocessing with remarkable effectiveness.

In conclusion, weekly microbiologic controls must be undertaken to ensure the necessary quality of water and dialysate. Complete disinfection of the system on a weekly basis is the minimal preventive procedure to be established. Daily disinfection of the dialysis machine should also be carried out unless concurrent situations suggest a more intensive policy. Cartridge filters and ion-exchange resins must be monitored and changed or regenerated according to the manufacturer's instructions. Charcoal filters must be periodically checked, as well as chloramine levels in treated water.

High-temperature of vapor disinfection is another useful procedure to maintain the system free of contamination. This approach is mostly used when stainless steel piping and a "clean" vapor generator are available.

CONCLUSIONS

In summary, it appears evident today that maintaining the quality of dialysis solutions is a complex and multifactorial problem. The use of higher dialysis flow rates and the increasing number of high-flux dialysis procedures necessitate a high degree of attention to the quality of water treatment and the final dialysate preparation. A refined water delivery must be ensured, according to the AAMI recommendations, and continuous quality control must be provided. The microbiologic purity of dialysate cannot be neglected when newer, highly biocompatible treatments are clinically required. Therefore, despite the small number of clinically evident adverse dialysis reactions reported, as compared with the total amount of dialysis delivered, continuous surveillance of dialysate quality must be provided in order to reduce the frequency of such events to the minimum. On the other hand, a more sophisticated approach should also be considered in order to avoid long-term complications related to subclinical chronic immunostimulation of the dialysis patient. All factors responsible for adverse effects on patients should be considered and avoided in a continuous search for the most biocompatible treatment.

REFERENCES

1. Bommer J, Ritz E: Water quality: a neglected problem in hemodialysis. Nephron 46:1, 1987
2. Keshaviah P, Luehmann D, Ilstrup K, Collins A: Technical requirements for rapid high efficiency therapies. Artif Organs 3:189, 1987
3. Raij L, Shapiro FL, Michael F: Endotoxemia in febrile reactions during hemodialysis. Kidney Int 4:57, 1973
4. Graf H, Watzke H, Stanek HP et al: Bacterial contamination of dialysate in dialysis-associated endotoxemia. Blood Purif 5:284, 1987
5. Canaud B, Peyronnet P, Annynot AM, et al: Ultrapure water: a need for future dialysis, abstracted. EDTA Abstracts, 1986.
6. Colton CK: Analysis of membrane processes for blood purification. Blood Purif 5:202, 1987
7. Keshaviah P, Luehman F, Shapiro F, Compty C: Investigation of the risks and hazards associated with hemodialysis system. (Technical Report Contract 223-78-5046) U.S. Food and Drug Administration, Bureau of Medical Devices, Silver Spring, MD, 1980
8. Kjellestrand CM, Eaton JW, Yawata Y et al: Hemolysis in dialysed patients caused by chloramines. Nephron 13:427, 1974
9. Manzler AD, Schreiner AW: Copper induced acute hemolytic anemia. Ann Intern Med 73:409, 1970
10. Webster JD, Parker TF, Alfrey AC et al: Acute nickel intoxication by dialysis. Ann Intern Med 92:631, 1980
11. Gallery EDM, Blomfield J, Dixon SR: Acute zinc toxicity in hemodialysis. Br Med J 4:331, 1972
12. Scanziani R: La qualità delle acque nel trattamento dialitico. Dial Oggi 25:37, 1989
13. Kjellstrand CM: Toxicity of material and medications used in dialysis. Trans Am Soc Artif Intern Organs 24:764, 1978
14. Mion C, Canaud B, Francesqui MP et al: Bicarbonate (HCO_3) concentrate (CONC). A hidden source of microbial contamination of dialysis fluid. Blood Purif 5:299, 1987

15. Ebben JP, Hirsch DN, Luehmann DA et al: Microbiological contamination of liquid bicarbonate concentrate (LBC) for hemodialysis (HD). ASAIO Trans 33(3):269, 1987
16. Man NK, Ciancioni C, Guyomard S et al: Risks and hazards of contaminated dialysate associated with high-flux membrane. Prev Nephrol 227, 1987
17. Port FK, VanDeKerkhove KM, Kunkel SL, Kluger MH: The role of dialysate in the stimulation of interleukin-1 production during clinical hemodialysis. Am J Kidney Dis 10(2):118, 1987
18. Canaud B, Nguyen QV, Kaaki M et al: Bicarbonate hemodiafiltration with in line production of substitution fluid: short dialysis of high-efficiency in uncompliant patients and the elderly. Blood Purif 6:348, 1988
19. Von Albertini B, Miller JH, Gardner PW, Shinaberger JH: High-flux hemodiafiltration: under six hours/week treatment. ASAIO Trans 30:227, 1984
20. Ronco C, Brendolan A, Bragantini L et al: Technical and clinical evaulation of different short dialysis techniques. Contrib Nephrol 61:46, 1988
21. Bernick JJ, Port FK, Favero MS, Brown DG: Bacterial and endotoxin permeability of hemodialysis membranes. Kidney Int 16:491, 1979
22. Dinarello CA, Kreuger JM: Induction of interleukin-1 by synthetic and naturally occurring muramyl peptides. FASEB J 45:2534, 1986
23. Ronco C: Backfiltration in clinical dialysis: nature of the phenomenon and possible solutions. J Artif Organs 13:11, 1990
24. Ronco C: La backfiltration in dialisi: natura idraulica del fenomeno, risvolti clinici e possibili approcci al problema. p. 95. In: Attualità Nefrologiche e Dialitiche '88. Vol. 20. Wichtig, Milan, 1989
25. Maggiore Q, Pizzarelli F, Sisca S et al: Vascular stability and heat in dialysis patients. Contrib Nephrol 41:398, 1984
26. Alfrey AC: Dialysis encephalopathy. Kidney Int 18 (suppl. 29): S53, 1986
27. Alfrey AC, Legendre GR, Kaehny WD: The dialysis encephalopathy syndrome. Possible aluminium intoxication. N Engl J Med 294:184, 1976
28. Salvadeo A, Minoia C, Segagni S, Vill G: Trace metal changes in dialysis fluid and blood of patients on hemodialysis. Int J Artif Organs 2:17, 1979
29. Petersen NJ, Boyer KM, Carson LA, Favero MS: Pyrogenic reactions from inadequate disinfection of a dialysis fluid distribution system. Dial Transplant 7:56, 1978
30. Port FK, Bernick JJ: Pyrogen and endotoxin reactions during hemodialysis. Contrib Nephrol 36:100, 1983
31. Kimmel PL, Bosch JP: Effectiveness of renal fellowship training for subsequent clinical practice. Am J Kidney Dis 2:249, 1991
32. Bland LA, Favero MS: Microbial contamination control strategies for hemodialysis systems. Plant Technol Safety Management Ser No 3, 1989
33. Davis MK, Barrett SE, McGuire MJ: The change of water treatment methods from chlorine to chloramine by water districts. Contemp Dial 9:31, 1984

5

Newer Membranes: Cuprophane Versus Polysulfone Versus Polyacrylonitrile

Peter Konstantin

INTRODUCTION

In the 1960s, the decade during which routine chronic hemodialysis was introduced, cellulose membranes were the only type used in this treatment. However, the limitations of regenerated cellulose led scientists at the end of the decade to develop highly permeable membranes, such as Amicon's polysulfone and Rhône-Poulenc's polyacrylonitrile membranes, which provide improved elimination of high-molecular-weight uremic toxins, thus more directly imitating the function of the normal human kidney.

Further efforts have been made to improve standard hemodialysis by the development of synthetic, noncellulosic, and more biocompatible membrane materials. In the early 1980s these efforts led to the introduction of the Fresenius hydrophilic polysulfone membrane, possessing enhanced structural integrity together with high water and solute flow capacity and increased diffusive transport properties. The hydrophilic nature of this modified polysulfone membrane made it possible to use this membrane for high-flux hemodialysis and hemodiafiltration as well as for hemofiltration.

Together with these improved membranes, today's reliable balancing systems to control ultrafiltration have enabled high-flux dialysis to become a practical reality. The performance of a membrane in extracorporeal therapy for end-stage renal disease is determined by its structure, its overall mass transfer properties, and its blood compatibility.

MEMBRANE PROPERTIES

The membranes described here are manufactured in the form of capillary hollow fibers according to the phase inversion principle. The basic polymer, dissolved in a water- miscible solvent, is extruded with a core liquid to keep the lumen open (in the case of cuprophane) and/or to precipitate the hollow fiber from the inside out to form a specific pore structure (for polysulfone). By adjusting the spinning parameters (e.g., type and concentration of polymer, solvents, additives, temperature, and type of precipitation medium), it is possible to obtain membranes that differ in water flux and solute permeabilities (Table 5-1).

Most dialyzers today are still sterilized with ethylene oxide, which, if the equipment is not properly degassed, leaches out during hemodialysis and can cause hypersensitivity reactions. Up to now the only exception has been cuprophane, filled either with water or with excess glycerol. Also, not all membrane materials can be sterilized by radiation, and during γ-ray sterilization degradation of polymers or formation of radicals cannot be excluded. Recently, polysulfone has been introduced as the first steam-sterilized, non-glycerol-containing, dry high-flux filter, which eliminates the problem of leachable and residual ethylene oxide (Table 5-1).

Figures 5-1 to 5-3 show scanning electron micrographs of cuprophane, polyacrylonitrile, and polysulfone membranes. Cuprophane has a very dense homogeneous structure, the pores of which cannot be visualized even at the

Table 5-1. Comparison of Membrane Materials

	Polysulfone		Cuprophane	AN 69
	(High-flux)	(Low-flux)	(low-flux)	(high-flux)
Diameter (μm)	200	200	200	230
Wall thickness (μm)	40	40	8	40
Hydraulic permeability (ml/h/mmHg/m^2)	200	5	5	50
Pore filler	—	—	glyc, H_2O	glyc
Sterilization	Eto, steam	Eto	Eto, steam	Eto, γ-radiation

Abbreviations: glyc, glycerol, Eto, ethylene oxide.

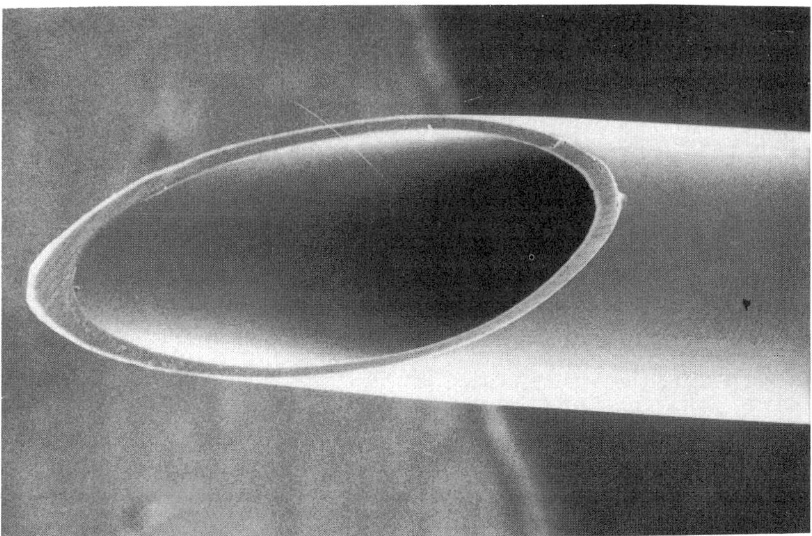

Fig. 5-1. Cross section of a cuprophane hollow fiber.

highest magnification of a scanning electron microscope. Polyacrylonitrile membrane AN69 is a copolymer of acrylonitrile and sodium methallylsulfonate, the structure of which is very much influenced by its charged methallylsulfonate commonomer. Whereas a pure polyacrylonitrile membrane has the large pores of an ultrafiltration membrane, this membrane shows a finely porous, homogeneous wall structure. Blending with polyvinylpyrrolidone[1] instead of chemical modification, as is done with polysulfone, is another way of altering the physical structure of a membrane. Instead of large, fingerlike pores,[1] this membrane exhibits the spongelike structure of a microfiltration membrane. The increased diffusive transport of solute associated with this structure enables this normally hydrophobic membrane material to be used in hemodiafiltration and high-flux dialysis. Also, this structure makes the membrane uniquely suitable for the removal of bacteria and pyrogens from dialysate. Because of the multiplicity of pores differing only slightly in size, surface deficiencies that may lead to a breakthrough in a regular ultrafilter with a fingerlike pore structure do not cause any such problem.

PARAMETERS INFLUENCING SOLUTE CLEARANCES

A low-flux membrane uses diffusion as the transport mechanism with the difference between the solute concentrations on the blood and dialysate sides as the driving force. Since the diffusion rate of a molecule is dependent on its size, larger molecules are cleared more slowly than smaller ones. This is

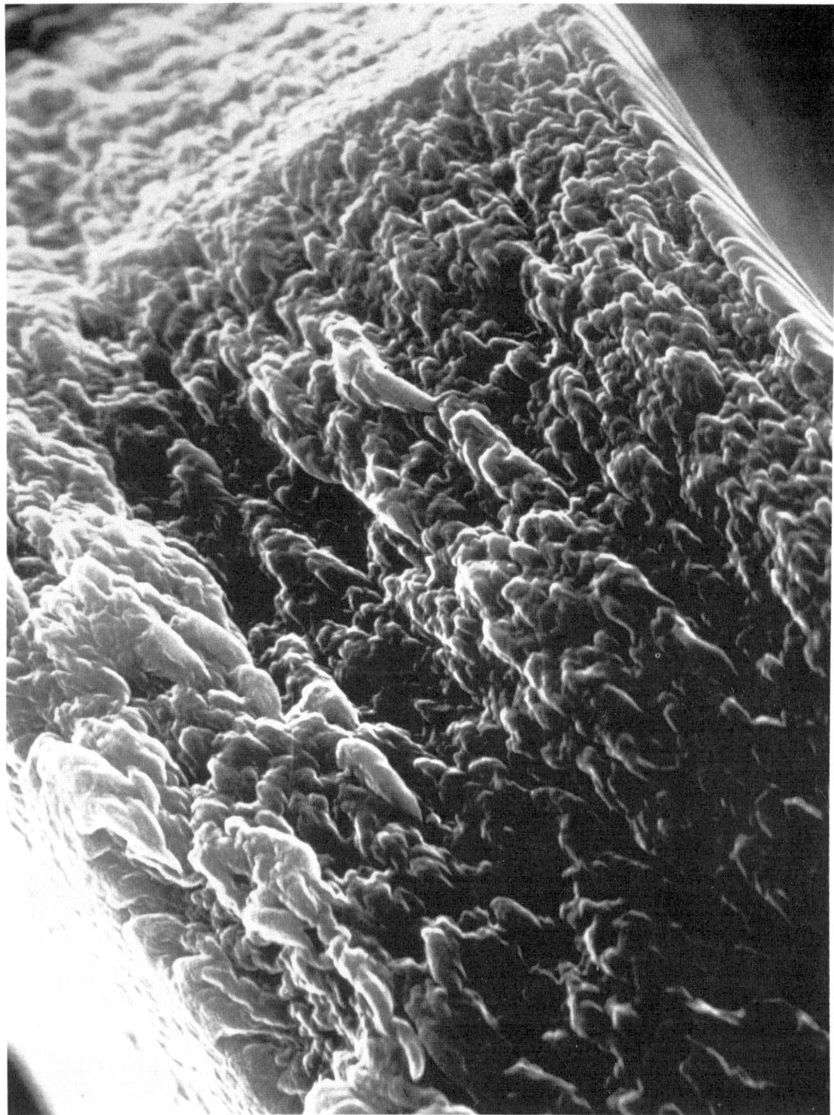

Fig. 5-2. Cross section of a polyacrylonitrile AN69 hollow fiber.

different for a high-flux membrane, for which convection is an additional driving force. As long as the molecular size of a solute is below the cutoff of the membrane, the clearance is only limited by the filtration rate; thus a 12,000 molecular weight molecule has the same clearance rate as urea, which has a molecular weight of 60. This is illustrated in Figure 5-4, showing the in vitro clearances of polysulfone low-flux and high-flux dialyzers with increasing surface areas. It can be recognized that for urea and creatinine there is very little performance difference between a polysulfone low-flux

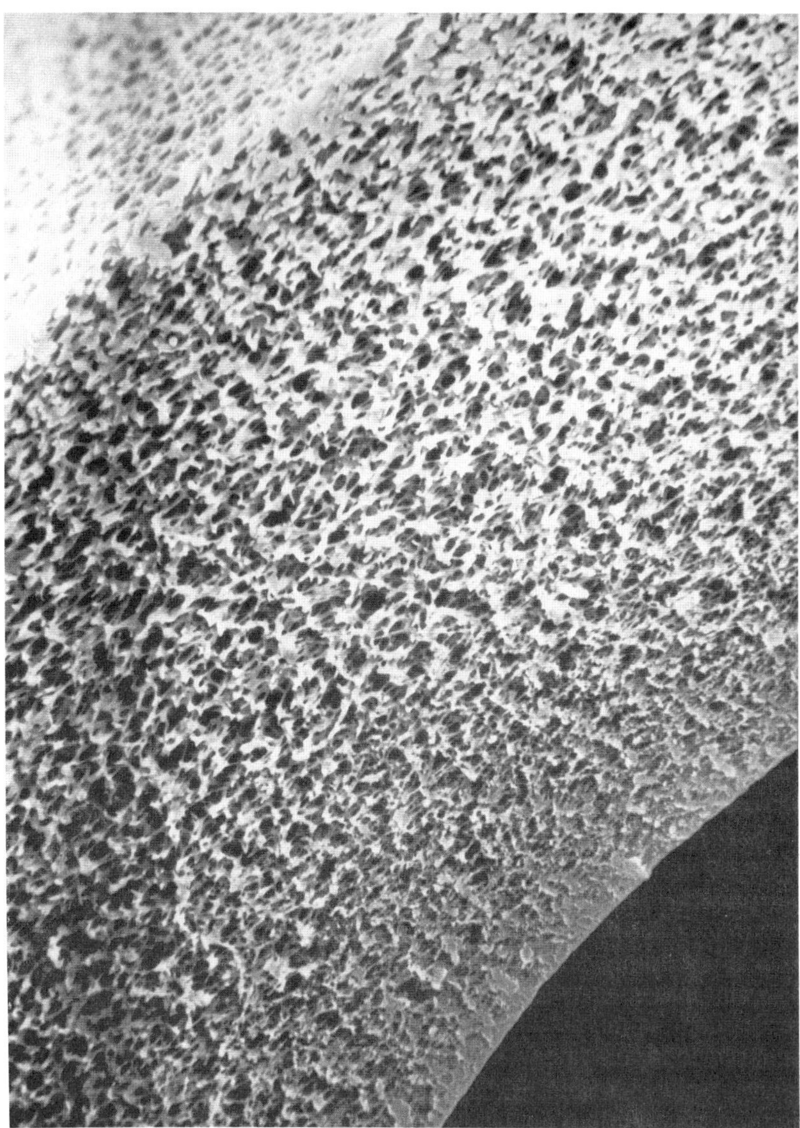

Fig. 5-3. Cross section of a polysulfone hollow fiber.

membrane and a high-flux 1.8-m^2 device. However, even with phosphate and to a greater extent with vitamin B_{12}, the convective contribution to the clearance plays a major role, and distinctive performance differences can be observed for low-flux and high-flux devices of equal surface areas. The same differences for clearance of high molecular weight solutes can be found with cellulosic membranes as described below in connection with aluminum and β_2-microglobulin removal.

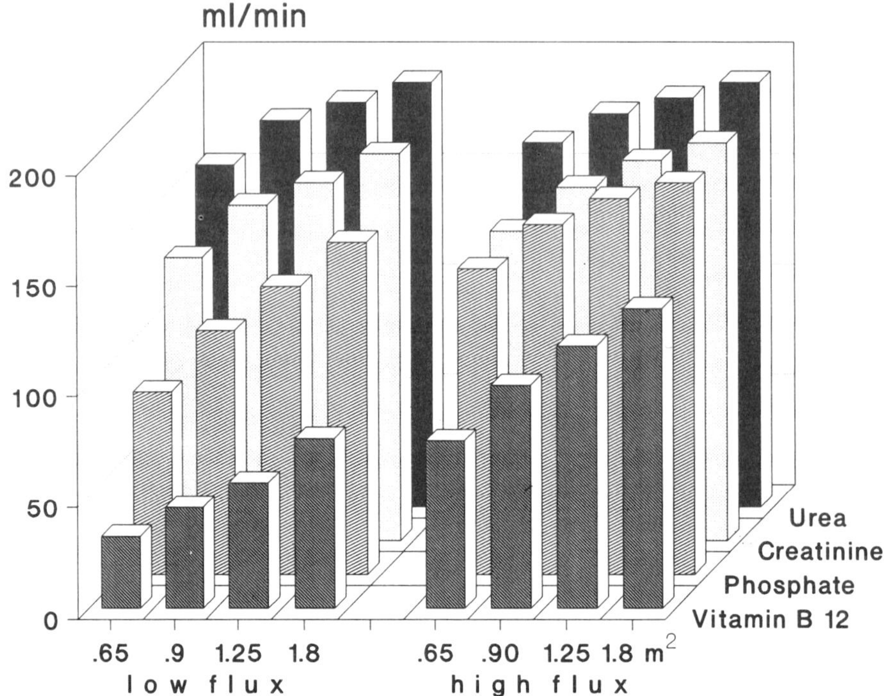

Fig. 5-4. Polysulfone in vitro clearances.

Ways to further improve solute clearance for a given membrane are shown in Figures 5-5 to 5-7. As stated before, the diffusive clearance is dependent upon the solute concentration difference between the blood and the dialysate side. If, therefore this concentration is decreased by increasing either the blood flow (Fig. 5-5) or the dialysate flow (Fig. 5-6), the concentration polarization at the membrane wall is diminished and thus an increase in low molecular weight substances can be observed. The only way in which removal of larger solutes such as inulin can be effected is by addition of ultrafiltration. This, of course, can be accomplished only with a high-flux membrane. Figure 5-7 depicts inulin clearance as a function of filtration rate and blood flow. The higher the filtration rate, the higher the clearance. Also, blood flow influences clearance until a plateau is reached, which is a result of concentration polarization on the blood side of the membrane.

ALUMINUM REMOVAL

The widespread long-term use of aluminum hydroxide as a phosphate binder in hemodialysis patients causes aluminum accumulation in the body and consequent clinical problems. Since plasma aluminum is primarily bound to transferrin (molecular weight 68,000) or to albumin, it is nondialyz-

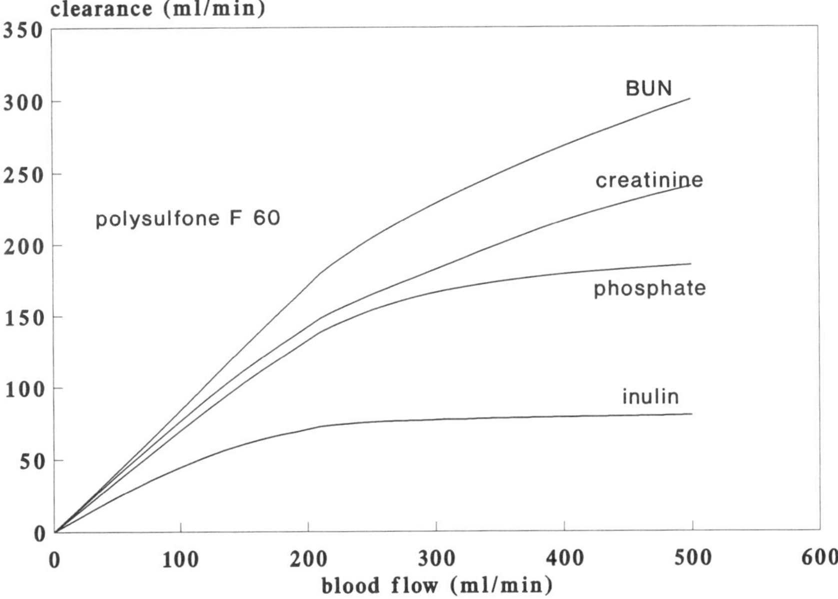

Fig. 5-5. Clearance versus blood flow.

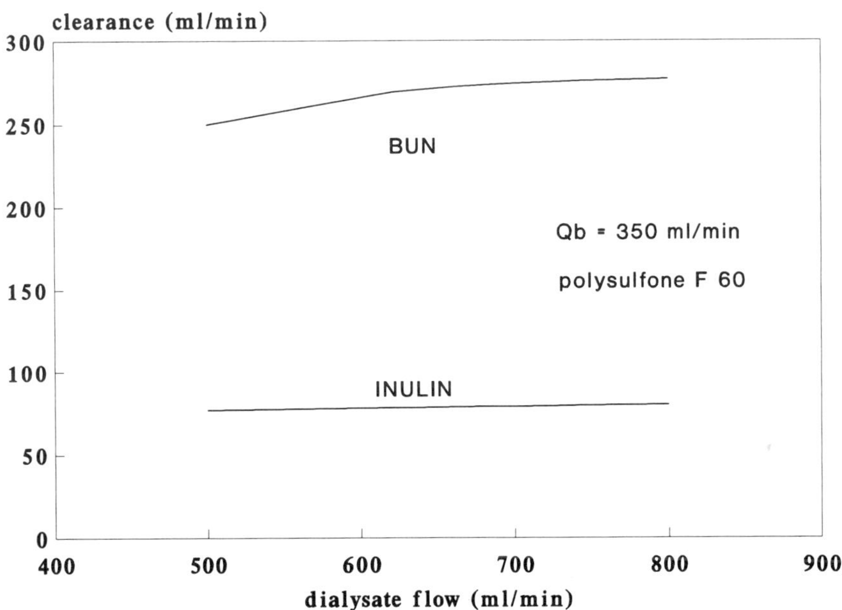

Fig. 5-6. BUN and inulin clearances as a function of dialysate flow.

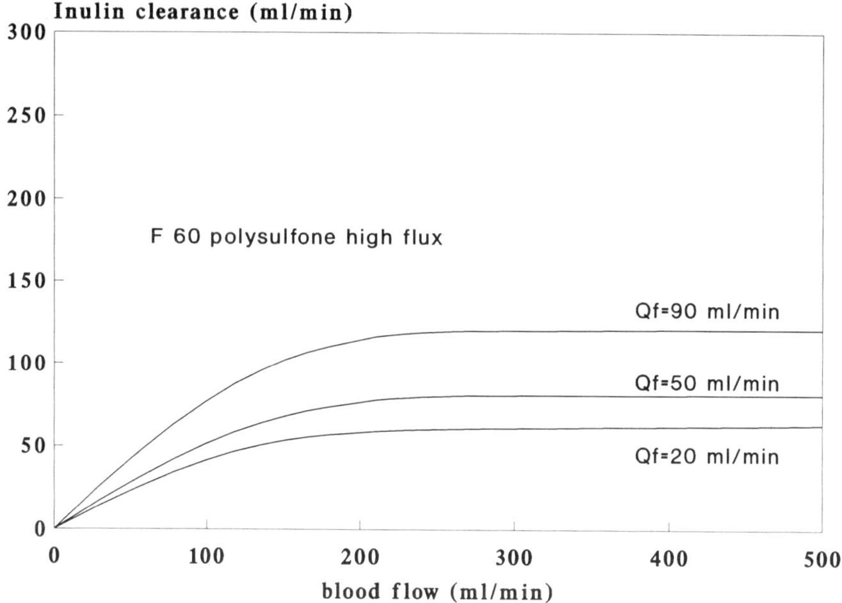

Fig. 5-7. Inulin clearance as a function of filtration rate.

able, and its removal by dialysis requires chelation with deferoxamine (DFO).

Several reports in the literature indicate that cuprophane dialysis removes only about 25 to 30 percent of the aluminum chelated, even though the mobilized aluminum is mainly found as aluminum deferoxamine with a molecular weight of 630. Use of activated carbon or of a high-flux dialyzer has therefore been suggested. Table 5-2 compares aluminum removal with a polyacrylonitrile AN69 device and with a charcoal filter. Similar removal rates were found, and it was concluded that because of lower costs and fewer side effects use of the high-flux dialyzer is to be preferred.[2]

Molitoris[3] made a comparative study of cuprophane and polysulfone dialyzers (Fig. 5-8). After DFO administration the aluminum plasma level rose

Table 5-2. Aluminum Removal by an AN69 Membrane and a Charcoal Filter

	Mean Aluminum Levels (μmol/L)	
	Charcoal (n = 14)	AN69 (n = 10)
Predialysis	186 ± 21	194 ± 30
Postdialysis	91 ± 25	109 ± 34
Aluminum removed	91 ± 17	84 ± 15

(Data from Valentijn.[2])

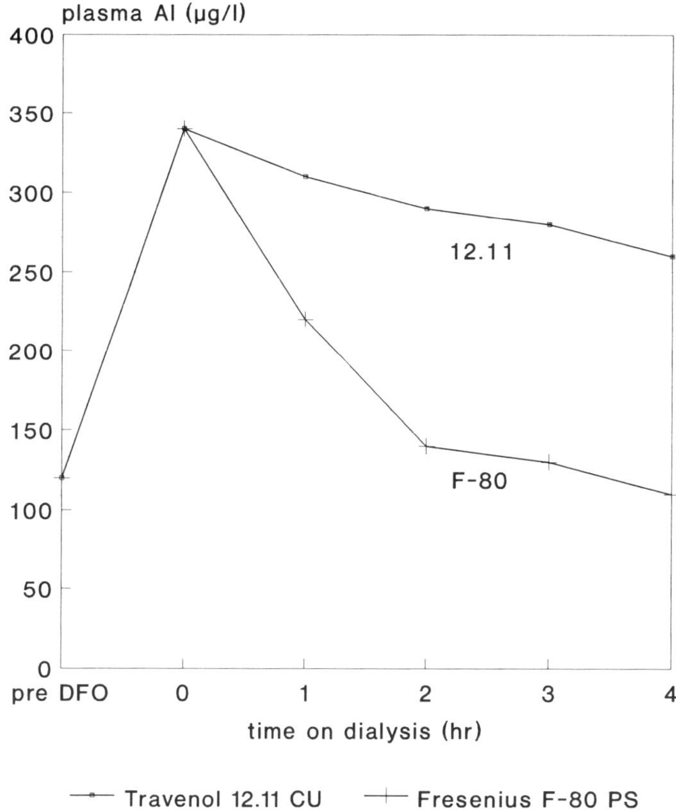

Fig. 5-8. Removal of DFO-chelated aluminum during hemodialysis with polysulfone (PS) and cuprophane (CU) dialyzers. (Data from Molitoris.[3])

from 120 to 330 μg/L. During cuprophane dialysis the plasma aluminum levels were only minimally reduced, whereas the 4-hour treatment with the polysulfone F 80 dialyzer returned plasma aluminum levels to pre-DFO values. In one patient aluminum removal was evaluated as a function of surface area for the Travenol 12.11 cuprophane dialyzer and the F40, F60, and F80 polysulfone devices (Fig. 5-9). The intradialytic half-times decreased from 484 to 276 minutes and from 108 to 99 minutes. These data prove that in contrast to a low-flux cellulosic membrane, high-flux membranes effect rapid removal of DFO-aluminum complex, thereby limiting DFO exposure and decreasing DFO-related side effects in hemodialysis patients.

β_2-MICROGLOBULIN REMOVAL

Dialysis-related amyloidosis is a severe and crippling complication of long-term dialysis. It usually appears after about 5 to 7 years of dialysis, presenting as carpal tunnel syndrome or as shoulder, hip, or knee abnor-

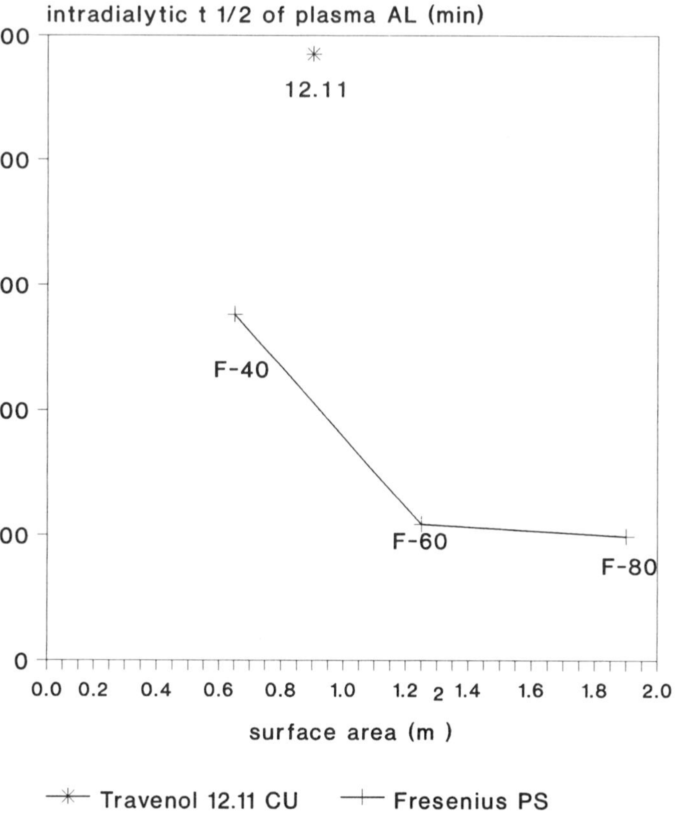

Fig. 5-9. Intradialytic half-times of plasma aluminum using cuprophane and polysulfone dialyzers of different surface area. (Data from Molitoris.[3])

malities. Clinical diagnosis is confirmed by radiology, biopsy, or more recently, by scanning of affected areas after injection of radiolabeled compound P or β_2-microglobulin. In 1985 Gejyo discovered that the precursor of the amyloid is β_2-microglobulin, a protein of 11,800 molecular weight, which is normally removed by glomerular filtration and proximal tubular reabsorption and proteolysis. Its normal generation rate is 1.0 to 2.0 g/wk, but there is some controversy over the generation rate of this molecule in hemodialysis patients. There are, however, direct experimental data indicating increased synthesis of β_2-microglobulin from lymphocytes after cuprophane dialysis in vivo or incubation with that membrane in vitro[4] (Fig. 5-10).

As renal function deteriorates, serum β_2-microglobulin levels rise progressively and tend to reach 20 to 30 times normal. Cuprophane dialysis does not remove β_2-microglobulin, and following its identification as the potential precursor of the amyloid, considerable interest has been focused on methods to remove it in order to prevent or at least delay the onset of dialysis-related amyloidosis.

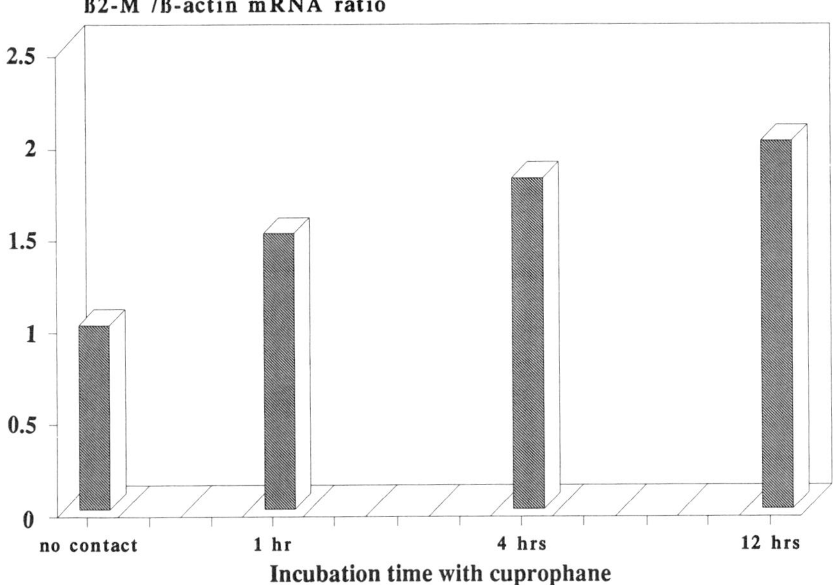

Fig. 5-10. Beta-2-microglobulin synthesis in lymphocytes incubated with cuprophane. (Data from Jahn.[4])

In one study five patients were subjected to three consecutive dialysis sessions with three different membranes—polysulfone low-flux, AN69 Filtral, and polysulfone high-flux (Fig. 5-11). Because of hemoconcentration dialysis on the polysulfone low-flux membrane resulted in an increase β_2-microglobulin level, but the AN69 membrane yielded a 20 percent reduction and the polysulfone high-flux membrane gave a 41 percent reduction.[5]

In an in vitro experiment, the same group used iodine 125-labeled β_2-microglobulin to determine how much of the amount cleared was removed by adsorption.[5] The results listed in Table 5-3, indicate that the AN69 membrane has the highest adsorptive capacity. Significant amounts were also found to be adsorbed by the high-flux polysulfone, whereas only insignificant amounts were adsorbed by the low-flux membrane. The explanation for this is that β_2-microglobulin, with a molecular weight of 12,000, is unable to penetrate the deeper layers of the low-flux polysulfone, whereas it is adsorbed in the deeper as well as the more superficial layers of the high-flux membrane wall.

BACK TRANSPORT

Back transport in a dialyzer consists of back diffusion, which occurs in low-flux as well as high-flux devices, and backfiltration, which is prevalent in high-flux devices but also occurs to a variable degree in any form of

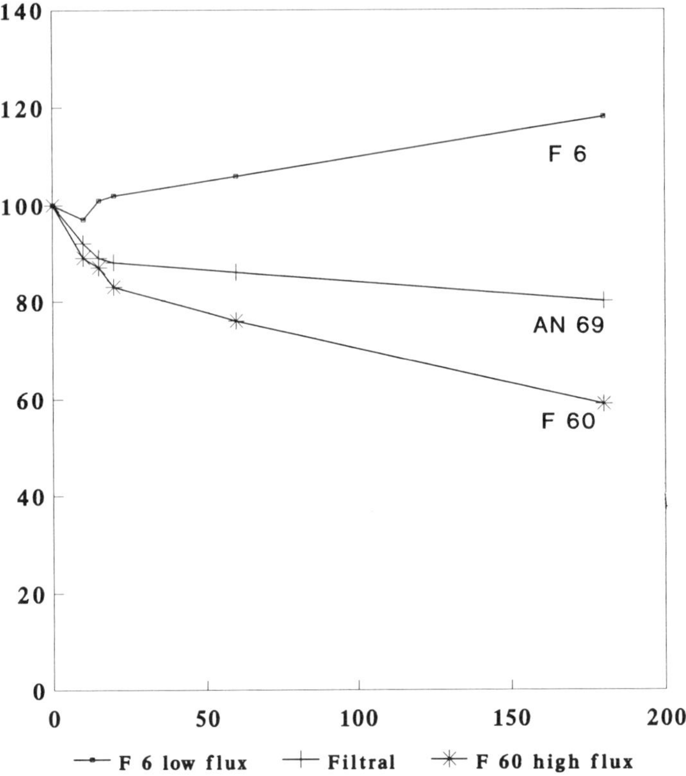

Fig. 5-11. Kinetics of serum β_2-microglobulin levels during dialysis with low-flux polysulfone, AN69 (Filtral), and high-flux polysulfone membranes. (Data from Goldman et al.[5])

Table 5-3. In Vitro Evaluation of β_2-Microglobulin Adsorption on Dialysis Membranes

Dialysis Membrane	Total Mass of β_2-M (mg)[a]	^{125}I-β_2-M Adsorbed (%)[b]	β_2-M Adsorbed (mg)
AN69	130	37	48
Polysulfone			
High-flux	105	18	19
Low-flux	120	<8	<10

Abbreviation: β_2-M, β_2-microglobulin.
[a] Amount of β_2-M in the plasma compartment at the beginning of the experiment.
[b] Percentage of ^{125}I-β_2-M adsorbed on the dialyser.
(Data from Goldman et al.[5])

hemodialysis unit, especially at low ultrafiltration rates. Lonnemann et al.[6] were able to show that not all dialyzers behaved in the same way following bacterial challenge. An in vitro closed-loop dialysis circuit was used, which contained 10 percent plasma in minimal essential media (MEM), a cell culture medium, in the blood compartment and MEM with *Pseudomonas maltophilia* filtrate in the dialysate compartment. Then after 2 hours, blood-side samples were taken and were incubated with monocytes, and the amount of tumor necrosis factor produced from these monocytes was measured by radioimmune assay (RIA). The results of a series of dialyzer challenges are shown in Figure 5-12. One sees that among the high-flux membranes, polysulfone did not leak in response to this challenge, as compared with to AN69 and cellulose triacetate (CIA). In addition, cuprophane, the tightest membrane with the lowest molecular weight cutoff (less than 8,000) appears to leak the most. This establishes as a first rule that not all high-flux dialyzers leak bacterial products under test conditions. Second, cuprophane leaks more easily than high-flux membranes.

Further evidence supporting the safety of polysulfone may be derived from the work of Schindler and Dinarello,[7] who challenged polysulfone dialyzers with *Pseudomonas aeruginosa* bacterial filtrate by pumping it through the dialyzer used as an ultrafilter. Even though the challenge was enormous, no breakthrough was seen in the postfilter sample, taken after 4 L of challenge material had been pumped through, until a 1 : 10 dilution of the broth was used, which resulted in an endotoxin concentration in the microgram range and minimal breakthrough (Fig. 5-13). Use of a cut hollow fiber device, with no surface intactness, yielded similar results.

Thus, factors other than surface intactness and pore size seem to play a role when polysulfone is used in bacterial challenge experiments. One factor is probably adsorption, which is related to the chemical structure of polymer used in membrane manufacture. We assume that double and triple bonds such as are present in the benzene rings of polysulfone or the nitrile group

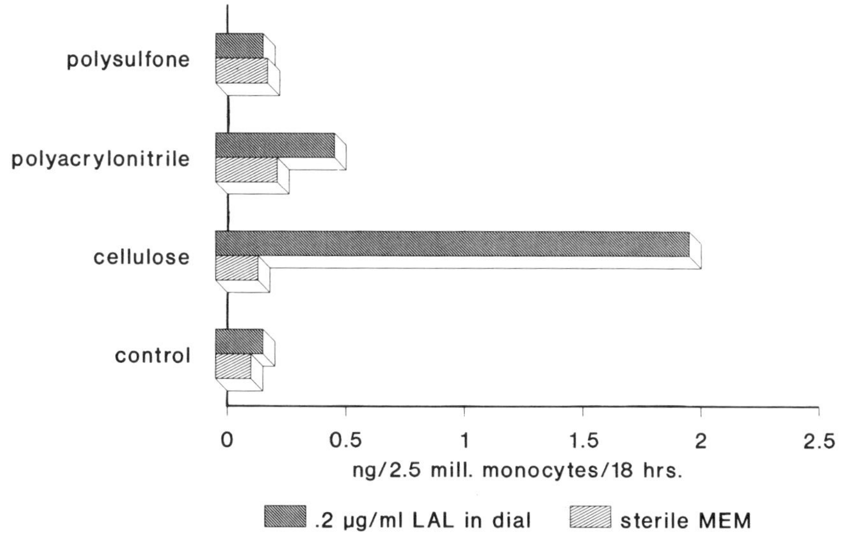

Fig. 5-12. The permeability of dialyzer membranes to tumor necrosis factor alpha-inducing substances. (Data from Lonnemann et al.[6])

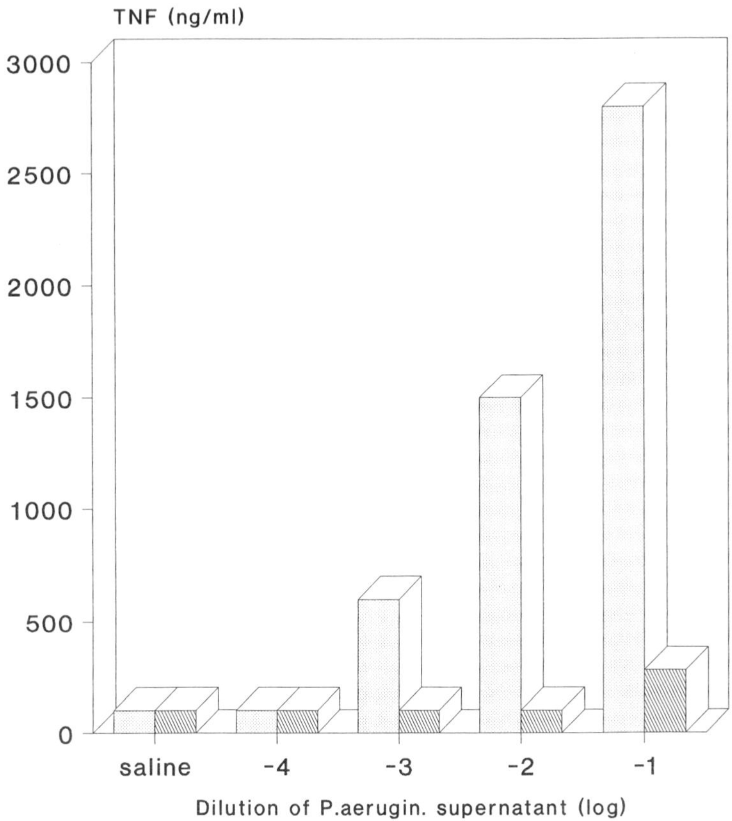

Fig. 5-13. Production of tumor necrosis factor (TNF) by peripheral blood monocytes incubated with pre- and post-*Pseudomonas aeruginosa* filtrate (postfilter samples taken after 4 L). (Data from Schindler and Dinarello.[7])

of polyacrylonitrile, by producing strong van der Waals forces via the pi electrons, are responsible for the better adsorptive properties of these membranes as compared with cuprophane.

In summary, it may be noted that in spite of back filtration, pyrogenic material does not seem to cross high-flux membranes as easily as cellulosic membranes. Furthermore, despite the potential for backfiltration, no evidence of untoward clinical effects, except for allergic reactions to polyacrylonitrile AN69 membrane and to the use of ACE inhibitors,[8] has been reported despite the wide use of these open membranes. Von Albertini and Bosch[9] reports that in over 10,000 high-flux treatments with or without on-line dialysate filtration, not a single case of sepsis or pyrogenic reaction was observed that was attributable to the high-flux polysulfone membrane used.

CONCLUSION

Most patients undergoing long-term dialysis have survived with cuprophane dialysis, but these patients suffer from a variety of symptoms including bone disease and malnutrition. There is no definite proof, but there can be hope, that synthetic high-permeability membranes may improve hemodialysis patients' quality of life and may reduce untoward complications of long-term dialysis treatment. If one believes that clearance of small solute molecules is all that matters, there is, of course, no need to select a more expensive synthetic high-flux membrane. If however, one believes that molecules in the higher molecular weight range, such as β_2-microglobulin, should also be removed, there is no choice other than to select a synthetic high-flux membrane to combine biocompatibility with better solute removal.

REFERENCES

1. Goehl H, Konstantin P: Membranes and filters for hemofiltration. p. 41. In Henderson LW (ed): Hemofiltration. Springer-Verlag, Berlin, 1986
2. Valentijn RM: Comparison of aluminum removal between AN69-S membrane and a charcoal filter, abstracted. Eur Dial Transplant Assoc, 1985
3. Molitoris BA: Rapid removal of DFO-chelated aluminum during hemodialysis using polysulfone dialyzers. Kidney Int 34:98, 1988
4. Jahn B: Beta$_2$-microglobulin synthesis in lymphocytes by cuprophan. Kidney Int 4:285, 1991
5. Goldman M, Nortier J, Dhaene M et al: Fate of beta-2-microglobulin during dialysis on polysulfone and AN 69 membranes. Contrib Nephrol 74:127, 1989
6. Lonnemann G, Behme TC, Lenze B et al: The permeability of dialyzer membranes to TNF alpha-inducing substances derived from water bacteria. Kidney Int (in press) 1992
7. Schindler R, Dinarello C: Ultrafiltration to remove endotoxins and other cytokine-inducing materials. Biotechniques 8:408, 1990
8. Parnes EL, Shapiro WB: Anaphylactoid reactions in hemodialysis patients treated with the AN69 dialyzer. Kidney Int 40:1148, 1991
9. Von Albertini B, Bosch JP: Short hemodialysis. Am J Nephrol 11:169, 1991

6

Ultrafiltration Control

George W. Buffaloe

INTRODUCTION

The requirement for fluid removal is an integral part of hemodialysis therapy. Whereas the absolute amounts of fluid to be removed from patients by thrice weekly hemodialysis treatments have not changed since the beginning of chronic treatment, the rate and control of fluid removal have changed significantly owing to shorter treatment times and higher-efficiency dialyzers with larger ultrafiltration coefficients. The appropriate level of ultrafiltration rate control in today's high-efficiency hemodialysis therapies is achieved by either direct control of transmembrane pressure or control of volumetric flow rates into and out of the hemodialyzer.

BACKGROUND

Fluid consisting of water, electrolytes, and other plasma constituents is removed from the patient by the action of a differential hydraulic pressure across the semipermeable membrane in the hemodialyzer. The hydraulic permeability of the dialyzer, that is, the ability of the dialyzer membrane to allow passage of fluid, is called the *ultrafiltration coefficient* (Kuf), with units of milliliters per hour per millimeter of mercury. The hydraulic pressure gradient between the blood compartment and the dialysate compartment of the dialyzer is called the *average transmembrane pressure* (measured in millimeters of mercury) and is usually calculated by taking the difference between the average blood-side pressure and the dialysate-side pressure, assuming a linear pressure drop across the inlet and outlet of the two compartments. The ultrafiltration rate in milliliters per hour is the product of the dialyzer Kuf and the transmembrane pressure. In routine conventional dialysis, the required transmembrane pressure is calculated by dividing the desired ultrafiltration rate by the dialyzer ultrafiltration coefficient, and then appropriate dialysate pressure setting is then calculated by subtracting the venous pressure from the required transmembrane pressure.

In principle, ultrafiltration control appears straightforward; in reality, however, control of the parameters from which the ultrafiltration rate is derived has proved challenging. The dialyzer Kuf can vary as a result of membrane manufacturing variability, and the clinical control of transmembrane pressure can be difficult owing to venous pressure fluctuations. Early dialysis equipment provided only pressure monitoring and control, usually incomplete, from which required transmembrane pressures could be established. Later equipment could actually measure ultrafiltration rates during periodic bypass of dialysate flow, and some equipment provided an estimate of the dialyzer's ultrafiltration coefficient. Although these improvements added predictability to ultrafiltration control, quite often patients still required periodic weighing during treatment in order to achieve clinically acceptable control of fluid losses.

The first ultrafiltration control equipment appeared in the 1970s for use with high-Kuf synthetic (noncellulosic) membrane dialyzers. Today a variety of equipment is available for clinically acceptable control of fluid removal from patients in various high-efficiency therapy regimes.

ULTRAFILTRATION CONTROL CIRCUITS

Because of the many variables that determine dialyzer transmembrane pressure, which in turn determines the ultrafiltration rate, current equipment designed for high-efficiency dialysis controls ultrafiltration rates either by monitoring dialysate flow rates into and out of the dialyzer, with feedback control of the transmembrane pressure, or by directly controlling these dialysate flow rates volumetrically. Accurate control of fluid removal from the patient's blood passing through the dialyzer would be relatively simple from a technological viewpoint if not for the requirement that dialysate flow must achieve the necessary uremic toxin removal by diffusive transport. This requirement of dialytic therapy imposes a large dialysate flow rate of 500 to 800 ml/min onto a small ultrafiltration flow rate of 10 to 30 ml/min.

Flow Rate Monitor

Flow rate monitors control ultrafiltration rate by measuring dialysate flow rates into and out of the dialyzer and controlling the dialysate pressure to achieve the desired ultrafiltration rate (Fig. 6-1). This approach requires a feedback or servo-control loop in which the ultrafiltration rate (i.e., the difference between the dialysate outflow rate and inflow rate) is measured and the dialysate pressure is regulated in order to achieve the appropriate transmembrane pressure. Two examples of this design approach in hemodialysis equipment are the Baxter 550 (Baxter, Deerfield, IL), which monitors the dialysate flow rates with bearingless rotary flowmeters, and the Gambro AK-10 (CGH Medical, Lakewood, CO), which uses a differential electromag-

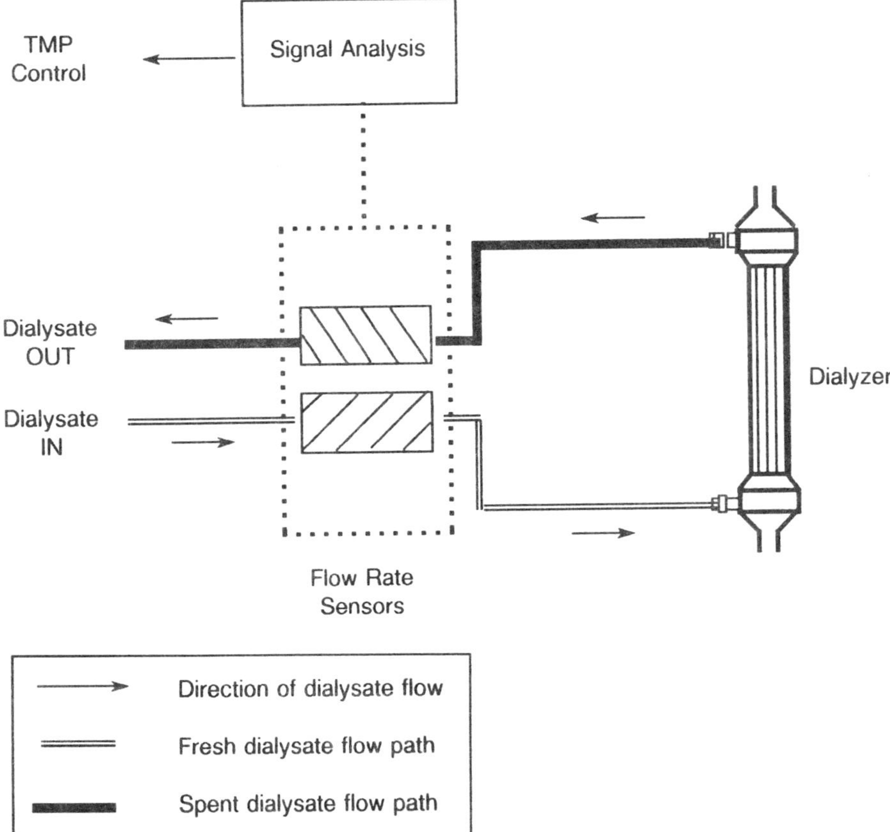

Fig. 6-1. Flow rate monitor.

netic flowmeter. The clinical performance of equipment designed by this approach is a function of the accuracy and frequency with which dialysate flow rates are measured and the accuracy with which transmembrane pressure is controlled.

Recirculation Loop

The recirculation loop (Fig. 6-2) is the simplest of the volumetric control circuits. A constant volume of dialysate in a noncompliant, recirculating hydraulic circuit is pumped at a selected dialysate flow rate and an ultrafiltration pump removes fluid from the loop at a fixed rate equal to the desired ultrafiltration rate. The volume removed from the loop is replaced by an identical volume of fluid, which is transported out of the patient's blood, through the dialyzer membrane, and into the dialysate compartment, which is part of the recirculating dialysate loop. It is apparent that the ultrafiltration pump could be located on the dialysate line either entering or leaving the dialyzer, since the circuit volume is constant.

All volumetric flow rate control designs are functional closed loops and rely on controlled removal of fluid from the loop to control fluid removal from the patient. Early recirculation loop designs used a large volume of

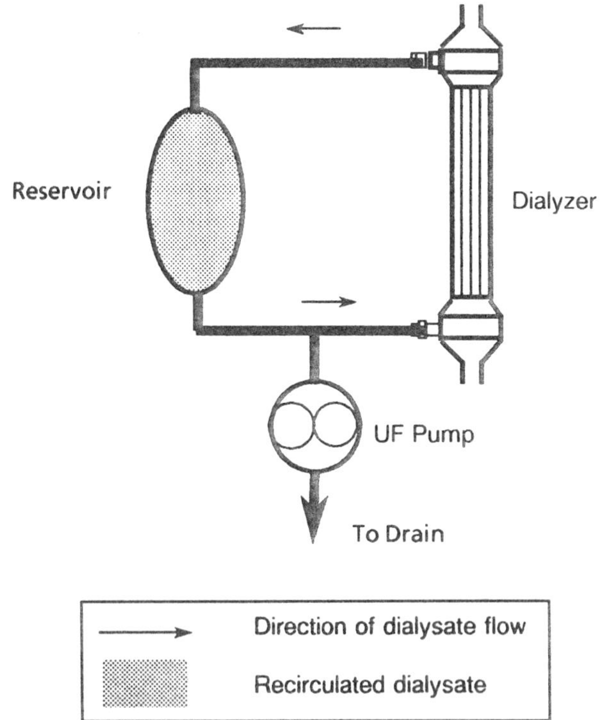

Fig. 6-2. Recirculation loop.

recirculating dialysate for an entire treatment. An example of this design was the Rhône-Poulenc Rhodial, which had a recirculation volume of 75 L. The primary disadvantage of this approach was the relative inefficiency of removing uremic toxins owing to their buildup in the recirculating dialysate loop and the consequent decrease in diffusive transport of these uremic toxins from the patient's blood.

Recirculation Loop with Dialysate Replacement

The design shown in Figure 6-3 is basically another form of a recirculation loop; however, there is a low volume of fluid in the reservoir, which is replaced periodically with fresh dialysate. This replacement is accomplished by means of valves which isolate the dialysate reservoir from the dialyzer. The spent dialysate in the reservoir is replaced with fresh dialysate at a rapid flow rate at predetermined intervals. The valve positions in Figure 6-3A represent recirculating flow through the dialyzer. Periodically, the valve positions are switched (Fig. 6-3B), and the spent dialysate in the reservoir is rapidly replaced with fresh dialysate. This approach addresses the inefficiency of toxin removal due to their buildup in the dialysate loop (as in the circuit of Figure 6-2); and it thus makes it possible to achieve near continuous flow through the dialyzer and to achieve toxin removal efficiencies approaching those of continuous, single-pass dialysate flow. An example of equipment utilizing this design approach is the Hospal Monitral (CGH Medical, Lakewood, CO).

Single Balance Chamber

In the design shown in Figure 6-4, the reservoir is basically transformed into a balance chamber with the insertion of a flexible diaphragm, which separates the incoming fresh dialysate from the outgoing spent dialysate. Figure 6-4A shows fresh dialysate flowing through the dialyzer, with spent dialysate filling the balance chamber. Figure 6-4B shows the filling of the balance chamber with fresh dialysate, with simultaneous expulsion of spent dialysate to the drain. This design requires intermittent flow through the dialyzer; thus overall toxin removal from the patient is compromised.

Dual Balance Chambers

The design shown in Figure 6-5 uses two balance chambers to approach a continuous flow of dialysate through the dialyzer. Figure 6-5A shows the valve positions when chamber 1 supplies fresh dialysate to the dialyzer, and Figure 6-5B shows the valve positions when chamber 2 supplies the fresh dialysate. This alternating valve switching pattern has the potential for continuously supplying fresh dialysate to the dialyzer, depending on the

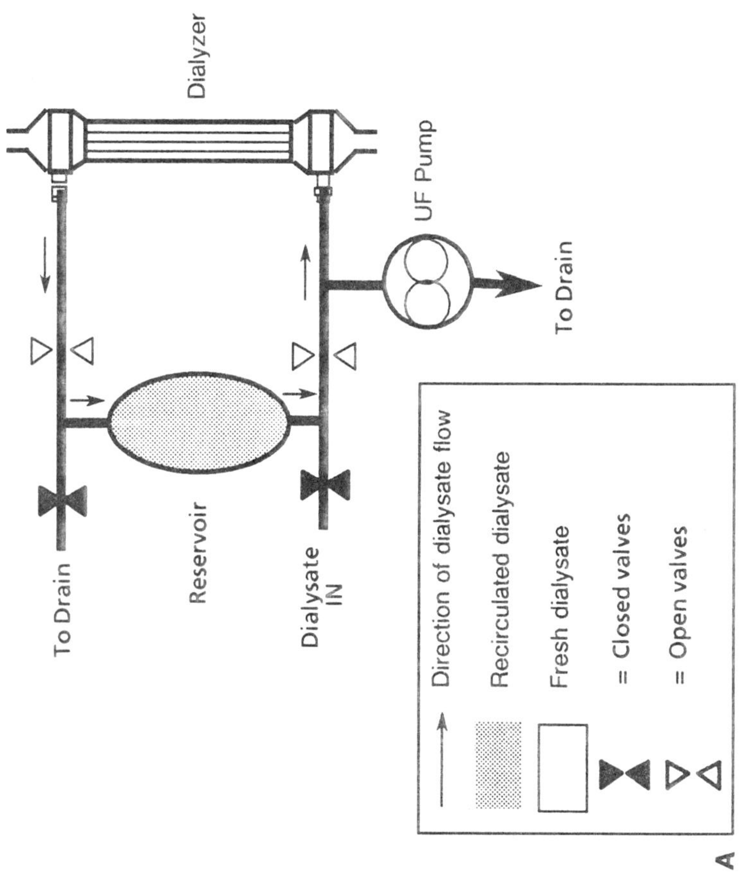

Dialyzer
UF Pump
To Drain
To Drain
Reservoir
Dialysate IN
Direction of dialysate flow
Recirculated dialysate
Fresh dialysate
= Closed valves
= Open valves
A

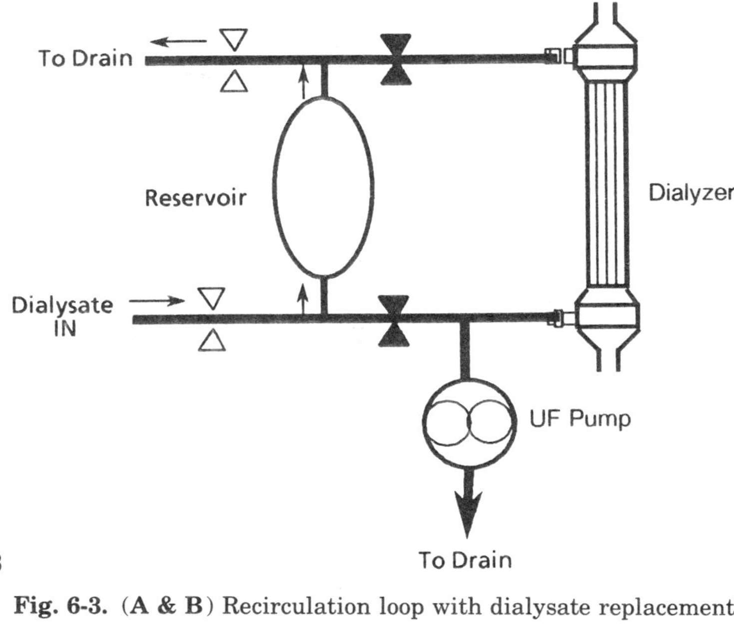

Fig. 6-3. (**A & B**) Recirculation loop with dialysate replacement.

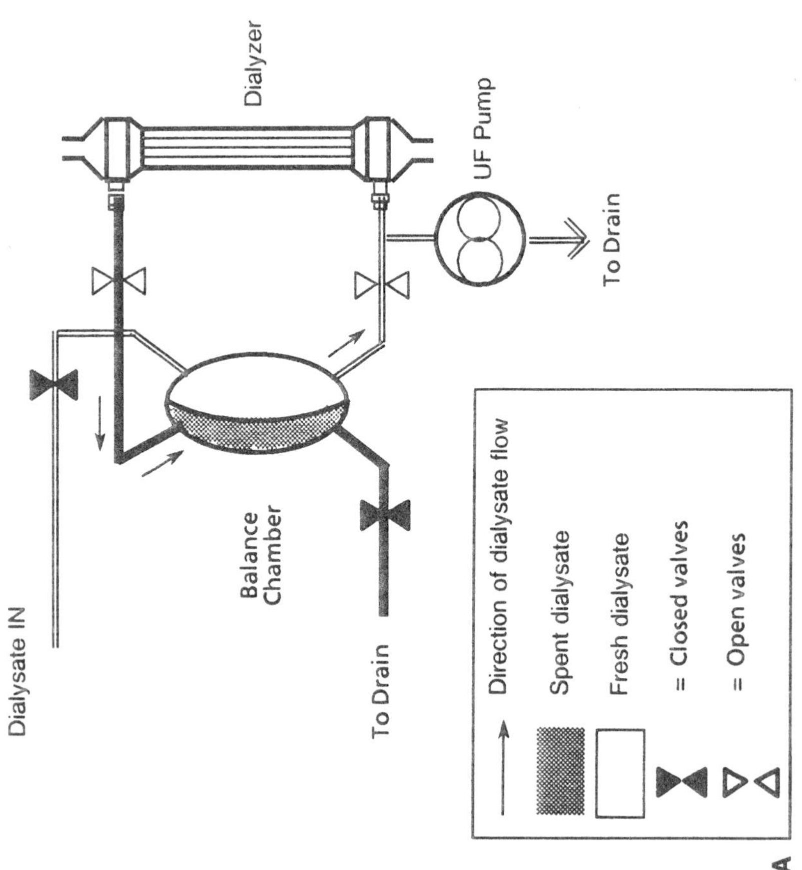
Dialysate IN
Balance
Chamber
To Drain
Dialyzer
UF Pump
To Drain
Direction of dialysate flow
Spent dialysate
Fresh dialysate
= Closed valves
= Open valves
A

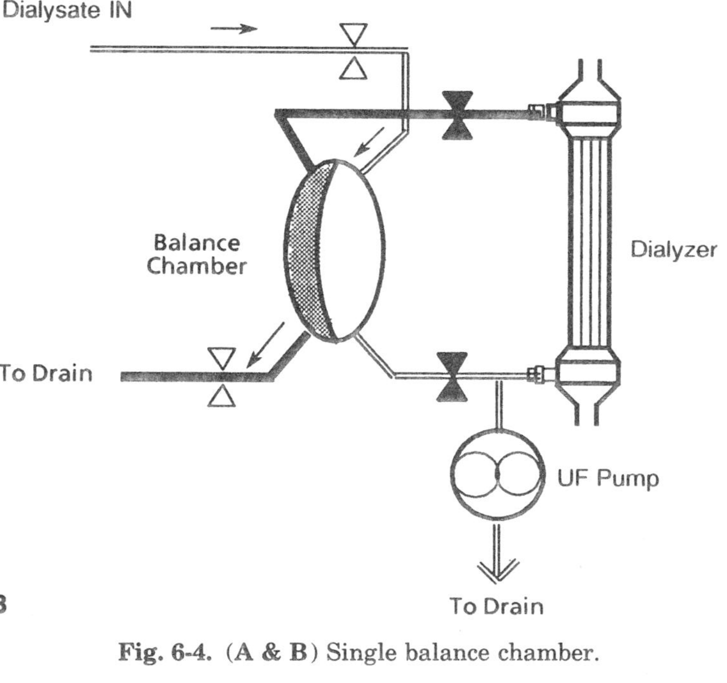

Fig. 6-4. (**A & B**) Single balance chamber.

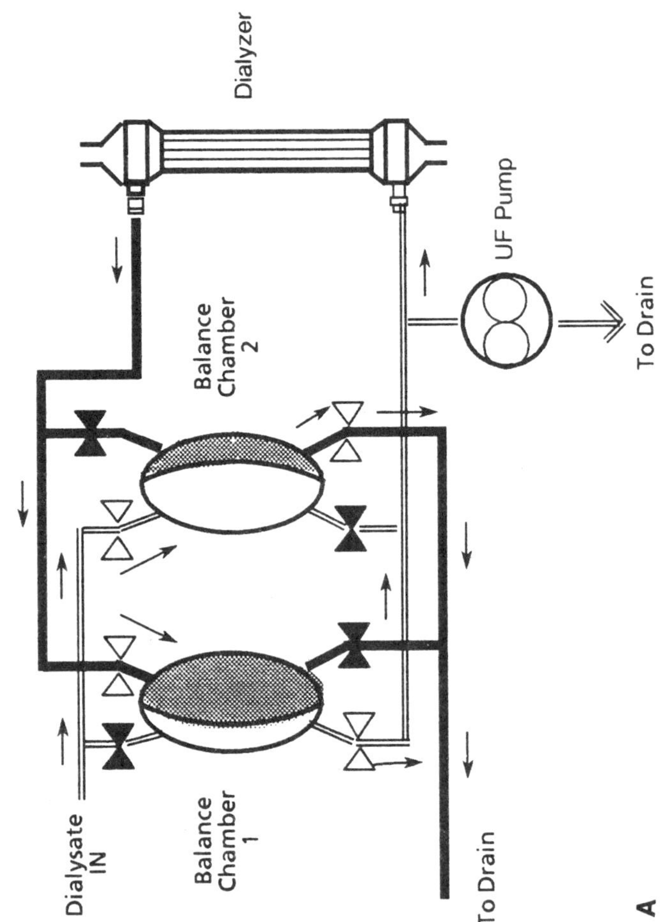
Dialyzer
Balance Chamber 2
UF Pump
To Drain
Dialysate IN
Balance Chamber 1
To Drain
A

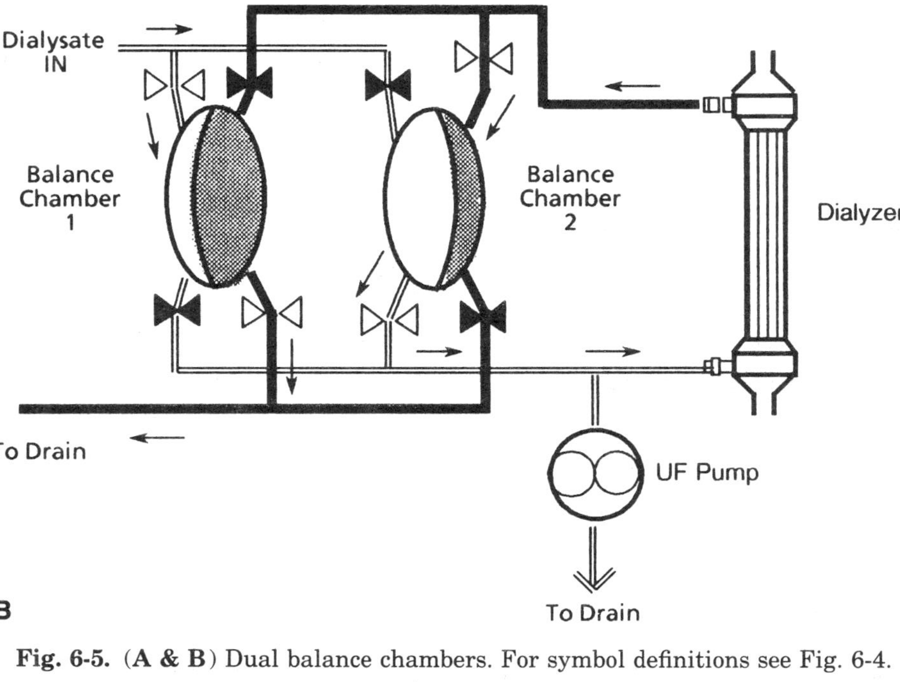

Fig. 6-5. (**A & B**) Dual balance chambers. For symbol definitions see Fig. 6-4.

design of the flow-sensing and valve-switching mechanisms. In this design the accuracy of control of ultrafiltration rates is relatively independent of the Kuf of the dialyzer and more dependent on the overall function of the hydraulic circuit. Examples of this design include the COBE Centrysystem 2 and Centrysystem 3 (CGH Medical, Lakewood, CO), the Fresenius 2008 (Fresenius USA, Concord, CA), and the Drake Willock 4800F (CD Medical, Miami, FL).

7

High-Efficiency Treatments Using Conventional Equipment

Allan J. Collins

INTRODUCTION

Shortened dialysis treatments have continued to be used in the clinical setting since their introduction in 1985.[1-6] Considerable experience has been gained since then with such shortened dialysis treatment in terms of adequacy of total dialysis delivery and the technical requirement needed for its success.[7] It is estimated that approximately 50 percent of patients treated in the United States undergo dialysis for less than 3 hours. There has been concern, however, over the general applicability of reduced treatment time and its impact on the survival of patients in the United States. This chapter reviews basic principles of high-efficiency hemodialysis therapy; optimal therapy prescriptions and delivery; technical considerations, particularly focused on bicarbonate concentrate; and long-term survival results.

DEFINITION OF HIGH-EFFICIENCY THERAPIES

Various definitions of shortened treatment time in the past have centered on dialysis treatments of less than 3 hours (Table 7-1). Alternatively, simplified definitions include blood flow rates greater than 300 ml/min and urea clearances greater than 200 ml/min. This urea clearance was typical for a cuprophane hollow-fiber dialyzer with a 250 ml/min blood flow rate, used in clinical practice between the late 1970s and early 1980s. Additional definitions, which yield relative efficiency of solute removal, center on either the urea clearance divided by body weight in kilograms or the urea clearance divided by volume of urea distribution. These latter two definitions provide a more reasonable comparison relative to the kinetic parameters used to remove the solutes. Previously, Kjellstrand and associates and Kaiser and co-workers had indicated that in both pediatric and adult settings, the limitations of acetate tolerance for efficiency of dialysis are defined by a ratio of urea clearance to body weight that is less than or equal to 3.0 ml/min/kg.[8-11] Adjustments for an average body weight and a urea distribution volume of approximately 58 percent yields a urea clearance/urea distribution volume ratio of approximately 5.2 ml/min per liter of total body water. With this particular definition, treatments that exceed this level would be considered highly efficient therapies.

Table 7-1. Definition of Highly Efficient Dialysis

Treatment time under 3 hours
Blood flow rate greater than 300 ml/min
Urea clearance greater than 200 ml/min
K/wt greater than 3.0 ml/min/kg
K/V greater than 5.2 ml/min/kg total body weight

Table 7-2. Highly Efficient Treatments ($Kt/V < 1.0$)

Year	K/wt	Kt/V
Hemofiltration		
1981[22]	3.16	0.66
1981[23]	4.30	0.89
Hemodiafiltration		
1983[24]	3.46	0.63
1984[4]	4.69	0.93

A number of authors have published early experiences with high-efficiency treatments, and the reader is referred to the references indicated for background information and previous review articles.[4,5,12] More recently, from 1981 through 1987, highly efficient therapies have been carried out by a number of authors; however, total dialysis therapy, delivered as quantitated by Kt/V (where K is dialyzer urea clearance, t is dialysis time, and V is volume of distribution of urea), has been marginal if not inadequate for survival (Table 7-2). In the most recent interval high-flux and high-efficiency therapies have delivered Kt/Vs in the range of 1.0 to 1.3 (Table 7-3). These early attempts have had long-term success with Kt/Vs greater than 1.0. The optimal Kt/V may, in fact, be higher.

THERAPY PRESCRIPTION

Unfortunately, some shortened dialysis treatment regimens simply reduce treatment time without compensating for lost urea removal, thereby delivering less overall dialysis. Urea kinetic modeling and the use of urea index Kt/V, first proposed by Gotch and Sargent in the reanalysis of the National Cooperative Dialysis Study, have allowed a more rational basis for prescribing and monitoring dialysis therapy.[13] Gotch and Sargent showed a relationship between the high incidence of therapy failure in the National Cooperative Dialysis Study and a Kt/V of less than 0.8. They also pointed out a lower incidence of failure when the urea index ranged between 1.0 and 1.4. A number of other authors have also demonstrated that low Kt/Vs in patients without complications are associated with increased morbidity.[7] The exact

Table 7-3. Highly Efficient Treatments ($Kt/V \geq 1.0$)

Year	K/wt	Kt/V
High-Efficiency Dialysis		
1984[1,3]	4.14	1.22
1985[14]	6.9	1.43
1987[25]	4.5	1.3
High-Flux Dialysis		
1986[26]	3.98	1.03
1986[6]	4.14	1.00

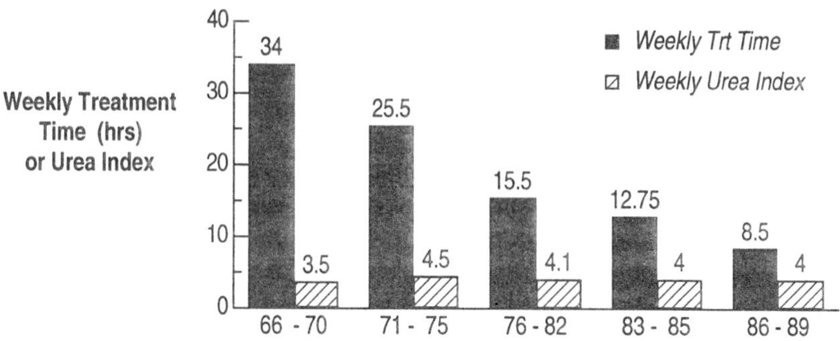

Fig. 7-1. Comparison of weekly treatment times and weekly urea index in nondiabetic hemodialysis patients without complications, 1966 to 1988.

Kt/V level to be delivered to patients once 1.0 is reached, however, has been controversial. The survival rate in the Regional Kidney Disease Program in Minneapolis has been excellent, with a Kt/V averaging 1.33 per treatment from 1966 to 1989. Figure 7-1 shows the average weekly treatment time and average weekly urea index during the interval as noted. The average weekly Kt/V for all patients has been fairly constant at 4.0. A detailed analysis of varying levels of Kt/V will be presented later in the survival analysis. In summary, it appears that the minimum Kt/V to be prescribed and delivered for dialysis therapy would be 1.0, although some investigators suggest that higher Kt/Vs may be advantageous.

TECHNICAL REQUIREMENTS FOR DELIVERY OF HIGH-EFFICIENCY THERAPIES

The delivery of an adequate dialysis treatment is highly dependent on adequate solute removal, adequate fluid removal, and the stability of the treatment. Adequate solute removal has previously been defined as a Kt/V greater than 1, while adequate fluid removal is linked to the patient's ability to shift fluid from the extravascular to the intravascular space. In our experience with isolated ultrafiltration, patients can usually tolerate between 25 and 35 ml/min of ultrafiltration, which is equivalent to approximately 1.5 to 2.1 kg/h. In the past, acetate dialysate with high ultrafiltration rates was associated with nausea, vomiting, and hypotension. With bicarbonate dialysate, however, these ultrafiltration rates are achievable with extremely low levels of nausea, vomiting, and headache and reduced levels of hypotension as compared with standard acetate therapy.[1,2] Additional aspects of solute removal are concerned with dialysate composition. Many authors have used sodium levels between 140 and 145 mEq/L, a dialysate bicarbonate buffer of 35 mEq/L, and 4.5 mEq/L of acid concentrate.[4,5,7,14] The combination, then, of an adequate therapy prescription and a bicarbonate dialysate with a sodium content of approximately 142 mEq/L should provide the basic components of therapy.

DIALYZER EFFICIENCY

The relationship between urea clearance and blood flow rate is highly dependent on permeability and on the area-mass transfer coefficient product (KoA) of the dialyzer. Standard-efficiency dialyzers yield average blood urea nitrogen (BUN) clearances of 190 to 200 ml/min with a blood flow rate of 250 ml/min, providing a KoA value of approximately 500. High-efficiency and high-flux dialyzers, typically with cellulose acetate, polysulfone, or cuprammonium membranes, have mass transfer coefficients between 800 and 1,000. These later dialyzers, with the higher blood flow rates of approximately 300 to 400 ml/min, yield 20 to 25 percent additional clearance compared to the low mass transfer coefficient dialyzers. In addition, dialyzer performance can be increased by 8 to 12 percent by increasing the dialysate flow from 500 ml/min to between 700 and 1,000 ml/min. When increased above 700 ml/min, however, this flow rate is also associated with increased cost of concentrate, which must be taken into consideration.

To achieve higher clearances on the higher-performance dialyzers, increased blood flow rates are used. The delivered blood flow rate, however, is highly dependent on the blood pump design, the resiliency of the tubing segments in the blood pump, and the adequacy of pressure drops across the fistula needle. Negative pressure that develops in the arterial line between the needle and the blood pump is associated with partial collapse of the tubing segment in the pump, resulting in a reduced blood flow rate. Figure 7-2 shows the relative decrease of delivered blood flow rate during a 3-hour dialysis treatment with increasing negative pressure. The critical line usually has an average pressure of −50 to −150 mmHg at a 400 ml/min blood flow rate. When the blood pump setting is maintained for 3 hours of treatment, the effective blood flow rate decreases by approximately 8 percent secondary to the negative pressure and to loss of resilience of the pump segment.

The delivered blood flow rate is also highly dependent on occlusion of the blood pump and the durometer of the tubing pump segment. This blood flow rate is one aspect of delivering an adequate treatment, but the capacity of the blood access is equally important. Typical access flows are between 500 ml/min and 1 L/min, and therefore high blood flow rates may stress the capability of the access to deliver adequate blood flow to the extracorporeal circuit for dialysis. Access recirculation studies are required when the higher blood rate, used to ensure the prescribed blood flow rate, does not exceed the access capability. Schwab et al.[15] and others have shown that recirculation in the access is highly associated with increasing negative pressure in standard dialysis, but that this correlation is not as close for dialyzers that use high blood flow rates. Therefore, use of the dialyzer-circuit venous pressure at

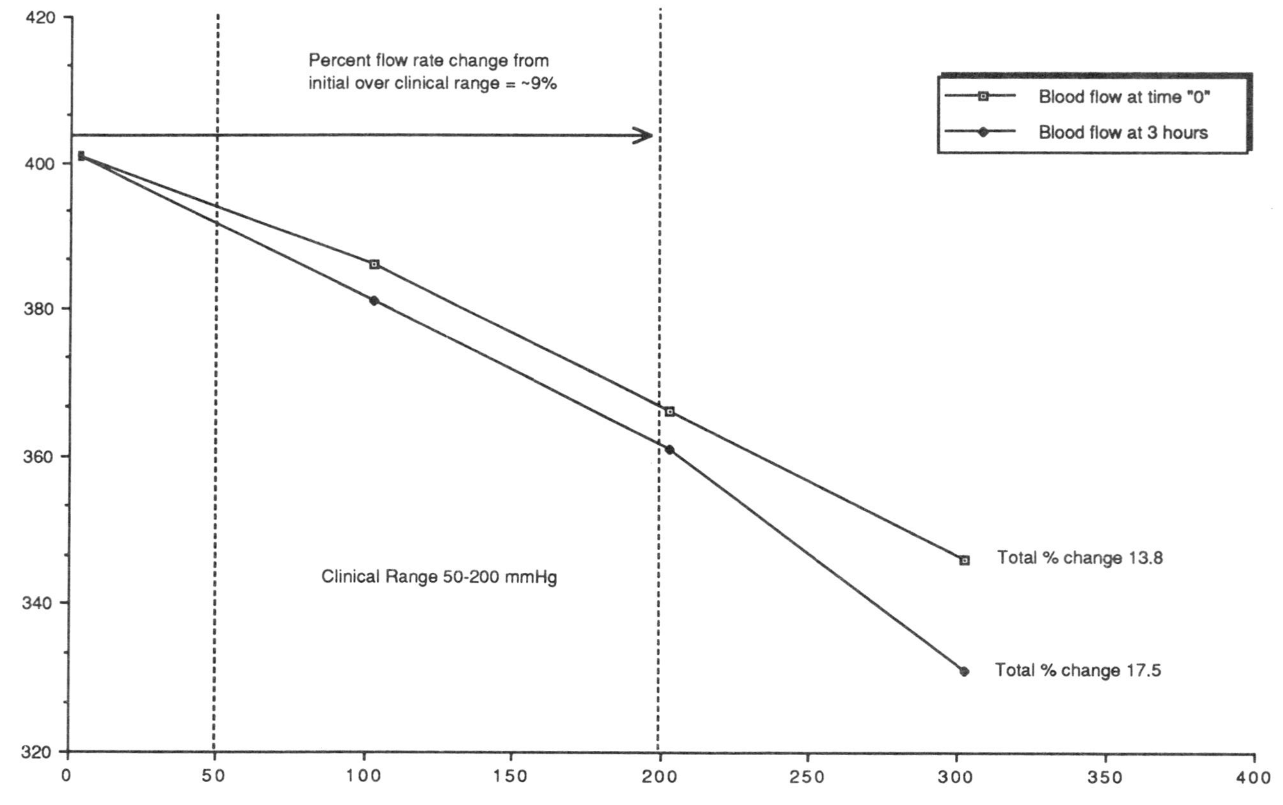

Fig. 7-2. Blood flow versus prepump negative pressure, at a 400 ml/min blood flow rate.

high blood flow rates to indicate possible recirculation is problematic in view of the increased pressure drop across the fistula needle. Examination of the sources of pressure in the dialysis circuit will give some insight into the difficulties in interpreting the venous pressure. An arterial restriction in the access would lower the mean pressure in the access and predispose to recirculation. If the abnormalities are located on the venous side, with venous stenosis associated with an open arterial system, high mean arterial pressure within the access will result, along with increased venous pressure noted on the venous monitor. In this latter circumstance, an elevated pressure would be associated with recirculation. Additionally, the recirculation would lead to a reduced effective clearance and a reduced delivered Kt/V index. If the therapy delivered is significantly less than that prescribed, the access recirculation should be calculated to determine the cause of the gap between the prescribed and delivered therapy.

Some technical considerations are important to recognize when drawing pre- and postdialysis blood samples for quantification of dialysis therapy. Drawing of the predialysis blood sample is usually without any significant problems since the extracorporeal circuit has not been completed. However, there are some technical difficulties in obtaining an accurate postdialysis sample that has not been falsely lowered by recirculation. In my group's own experience, the postdialysis blood sample is best drawn immediately after discontinuation of the treatment with the blood pump stopped. A waiting period of 2 to 3 minutes should be observed to allow the access recirculation to be swept out after the blood pump is stopped. Drawing of the postdialysis sample from the arterial fistula needle, after flushing the fistula needle multiple times to remove potentially recirculated blood, is also important. This sample is drawn before the rinse-back to eliminate any possible immediate dilutional effects from the 300 to 500 ml of saline that is used during the rinse procedure. In this manner, a postdialysis blood sample can be drawn with good reproducibility. Another confounding factor occurs in patients who have considerable rebound because of poor cellular urea transport from the intracellular to the extracellular space. Persistently high, greater than prescribed Kt/Vs are usually associated with two phenomena: the two-pool effect, which gives a falsely low postdialysis urea nitrogen level, and the inadequately drawn postdialysis sample. Therefore, access recirculation and delivered therapy are closely linked.

ULTRAFILTRATION CONTROL SYSTEMS

The monitoring systems that have been placed in dialysis equipment have improved the safety and efficacy of delivery systems in the areas of conductivity, temperature, blood leak detection, and air detector systems. Ultrafiltration control systems, which were introduced in dialysis machines in the mid-1980s, have provided increased stability of ultrafiltration and predictability of fluid removal during the dialysis treatment. Two basic systems are used to achieve this ultrafiltration control. The first is a mechanical-based system, which has a matched bellows pumps in a multiple valving system, allowing the dialysate inflow and outflow to be matched with a separate ultrafiltration control pump. This pump generates the necessary transmembrane pressure to achieve the appropriate weight loss per minute prescribed for the treatment. Examples of this type of equipment include Monitrol (Hospal Medical Corp., Edison, NJ); Cobe System Three (CGH Medical Lakewood, CO); Litton CO Frezeni S2008 (Fresenius Corp., Concorde, CA); and System 1000 (Althin Inc., Portland, OR). An alternative system is sensor-based, using computer control of dialysate inflow and outflow pumps. The computerized system has sophisticated sensors to determine dialysate flow, using a microprocessor to calculate the differential for dialysate inflow and outflow and thus generate the necessary transmembrane pressure to achieve the desired ultrafiltration rate.

Both ultrafiltration control systems, the closed-loop valvular type and the sensor-based system, have advantages and disadvantages relative to reliability and performance. In the sensor-based systems particular debris large enough to enter the sensors can disrupt flow, or microbiologic byproducts such as polysaccharide alginate, which is excreted by bacteria and known as *biofilm,* can build up in the sensors and disrupt the flow paths. In the hydraulic-based systems the integrity of valves and pumping mechanisms as well as of membranes between pumping chambers can be disrupted by precipitates and biofilm deposits, which cause malfunctions. In addition, on the dialysate outflow side, microbiologic overgrowth tends to be promoted secondary to the availability not only of glucose but also of nitrogenous waste products from the patient. This can promote differential bacterial growth on the outflow side compared with the inflow side. Appropriate cleaning and maintenance procedures, however, can alleviate all the above-mentioned problems with both the sensor-based and valvular-based systems. In each system adequate control of dialysate pH reduces the possibility of calcium carbonate precipitation. In addition, acid rinsing of the dialysate flow paths can be used to dissolve calcium carbonate. Bleaching of equipment disrupts the microbiologic biofilm deposits within the dialysate flow path, valves, and sensors, thereby maintaining valve and flow sensor function. Equipment manufacturers have developed appropriate procedures for acid rinsing of machines as well as appropriate bleach and disinfectant procedures to provide adequate reliability.

DIALYSATE CONCENTRATE

Successful clinical application of high-efficiency therapies has been linked to the use of bicarbonate dialysate, which as compared with acetate, has reduced interdialytic symptoms and hypotension. Large-scale bicarbonate use within dialysis units entails a number of technical issues that need to be addressed to ensure safety and efficacy. The proportioning systems for bicarbonate dialysate, for instance, increase the complexity of the circuit and require monitoring systems to ensure proper proportioning. Bicarbonate concentrate proportioning can be controlled by pH monitoring to help prevent precipitation. Additionally, safety systems are necessary to ensure that concentrates are appropriately dispensed to deliver a dialysate with the proper concentrations of constituents. Adequate safety systems have been developed by a number of manufacturers, either by color coding or by key-locking systems to ensure that the concentrate containers are not attached to the wrong proportioners.

MICROBIOLOGY OF BICARBONATE DIALYSATE

Microbiologic contamination of bicarbonate concentrate has been identified as a major issue in dialysis units by Ebben et al.[16] and Bland et al.[17] The challenges in the clinical setting are to control the microbiology and to provide adequate safety relative to endotoxin levels in the dialysate. The growth characteristics of the bacteria involved in bicarbonate concentrate contamination have been identified and appear to be from gram-negative halophilic rods, which require sodium chloride or sodium bicarbonate for growth, unlike water organisms, which require no sodium chloride to grow. The culture medium providing the best yields for bicarbonate concentrate organisms contains sodium chloride, which is provided in tryptic soy agar, in contrast to the standard medium used to culture pure water organisms, which contains no sodium chloride. Manufacturers have produced commercial sampler systems with different types of media to culture these organisms on a routine basis.

An additional area of concern about growth characteristics of these bacteria is whether the containers holding the concentrate have been cleaned and disinfected prior to introduction of a new batch of concentrate and whether concentrate is saved from day to day. Ebben et al.[16] have shown that with clean and disinfected containers, the latent period for bacterial growth is 3 to 5 days, with an exponential growth phase occurring at 5 to 8 days and maximal levels reached within 10 days.[16] If a previously contaminated container is used to make up fresh bicarbonate concentrate, the latency phase is only 1 day, the exponential phase is 2 to 3 days, and maximal levels of 10^5 to 10^6 colony-forming units per milliliter are reached by 4 days. These growth characteristics provide the rationale for cleaning and disinfecting containers for bicarbonate concentrate so as to ensure adequate control of microbiology. When these procedures are put into practice, bacterial overgrowth can be kept within appropriate limits.

Bacterial overgrowth can cause obstruction of the outflow stream and drain system within the dialysis units. Air gapping of the outflow dialysate line prior to entrance into the drain system at the station prevents back contamination from overgrowth within the pitched drain pipes. Investigation within the drain system of the Regional Kidney Disease Program's dialysis unit has shown heavy overgrowth in drains with bicarbonate dialysate and extensive biofilm deposition within the drain systems. This is a particular difficulty in drain systems constructed with standard iron pipe as compared with those using polyvinylchloride piping. In certain circumstances in which the pitch of the piping allows only slow flow, Pyrex glass piping is required to reduce biofilm deposition because a smooth surface will reduce accumulation of bacterial and biofilm products. Routine cleaning and bleaching procedures carried out on a quarterly basis throughout the drain system are advisable to prevent retrograde contamination to the dialysis machines, as well as to eliminate clogging of the drain system by bacterial by-products.

HIGH-EFFICIENCY THERAPIES IN CLINICAL PRACTICE

In the early 1990s two major forms of high-efficiency therapy are in large-scale clinical practice, namely, high-efficiency hemodialysis and high-flux hemodialysis. High-efficiency dialyzers, as previously mentioned, typically have ultrafiltration coefficients less than 15 ml/h/mmHg, while these coefficients in high-flux dialyzers are greater than 15 ml/h/mmHg. In addition, criteria such as dialysis efficiency, as measured by the ratio of the dialyzer urea clearance K to total body water V, have been used to characterize efficiency. (Previously, a K/V ratio less than 5.2 corresponded to a K/W ratio [where W is body weight in kilograms] of 3.0.) This has been used by Kjellstrand and co-workers to characterize the limits of acetate tolerance.[8–10] More recently, more highly efficient therapies have provided K/W and K/V above 3.0 and 5.2, respectively. Typical newer therapies, both high-efficiency and high-flux, have a K/V of 6 to 7. Therapy prescription and the components required for adequate high-efficiency and high-flux dialysis have previously been described. Most successful applications have been based on a bicarbonate dialysate delivery system with ultrafiltration control mechanisms. In vivo therapy prescriptions have been proposed to center on a Kt/V ranging from 1.0 to 1.4. This is confirmed by kinetic modeling of midweek pre- and postdialysis BUN to ensure that the delivered therapy is within the previously indicated range. Some programs use higher Kt/Vs—a minimum of 1.2 for nondiabetics and a minimum of 1.4 for diabetics—as targets for optimal therapy. Once again, these programs use kinetic modeling of midweek pre- and postdialysis BUN to confirm adequate delivery of the therapy.

Survival of patients undergoing high-efficiency dialysis has recently been evaluated by a number of investigators and shown to be equal to or better than that of patients treated by standard acetate dialysis.[7,18,19] Both high-flux and high-efficiency dialysis have shown annual gross mortality rates considerably lower than the national rate—approximately 14 percent in data from the R.K. Davis Unit in San Francisco[21] and approximately 12 percent in data from the Minneapolis program. Additional risk factors have been identified for survival of hemodialysis patients that impact on nondiabetics receiving a prescribed Kt/V less than 1.2. These patients have a higher relative risk of death than those receiving a Kt/V greater than 1.2. In addition, diabetics with a prescribed dialysis regimen of Kt/V less than 1.4 have a higher relative risk of death than those with Kt/V greater than 1.4. The higher prescribed and delivered Kt/Vs reduce the relative risk of death by approximately 30 percent compared with the average U.S. data. If these data are confirmed in subsequent studies, the adequacy of dialysis will be determined by control of risks in the population and the total delivered therapy.

LIMITATIONS OF HIGH-EFFICIENCY THERAPIES

Fluid Removal

As dialysis treatment time is reduced, the rate of ultrafiltration is increased to compensate for the loss in treatment time. The use of bicarbonate dialysate and ultrafiltration control equipment has improved the predictability of fluid removal during the treatments. Typically, in our experience, the average patient may lose approximately 3 to 4 kg per 2.5- to 3-hour treatment with ultrafiltration rates ranging between 20 and 35 ml/min. The upper limit of patient stability appears to be a maximum of 2 kg/h of fluid removal.

Cardiovascular Stability

Initially, there were concerns as to whether or not cardiovascular stability would improve with high-efficiency therapies as compared with standard acetate dialysis.[1,2] The use of bicarbonate dialysate and ultrafiltration control systems have provided adequate systems to improve cardiovascular stability during the dialysis treatment, such that the rate of symptomatic hypotension is less than 8 percent and asymptomatic hypotension is an additional 5 to 8 percent. Overall, this is less than the total 20 to 25 percent hypotension seen with acetate dialysate. In this context, there is little contraindication to high-efficiency bicarbonate therapies relative to cardiovascular stability.

High Extracorporeal Blood Flow

The average blood flow rates of typical high-efficiency and high-flux therapies are between 350 and 400 ml/min. Artery collapse and access recirculation are clinical problems of major concern. Some investigators have reemphasized previous relationships between the elevation of venous pressure and access recirculation relative to the effect of the dialysis being delivered.[15] Recirculation studies can be performed by three basic dialysis techniques.

The first technique uses the single-pool assumptions with universal mixing of urea nitrogen in the single-body pool. The following formula shows that the recirculation rate R would be equal to

$$R = \frac{\text{pool solute concentrate} - \text{arterial solute concentrate}}{\text{pool solute concentrate} - \text{venous solute concentrate}}$$

In this application, the pool sample is drawn from a peripheral vein opposite the access arm. It should be noted that there is a difference between the arterialized sample coming into the arterial line of the dialysis circuit and the venous sample drawn from the opposite arm. Dilutional effects can occur, causing approximately a 5 to 10 percent inaccuracy in the recirculation measurement. This is because the high blood flow rate contributes a very low urea concentration to the venous circulation returning centrally and mixing with the total cardiac output. The return of blood with a very low urea nitrogen content tends to dilute the arterial sample that is feeding the arterial access, thereby giving a false impression of the difference between the venous pool sample and the arterial sample going into the dialyzer.

A second technique to potentially eliminate this problem is to take the pool sample from the arterial side of the circuit with the blood pump turned off for approximately 1 minute. This allows the access to clear of recirculated blood, thereby giving a truer arterial sample feeding the access. The one limitation of this approach is that the arterial concentration entering the access will begin to rise slightly owing to the stopping of the blood pump, thus eliminating the return to the central circulation of a high blood flow rate with a low urea concentration. This system, however, seems to cause much less error, since the sequence of collecting the arterial and venous blood samples involves starting the blood pump after the arterial sample is obtained.

The third method that has been proposed leaves the extracorporeal circuit intact and occludes the access between the arterial and venous needles to draw the arterial pool sample. In this way the dialysis circuit is not interrupted, nor is the rate of high blood flow return with a low urea concentration in the central circulation. This last technique may have some operational problems, as the fistula needles may not be adequately separated, and occlusion between the needles can thus occur without causing collapse of the arterial line secondary to needle suction against the access wall. In summary, the two latter techniques, which involve either stopping the blood pump or producing an occlusion between the extracorporeal circuit needles, yield more accurate sampling and eliminate difficulties with central mixing of low-urea blood, which would thereby violate the single-pool assumptions. High blood flow rates with high rates of urea removal can exceed the transfer coefficients from intracellular to extracellular space for solute removal. This is the basis for two-pool kinetic modeling as proposed by Ilstrup et al.[20] Techniques for handling these particular problems are outlined in the previous chapters. Finally, to achieve high extracorporeal blood flow rates, needle diameter and length are important considerations. Typical clinical applications use 15-gauge, ultra-thin-walled needles approximately 1 inch in length. For blood flow rates exceeding 400 ml/min, 14-gauge needles may also be used, but these may have limitations relative to long-term survival of the blood access.

FUTURE DEVELOPMENTS

The critical issue central to all dialysis therapy is delivery of an adequate therapy prescription. New techniques need to be developed to adequately predict the difference between single-pool and two-pool urea kinetic modeling, which appears to be a common phenomenon occurring in dialysis patients who are treated with high-flux and high-efficiency therapies. Adequate delivery of the dialysate prescription clearly appears to affect the long-term survival of both diabetic and nondiabetic patients and, therefore, aggressive monitoring of this on a routine basis in dialysis equipment should be developed. Extremely high-efficiency and high-flux dialyzers with surface areas greater than 2 m^2 are not available at this time but will probably be necessary in order to continue providing adequate treatments with efficient delivery that meet the operational needs of the dialysis programs.

CONCLUSIONS

High-efficiency and high-flux therapies have been applied in the clinical setting since 1985 and have shown excellent results relative to stability of dialysis treatments, adequacy of therapy delivered, and safety of the basic procedures. Therapy prescription continues to be a critical issue and needs to be addressed not only on the basis of in vitro data but also by in vivo therapy confirmation. Careful attention to bicarbonate concentrate and its tendency for microbiologic overgrowth are important clinical requirements. When attention is paid to the details of therapy prescription, dialysate composition, control of bicarbonate concentrate contamination, and good maintenance of dialysis machines, a successful program can be achieved and maintained.

REFERENCES

1. Collins A, Keshaviah P, Berkseth R et al: Short efficient hemodialysis with reduced symptoms. Kidney Int 27:158, 1985
2. Keshaviah P, Collins A: Rapid high-efficiency bicarbonate hemodialysis. Trans Am Soc Artif Intern Organs 32:17, 1986
3. Collins A, Ilstrup K, Hanson G et al: Rapid high-efficiency hemodialysis. Artif Organs 10:185, 1986

4. Von Albertini B, Miller J, Gardner P, Shinaberger J: High flux hemodiafiltration: under six hours/week treatment. Trans Am Soc Artif Intern Organs 30:227, 1984
5. Wauters J, Pansiot S, Horisberger J: Short haemodialysis long-term results. Nephrol Dial Transplant 20:139, 1983
6. Keen M, Evans M, Gotch F: Comparison of morbidity in high flux dialysis. Kidney Int 31:235, 1987
7. Levin N, Dumler F, Zasuwa G, Stalla K: Mortality comparison between conventional and high flux dialysis. J Am Soc Nephrol 1:365, 1990
8. Kjellstrand C, Shideman J, Santiago E et al: Technical advances in hemodialysis of very small pediatric patients. Proc Clin Dial Transplant Forum 1:124, 1971
9. Kjellstrand C, Mauer S, Buselmeier T et al: Haemodialysis of premature and newborn babies. Nephrol Dial Transplant 10:349, 1973
10. Kaiser B, Potter D, Bryant R et al: Acid-base changes and acetate metabolism during routine and high-efficiency hemodialysis in children. Kidney Int 19:70, 1981
11. Bosl R, Shideman J, Meyer R et al: Effects and complications of high efficiency dialyzers. Nephron 15:151, 1975
12. Nissenson A, Fine R, Gentile D (eds): Clinical Dialysis. 2nd Ed. Appleton-Century-Crofts, East Norwalk, CT, 1990
13. Gotch F, Sargent J: A mechanistic analysis of the National Cooperative Dialysis Study (NCDS). Kidney Int 28:526, 1985
14. Rotellar E, Martinez E, Samso J et al: Why dialyze more than 6 hours a week. Trans Am Soc Artif Intern Organs 31:538, 1985
15. Schwab S, Lambert M, Collins D et al: Fistula dysfunction: effect on rapid hemodialysis. J Am Soc Nephrol 2:350, 1991
16. Ebben J, Hirsch D, Luehmann D et al: Microbiologic contamination of liquid bicarbonate concentrate for hemodialysis. ASAIO Trans 33:269, 1987
17. Bland L, Ridgeway M, Agnero S et al: Potential bacteriologic and endotoxin hazards associated with liquid bicarbonate concentrate. ASAIO Trans 33:542, 1987
18. Collins A, Liao M, Umen A et al: High-efficiency bicarbonate hemodialysis (HEBH) has a lower risk of death than standard acetate dialysis, abstracted. J Am Soc Nephrol 2:318, 1991
19. Collins A, Liao M, Umen A et al: Diabetic (DM) hemodialysis (HD) patients (PTS) treated with a high KT/V have a lower risk of death than standard (STD) KT/V, abstracted. J Am Soc Nephrol 2:318, 1991
20. Ilstrup K, Hanson G, Shapiro W, Keshaviah P: Examining the foundations of urea kinetics. Trans Am Soc Artif Intern Organs 31:164, 1985
21. Gotch F, Uehlinger D: Mortality Rate in U.S. Dialysis Patients. Dial Transplant. Vol. 20, No. 5, May 1991
22. Shaldon S, Beau M, Deschodt G, Mion C: Mixed hemofiltration (MHF): 18 months experience with ultrashort treatment time. Trans Am Soc Artif Intern Organs 27:610, 1981
23. Dongradi G, Haas T, Villeboeuf F, Fendler J: High-efficiency haemofiltration (ultrafiltration of more than 250 ml/min for two hours) in eight uraemic patients. Proc Eur Dial Transplant Assoc 18:176, 1981
24. Wizemann V, Kramer W, Knopp G et al: Ultrashort hemodiafiltration: efficiency and hemodynamic tolerance. Clin Nephrol 19:24, 1983
25. Keshaviah P, Collins A: High-efficiency hemodialysis. p. 109. In: D'Amico G, Colasanti G (eds): Contributions to Nephrology. Vol. 69. S Karger, 1989.
26. Campbell J, Dumber F, Stalla K, Levin N: High-flux shorttime hemodialysis: initial clinical experience. Kidney Int 31:229, 1987

8

High-Flux Hemodialysis

Sergio R. Acchiardo

INTRODUCTION

Many attempts have been made to reduce dialysis time by using high blood flows and large-area dialyzers.[1–4] In these studies acetate was usually used in the dialysate, and patients were followed for periods of 6 months to 6 years. In general, no differences were found between conventional and short dialysis. However, one study reported some problems with short dialysis,[5] including maintaining a water balance, maintaining adequate blood pressure control, maintaining adequate pedialysis serum potassium and phosphorus levels, and symptoms suggestive of peripheral neuropathy, such as itching, tingling, and numbness of the hands and feet.

In 1982 Kramer et al.[6] questioned the long-term safety of short hemodialysis. They reported an increased cardiovascular mortality in patients 55 years or older subjected to dialysis for 4 hours three times per week or less. Using advances in dialysis such as bicarbonate dialysate, ultrafiltration control systems, high blood flow rates, and dialyzers with large surface areas, several investigators have reported on their experiences with high-flux hemodiafiltration, rapid high-efficiency bicarbonate hemodialysis, and short dialysis.[7–10] In 1986 the first experiences with high-flux dialysis using polysulfone membranes, bicarbonate dialysate, high blood and dialysate flow, sodium modeling, and control ultrafiltration were reported.[11,12] The increased use of high-flux dialysis creates a need to discuss its indications, the essential elements involved, dialysis prescription, and potential benefits and problems.

CRITERIA FOR HIGH-FLUX DIALYSIS

Two forms of rapid dialysis have been more commonly used: rapid high-efficiency bicarbonate hemodialysis and high-flux hemodialysis. Both techniques use a dialyzer with high urea clearance (250 to 400 ml/min) and a high ultrafiltration coefficient. They also require an increase in blood and dialysate flow. The main difference between these therapies is the type of membrane used. Investigators have attempted to find a more permeable dialyzer membrane, which mimics glomerular permeability. Under normal conditions, substances with a molecular weight of 18 to 60,000 are filtered at the level of the glomeruli. In 1985 German investigators introduced a new polysulfone membrane with a high clearance for solutes of low and middle molecular weight (up to 5,000).[13] The membrane had a high biocompatibility as evaluated by leukocytes, thrombocytes, and complement levels. According to studies by Rockel et al., the in vivo cutoff of the polysulfone membrane is comparable with that of the peritoneum.[14]

We define high-flux dialysis as a method that uses a blood flow of 400 ml/min or greater, a dialysate flow of 700 to 800 ml/min, a biocompatible membrane with high permeability for solutes of low and middle molecular weight, a bicarbonate bath, variable sodium concentration in the dialysate, and volumetric ultrafiltration control.

Patient Selection

Basic requirements in selecting patients for high-flux dialysis are (1) a vascular access that can deliver at least 400 ml/min, (2) stable cardiac status, and (3) weight gain compliance of less than 5 kg between dialyses. A high rate of hypotensive episodes on conventional dialysis was not considered as a contraindication for high-flux treatment. As my experience has increased, I have become more liberal in the selection of patients. At present, 20 percent of my patients are diabetics, and many have coronary artery disease. The main limitation to the procedure has been excessive weight gain between dialyses. Of 60 patients undergoing high-flux dialysis, 10 (17 percent) have failed the therapy because of this problem. A small number of patients failed because of vascular access problems and recirculation. No disequilibrium syndrome has been observed in these patients.

COMPONENTS OF HIGH-FLUX DIALYSIS

The Dialyzer

For high-flux dialysis, the dialyzer must provide a high urea clearance (250 to 400 ml/min) suitable for a short treatment. The use of a biocompatible membrane such as a polysulfone, polyacrylonitrile, or cellulose triacetate membrane provides an increased clearance for substances of middle molecular weight and a substantial β_2-microglobulin removal (Table 8-1). In my institution's dialysis unit we have mainly used the Fresenius Hemoflow dialyzers F60 and F80, with surface areas of 1.25 and 1.80 m^2, respectively.

Table 8–1. Characteristics of Eight High-Flux Dialyzers

Manufacturer	Dialyzer Model	Membrane	Surface Area (m^2)	KuF (ml/h/ mmHg)	Urea Clearance, Q_B (ml/min) 200	300	400	Vitamin B12, Q_B 200 ml/min
Asahi	PAN-200	PAN	1.40	42	164	199	229	103
Baxter	CT 110G	CT	1.10	22	170	228	265	109
Baxter	CT 190G	CT	1.90	36	174	239	282	137
CD Medical	DuoFlux	CA	1.40	23	171	230	258	88
Fresenius	F-60	Polysulfone	1.25	40	164	213	243	118
Fresenius	F-80	Polysulfone	1.80	60	175	243	289	136
Hospal	300-S	AN69	1.15	20	156	201	243	74
Renal System	HDF 1350	Polysulfone	1.35	25	179	210	250	99

Abbreviations: KuF, ultrafiltration coefficient; Q_B, blood flow; PAN, polyacrylonitrile; CT, cellulose triacetate; CA, cellulose acetate.

The blood flow used in conventional dialysis was increased to a least 400 ml/min for high-flux dialysis (we use 15-gauge, 1.25-inch needles). We also increased the dialysate flow to 800 ml/min.

Reliable reuse equipment is necessary. Manual and automated methods are available for reprocessing the dialyzers. We have mainly used the Seratronic DRS-4 Dialyzer Reprocessing System, which uses reverse osmosis (RO) water; the blood compartment is cleaned with hydrogen peroxide, followed by reverse ultrafiltration and flushing with RO water. Our average number of uses is about 12. The overall permeability-area product (KoA) for urea, calculated at the 1st, 5th, 10th, 15th, and 20th use, decreased by 8 percent after 10 uses and 17 percent after 20 uses.

Water Treatment

Water treatment is particularly important in high-flux dialysis since pyrogenic reactions are more frequently observed with the use of bicarbonate-containing dialysis solutions and high-flux membranes. Recommendations for minimum water purity standards have been published by the Association for the Advancement of Medical Instrumentation[15] and should be strictly enforced.

Bicarbonate Bath

Disagreement exists about the cardiodepressor effect of acetate, but the peripheral vasodilation caused by acetate is clearly established. However, a consensus exists about the use of bicarbonate as a physiologic buffer, which is better tolerated than acetate and is associated less intradialytic morbidity. The incidence of nausea and vomiting has been considerably decreased as compared with conventional dialysis using an acetate bath. The effect of bicarbonate on the incidence of cramps is questionable. High-efficiency dialyzers and short dialysis time make the use of bicarbonate mandatory to avoid the danger of exceeding the maximum acetate utilization capacity. Unfortunately, liquid bicarbonate concentrate is a primary source of bacterial contamination. A survey conducted by the Centers for Disease Control[16] found that dialysis centers practicing high-flux dialysis were more likely to report pyrogenic reactions than centers practicing conventional dialysis (19 versus 12 percent $P > .01$). Furthermore, among centers reusing high-flux dialyzers, the reported number of pyrogenic reactions significantly increased with increase in the average number of times that the dialyzer was reused.

Sodium Modeling

Sodium modeling provides the capacity to increase the sodium concentration of the dialysate early in dialysis to counteract the transcellular urea gradient. Patients on high-flux dialysis with sodium modeling had fewer hypotensive episodes and cramps than patients not on the program.[17] They did not have an increase in thirst, episodes of fluid overload, or hypertension.

Automatic Ultrafiltration Control

Use of dialyzers with a high ultrafiltration coefficient requires precise ultrafiltration control. We use a Fresenius A2008D, which provides volumetric ultrafiltration control up to a maximum rate of 3,000 ml/h. One available method to control ultrafiltration is so-called volumetric ultrafiltration, which uses either the principle of matched pumps for fresh and spent dialysis fluid or the principle of a closed circuit (balancing chamber) to equalize the fluid flow into and from the dialyzer. Volumetric ultrafiltration is incorporated into several dialysis machines, including the Hospal, the Cobe Centry 3, the Drake 480, and the Fresenius 2008. This system permits the safe use of dialyzers with a high ultrafiltration coefficient. Another group of dialysis machines uses an ultrafiltration control system with flow sensors and a microprocessor to measure dialysate inflow and outflow and to adjust the transmembrane pressure to achieve the desired ultrafiltration rate (these include the Cobe Centry 2000, Travenol machines with advance ultrafiltration control, and the Gambro machine).

DIALYSIS PRESCRIPTION

Since the pathogenesis of uremia is not clearly understood, the characteristics of an adequate dialysis treatment are difficult to define. For patients transferred to high-flux dialysis solute and water removal should be equivalent to that provided by adequate conventional dialysis. Removal of all the interdialytic fluid gain is particularly important. One way to measure the adequacy of dialysis is the urea kinetic system described by Sargent and Gotch,[18] which was used to control the National Cooperative Dialysis Study.[19] From a mechanistic analysis of those data, Gotch defined the magnitude of the dialysis prescribed with respect to urea as Kt/V (where K is urea clearance of the dialyzer, t is dialysis time in minutes, and V is volume of distribution of urea).[20] The initial volume is calculated on the basis of the patient's surface area and sex. The definition of adequate dialysis is based on midweek predialysis blood urea nitrogen (BUN), protein catabolic rate, and Kt/V. A Kt/V of 1.0 to 1.3 has been recommended for patients undergoing high-flux dialysis who are eating 1 g protein/kg/d.[21]

Recently some investigators have pointed out that a two-compartment pool better reflects how the multiple compartments of the body behave than a single-compartment model, which introduces errors when prescribing high-flux dialysis. Gotch agrees that the single-pool urea slightly underestimates the volume and overestimates the protein catabolic rate.[20a] However, the errors at 2 hours were only 3 and 2 percent, respectively, compared with the 4-hour values, and these variations were not considered clinically important. When patients who have been undergoing conventional dialysis are transferred to high-flux dialysis, particular attention should be paid to the dialysis prescription, since the decrease in dialysis time makes fulfillment of the rest of the prescription, particularly blood flow, even more critical. Unfortunately, what is prescribed is not always delivered. Therefore knowledge of potential pitfalls in the dialysis treatment and how to avoid them is important. Recently a two-compartment pool has been proposed instead of the single compartment in order to better reflect the behavior of the multiple compartments of the body.

Dialyzer Urea Clearance

One of the technical requirements for high-flux is a urea clearance rate of 250 to 400 ml/min. The dialyzer urea clearance is used to calculate an adequate dialysis treatment, but it must be kept in mind that the manufacturer's in vitro clearance is usually 10 to 20 percent higher than the in vivo clearance. Furthermore, less than 30 percent of the in vivo clearances have been within 10 percent of the manufacturer's data. In vitro clearances are usually measured in water or in whole blood with a hematocrit of 25 percent. To replace clearance studies by mass transfer studies that obtain samples from the blood and the dialysate site is impractical. Great variability in different dialyzers that are reprocessed has also been shown to exist. This is true for cuprophane dialyzers (Terumo), but it could also apply to other dialyzers. Apparently, dialyzers are adversely affected by reprocessing.[22] First-use dialyzers have also shown unexpected substandard performances that are very worrisome, since their clearances are not checked routinely in clinical practice.[23]

Accurate Blood Flow

Blood pumps should be calibrated frequently to obtain an accurate blood flow. Owing to the high blood flows, negative pressure increases and actual blood flow decreases. At the higher blood flow rates, the actual blood flow delivery is as much as 20 percent lower than the prescribed delivery. One should therefore be aware of this phenomenon to prevent inadvertent underdialysis at high flow rates.[24] This decrease is usually more important with the development of hemoconcentration, which increases viscosity and thereby increases the negative arterial pressure even more. The ability of the tubing to reexpand fully between rapid compressions by the pump rollers is especially important when the negative arterial pressure exceeds 200 mmHg. Needle size is the limiting factor in the system.

Volume of Distribution

The volume of distribution should be calculated on the basis of weight, sex, and height,[25] since only 40 percent of the actual volume is within 56 to 60 percent of body weight. Alternatively, the volume of distribution can be calculated knowing the pre- and postdialysis BUN, clearance of the dialyzer, time on dialysis, and pre- and postdialysis body weight. If this calculated volume is not within 10 percent of the estimated volume, a problem in dialysis delivery is indicated.

Treatment Time

Actual time on dialysis should be recorded. Alarm interruptions should be taken into consideration as well as time for changes of clotting dialyzers. The treatment time is usually overestimated by the patient as well as by the staff.

Vascular Access Recirculation

One of the important factors in the success of high-flux dialysis is adequate vascular access blood flow. Recirculation will occur if the blood flow through the vascular access is insufficient to support the desired dialysis blood flow, resulting in an effective clearance lower than the dialyzer clearance.[26] The decrease in blood flow will result in an effective reduction of solute clearance.

Significant recirculation may be present even with low venous pressure. Of patients with more than 15 percent recirculation in one study, 86 percent had radiographically significant stenosis.[27] Overestimation of delivered blood flow, dialyzer dysfunction, and fistula recirculation affect the delivery of prescribed dialysis. These problems are magnified in high-flux dialysis. Calculation of the effective in vivo urea clearance is a valuable tool in detecting unexpected deficiencies in the delivery of the dialysis prescription. When the patient is started on high-flux dialysis, the vascular access should be checked for recirculation, and this check should be repeated every time the urea kinetics suggests the possibility of recirculation. In the presence of recirculation the delivery of adequate therapy can be seriously compromised. Recirculation is measured by the following formula:

$$\%R = [(P-A)/(P-V)]\ (100)$$

where R is recirculation and P is peripheral, A is arterial, and V is venous blood.

Calculation of Kt/V

Residual renal function plays an important role in the removal of solutes and should be taken into consideration in the calculation of Kt/V, which is usually prescribed on the basis of whole blood clearances even though changes in hematocrit will affect the clearance. These changes are usually small, but they can be compounded by other factors that also decrease effective blood flow.

Urea Rebound

Urea rebound is considered negligible in conventional dialysis and does not affect the reliability of single-pool urea kinetics.[19] The highest values of urea rebound (8.8 percent) were observed after procedures with the largest urea removal. An equilibration process rather than protein hypercatabolism seems to be responsible for the rebound. It is possible to minimize errors arising from application of a single-pool analysis by using a two-pool system.[28] Another way to alleviate the potential error is to increase Kt/V to ensure equivalent solute removal. To shorten dialysis time, higher blood flows are being used, which creates the possibility of increased urea rebound.

BACKFILTRATION

Bommer et al.[29] found no evidence for endotoxin transport across high-flux polysulfone membranes. These findings were corroborated by Van Haecke et al.,[30] who performed in vivo studies using *Pseudomonas*-produced toxins added to the dialysate of patients treated with large-pore polysulfone dialyzers (PS 600). However, other in vitro and in vivo studies have shown a significant passage of endotoxin across polysulfone membranes.[31] Endotoxins or their fragments can be transported by diffusion and convection across the intact high-flux membrane and reach the bloodstream, where they induce adverse effects in dialysis patients.[32] Clinical consequences of backfiltration vary from center to center and depend on the quality of dialysate,[33] since a main source of bacterial contamination is liquid bicarbonate concentrate. The occurrence of backfiltration has stressed the need for adequate water treatment and dialysate supplies. Centers using high-flux dialyzer membranes are more likely to report pyrogenic reactions, particularly when the dialyzers are reused.[16]

MORBIDITY AND MORTALITY

Several studies have shown a significant decrease in intradialytic morbidity with high-flux dialysis. The incidence of nausea, vomiting, and hypotension significantly decreased when patients formerly treated with acetate bath were started on bicarbonate dialysate therapy.[34] Since bicarbonate dialysate is an absolute requirement for high-flux dialysis, patients receiving this form of therapy benefit from its use. Furthemore, my colleagues and I observed a further significant decrease in hypotensive episodes as well as in muscle cramps in patients treated with sodium modeling.

Several investigators have reported improved survival of patients undergoing high-flux dialysis. In a retrospective study of 200 patients,[35] the calculated predicted-year survival was 96.6 percent. Levin et al.[36] reported their experience with high-flux dialysis in 172 patients. The mortality rate in these patients, adjusted for demographic variants, was 6 percent per year. My group's 4-year experience with high-flux dialysis, the yearly mortality rate was 4 percent.[37] Of our 60 patients, 18 percent were diabetics. Gotch and Uehlinger reported that 20 percent of their high-flux dialysis patients were diabetic and that the mortality rate was 14.2 percent.[38] Several factors are probably responsible for this decrease in mortality rate: more biocompatible membranes, the use of bicarbonate, precise control of ultrafiltration, and higher removal of middle-size molecules. Further studies involving larger numbers of patients followed for longer times are necessary to document this preliminary finding.

ADVANTAGES

β_2-Microglobulin

Evidence accumulated during the last few years indicates that β_2-microglobulin plays a role in the pathogenesis of several clinically important pathologic processes in chronic hemodialysis patients, including carpal tunnel syndrome and diseases of the bone and joints. β_2-Microglobulin has been shown to be the principal constituent of the amyloid deposits isolated from patients with bone or joint disease.[39] Its daily production has been calculated to be 150 to 200 mg. Patients undergoing high-flux dialysis with polysulfone membranes decreased their β_2-microglobulin levels by 43 percent. These dialyzers have been shown to remove 240 to 259 mg of β_2-microglobulin during hemofiltration of 20 L; however, the amount removed by high-flux dialysis has not been sufficient to avoid its accumulation.[40] The reuse of dialyzers and reprocessing have not affected the clearance of this substance. The removal of β_2-microglobulin in high-flux dialysis may affect the development of amyloidosis but to test this hypothesis, a long observation period (several years) is necessary. The prevention of complications associated with accumulation of β_2-microglobulin is important in judging the adequacy of dialysis.

Aluminum Clearance

Aluminum accumulation in hemodialysis patients has been associated with severe clinical problems, including bone disease,[41] encephalopathy,[42] and anemia.[43] High-flux dialyzers, especially polysulfone dialyzers, have a higher clearance for aluminum than conventional dialyzers. Molitoris et al.[44] demonstrated rapid and complete removal of deferroxamine (DFO)-chelated aluminum during a 4-hour hemodialysis with polysulfone dialyzers; thus, removal of DFO complexes was maximized and exposure to such complexes was minimized. These authors suggested the use of a Fesenius F-80 dialyzer in conjunction with reduced doses of DFO the day before dialysis in order to decrease DFO-related side effects in hemodialysis patients.

Lipids

The main lipid abnormality in uremia is hypertriglyceridemia, which occurs in 20 to 70 percent of dialysis patients. The most common lipoprotein pattern is type IV according to Frederickson's classification.[45]

Barth et al.[46] reported no significant changes in serum cholesterol, except for those attributed to hemoconcentration, but a lowering of serum triglycerides during dialysis with AN-69 membranes. They postulate that high-flux membranes may be more efficient in the removal of a high molecular weight inhibitor of lipoprotein lipase. Patients on high-flux dialysis using polysulfone or cellulose triacetate membranes had normal triglyceride levels and a normal high-density lipoprotein (HDL-2) in the face of diminished total HDL levels.[47] Levels of serum triglycerides in patients started on high-flux dialysis decreased after 6 months, as did levels of very low density and low-density lipoproteins, Apo C-III, and Apo C-III and the very low density to low-density lipoprotein ratio.[48]

Patients

Our patients like a short dialysis time because it interferes less with their life-styles. They reported that they were more active and less tired and "washed out" after dialysis. One-third of the patients stated that their appetites had increased, and half of the patients reported less nausea and vomiting. They tolerate dialysis better because of the use of bicarbonate, control ultrafiltration, more biocompatible membranes, and sodium modeling.

Provider Personnel

High-flux dialysis permits the treatment of a larger number of patients per day, thereby increasing efficiency by at least 30 percent. Most of our nurses perceived high-flux dialysis as a form of treatment that is well tolerated by the patients. Our nurses thought that their tasks were performed on schedule, but they finished the day more fatigued than usual and did not have enough time to teach the patients. The staff spent more time on machine setup, machine cleaning, and initiating and ending treatment, which left less time to interact with patients, but the staff spent less time treating complications. Personnel can be better utilized with high-flux procedures, since shortening dialysis time permits them to increase the number of patients from two to three per 10-hour shift.

CONCLUSIONS

High-flux hemodialysis provides an adequate treatment in a shorter time and is well tolerated by the patients and accepted by the staff. The main cause of failure is excessive interdialytic weight gain. It is obvious, therefore, that to optimally limit dialysis time, one must carefully assess the maximum tolerable ultrafiltration for each patient.

Mortality rate has been reported to be low; this needs corroboration with larger, randomized studies. Possible explanations of low mortality rate are biocompatible membranes, bicarbonate dialysate, control ultrafiltration, better clearances for substances of middle molecular weight, and sodium modeling.

REFERENCES

1. Man NK, Granger A, Rondon-Nucete M et al: One year follow-up of short dialysis with a membrane highly permeable to middle molecules. Proc Eur Dial Transplant Assoc 11:236, 1973
2. Cambi V, Savazzi G, Arisi L et al: Short dialysis schedules finally ready to become a routine? Proc Eur Dial Transplant Assoc 11:112, 1974
3. Maiorca R, Castellani A, Migozzi G et al: Short time personalized dialysis: good results in spite of high levels of small and middle molecules. Proc Eur Dial Transplant Assoc 11:146, 1974
4. Snyder D, Louis BM, Gorfien P et al: Clinical experience with long-term brief, "daily" hemodialysis. Proc Eur Dial Transplant Assoc 11:128, 1974
5. Alvarez-Ude F, Ward M, Elliot R et al: A comparison of short and long haemodialysis. Proc Eur Dial Transplant Assoc 12:606, 1975
6. Kramer P, Broyer M, Brunner FP et al: Combined report on regular dialysis and transplantation in Europe. Proc Eur Dial Transplant Assoc 19:4, 1982
7. Von Albertini B, Miller JH, Gardner PW et al: High-flux hemodiafiltration: under six hours/week treatment. Trans Am Soc Artif Intern Organs 30:227, 1984
8. Von Albertini B, Miller JH, Gardner PW et al: One year high-flux hemodiafiltration: 6 hrs/week, abstracted. J Am Soc Nephrol 18:78A, 1985
9. Rotellar E, Martinez ME, Plans A et al: Haemodialysis: only six hours once a week. Proc Eur Dial Transplant Assoc 22:312, 1985
10. Collins A, Ilstrup K, Hanson G et al: Rapid high-efficiency hemodialysis. Artif Organs 10:185, 1986
11. Acchiardo S, Burk L, Banister D: High-flux hemodialysis. Kidney Int 31:226, 1987
12. Campbell J, Dumler F, Stalla K et al: High-flux short time hemodialysis: initial experience. Kidney Int 31:229, 1987

13. Schneider H, Streicher E: Mass transfer characterization of a new polysulfone membrane. Artif Organs 9:180, 1985
14. Rockel A, Hertel J, Fiegel P et al: Permeability and secondary membrane formation of a high flux polysulfone hemofilter. Kidney Int 30:429, 1986
15. Association for the Advancement of Medical Instrumentation: American National Standards for Hemodialysis Systems. Assoc Adv Med Instrum, Arlington, VA 1982
16. Alter MJ, Favero MS, Moyer LA et al: Pyrogenic reactions in patients undergoing high-flux dialysis in the U.S., 1987–1989, abstracted. J Am Soc Nephrol 1:347, 1990
17. Acchiardo SR, Hayden AJ: Is Na^+ modeling necessary in high-flux dialysis? Trans Am Soc Artif Intern Organs 37(3):M135, 1991
18. Sargent JA, Gotch FA: The analysis of concentration dependence of uremic lesions in clinical studies. Kidney Int 7 (suppl 2):S35, 1975
19. Sargent JA: Control of dialysis by a single-pool urea model: the National Cooperative Dialysis Study. Kidney Int 23 (suppl 13):S19, 1983
20. Gotch FA: A mechanistic analysis of the National Cooperative Dialysis Study (NCDS). Kidney Int 28:526, 1985
20a. Sargent JA, Gotch FA: Principles and Biophysics of Dialysis. p. 107. In Maher JF (ed): Replacement of Renal Function by Dialysis. 3rd ed. Kluwer, Boston, 1989
21. Gotch FA, Keen M: The high-flux prescription, abstracted. Kidney Int 31:232, 1987
22. Delmez JA, Weerts CA, Hasamear PD et al: Severe dialyzer dysfunction undetectable by standard reprocessing validation tests. Kidney Int 36:478, 1989
23. Sargent JA: Shortfalls in the delivery of dialysis. Am J Kidney Dis 15:500, 1990
24. Schmidt DF, Schniepp BJ, Kurtz SB et al: Inaccurate blood flow rate during rapid hemodialysis. Am J Kidney Dis 17:34, 1991
25. Steffensen KA: Some determinations of the total body water in man by means of intravenous injections of urea. Acta Physiol Scand 13:282, 1947
26. Collins A, Hanson G, Berkseth R et al: Recirculation and effective clearances, abstracted. Kidney Int 33:219, 1988
27. Windus DW, Audrian J, Vanderson R et al: Optimization of high-efficiency hemodialysis by detection and correction of fistula dysfunction. Kidney Int 38:337, 1990
28. Pedrini LA, Zereik S, Rasmy S: Causes, kinetics, and clinical implications of post-hemodialysis urea rebound. Kidney Int 34:817, 1988
29. Bommer J, Becker KP, Urbaschek R et al: No evidence for endotoxin transfer across high flux polysulfone membranes. Clin Nephrol 27:278, 1987
30. Van Haecke E, Vanholder R, Ringoir S: Absence of in vivo endotoxin transfer from dialysate to blood through large pore dialyzers, abstracted. Kidney Int 37:322, 1990
31. Klinkman H, Falken Hagen D, Smollich BP: Investigation of the permeability of highly permeable polysulfone membranes for pyrogens. Contrib Nephrol 46:174, 1985
32. Man NK, Ciancioni C, Faivre J et al: Dialysis associated adverse reactions with high-flux membranes and microbial contamination of liquid bicarbonate concentrate. Contrib Nephrol 62:24, 1988
33. Baurmeister U, Travers M, Vienken J et al: Dialysate contamination and back filtration may limit the use of high-flux dialysis membranes. Trans Am Soc Artif Intern Organs 35:519, 1989

34. Hakim RM, Pontzer MA, Tilton D et al: Effects of acetate and bicarbonate dialysis in stable chronic dialysis patients. Kidney Int 28:535, 1985
35. Homberger JC, Chemew ME, Petersen J: Improved survival of patients on high-flux dialysis, abstracted. J Am Soc Nephrol 1:362, 1990
36. Levin NW, Dumler F, Zasuwa G et al: Mortality comparison between conventional and high flux dialysis, abstracted. J Am Soc Nephrol 1:365, 1990
37. Acchiardo S, Burk L, Moore L: Four years' experience with high-flux dialysis, abstracted. 11th Cong Nephrol, Tokyo, July 15–20, 1990, Program Abstr. p. 248A
38. Gotch FA, Uehlinger DE: Mortality rate in U.S. dialysis patients. Dial Transplant 20:255, 1991
39. Gejyo F, Odami S, Yamada T et al: β_2-microglobulin: a new form of amyloid protein associated with chronic hemodialysis. Kidney Int 30:385, 1986
40. Acchiardo S, Kraus AP, Jennings BR: β_2-microglobulin in patients with renal insufficiency. Am J Kidney Dis 13:70, 1989
41. Chan Y, Furlong TJ, Cornish CJ et al: Dialysis osteodystrophy: a study involving 94 patients. Medicine (Baltimore) 64:296, 1985
42. Alfrey AC: Dialysis encephalopathy syndrome. Annu Rev Med 29:93, 1978
43. Touam M, Martinez F, Lacour B et al: Aluminum induced, reversible microcytic anemia in chronic renal failure: clinical and experimental studies. Clin Nephrol 19:295, 1983
44. Molitoris BA, Alfrey AC, Alfrey PS et al: Rapid removal of DFO-chelated aluminum during hemodialysis using polysulfone dialyzers. Kidney Int 34:98, 1988
45. Chan MK, Varghese Z, Moorhead JF: Lipids abnormalities in uremia. Kidney Int 19:625, 1981
46. Barth RH, Zara AC, Berlyne GM: Reduction of serum triglycerides by heparin and high-flux hemodialysis membrane, abstracted. Kidney Int 37:288, 1990
47. Josephson MA, Fellner SK, Dasgupta A: Improved lipid profiles in patients on high flux hemodialysis, abstracted. J Am Soc Nephrol 1:363, 1990
48. Otsubo Y, Nagayama N, Harada R et al: The beneficial effect of high flux membrane on hemodialysis patients with hypertriglyceridemia, abstracted. J Am Soc Nephrol 1:371, 1990

9

Hemofiltration and Hemodiafiltration

Claudio Ronco

INTRODUCTION

The use of highly permeable membranes and the development of systems for ultrafiltration control have permitted application of a series of different treatments that represent possible alternatives to high-efficiency hemodialysis. These treatments using highly permeable membranes are schematically depicted in Figure 9-1. Hemofiltration, as well as hemodiafiltration and high-flux dialysis, can be performed with large, highly permeable dialyzers at high filtration rates. In the same figure the mechanism of transport in the different techniques is shown schematically. While hemofiltration is a completely convective therapy and requires pre- or post-treatment dilution to restore blood volume, hemodiafiltration and high-flux dialysis combine diffusion and convection.

In hemodiafiltration 9 to 12 L of ultrafiltrate are produced during a session and replaced in adequate amount with commercially prepared solutions. In

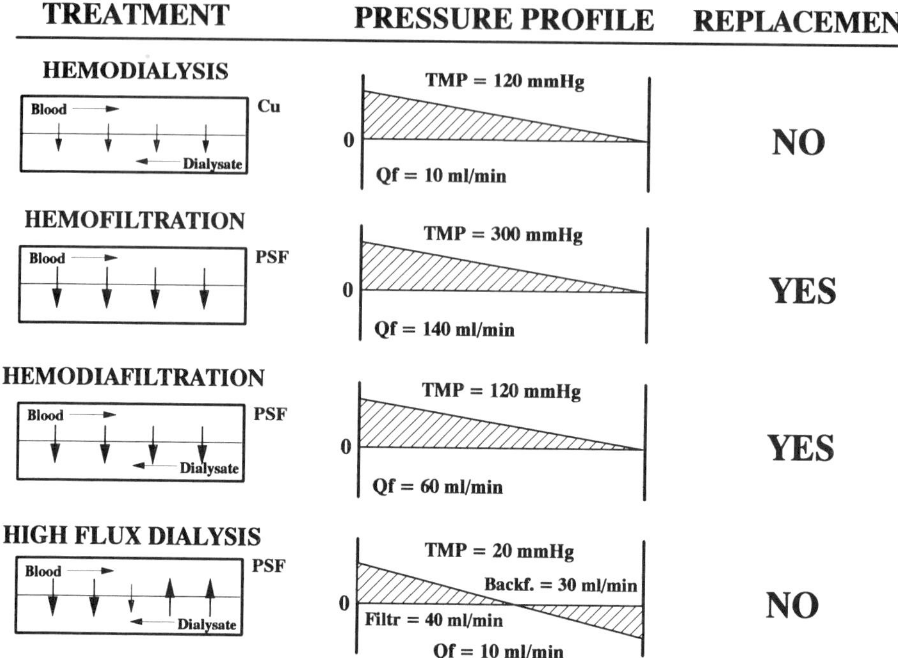

Fig. 9-1. Mechanism of operation of different dialysis techniques. In hemodialysis low-permeability (cuprophane) membranes are used, and diffusion is the mechanism of transport. The ultrafiltration rate is low and equals the patient's weight loss. There is no need for replacement. In hemofiltration highly permeable (polysulfone) membranes are used, and convection is the mechanism of transport. Replacement solution is necessary to maintain fluid balance. In hemodiafiltration convection and diffusion are combined, and highly permeable membranes are used. The pressure profile is constantly positive along the length of the dialyzer, and since the amount of ultrafiltration exceeds the patient's weight loss, reinfusion of replacement solution is necessary to balance the high filtration rates. High-flux dialysis also combines diffusion and convection, but the pressure profile is such that filtration takes place in the proximal part of the dialyzer and backfiltration in the distal part. In this case replacement solutions are not necessary, and net filtration equals the patient's weight loss.

the meantime, diffusion takes place because of the countercurrent dialysate flow, which provides an adequate gradient for solute transport. In high-flux dialysis, as in hemodiafiltration, convection is added to diffusion and ultrafiltration takes place in the proximal part of the dialyzer. The treatment, however, does not require reinfusion of replacement solution, since the fluid balance is achieved by backfiltration of dialysate in the distal part of the dialyzer. This mechanism is achieved by an accurate setting of the ultrafiltration control system, which regulates the net filtration rate according to the desired weight loss of the patient.

All these treatments provide better clearances for medium to large molecules as compared with standard hemodialysis, not only because of the higher permeability of the membrane and the larger pore size but also because medium to large solutes with poor diffusion coefficients are transported by a convective mechanism due to large amounts of ultrafiltration (Fig. 9-2).

Since high-flux dialysis has already been described in detail in Chapter 8 of this book, we briefly summarize below the characteristics of the hemofiltration and hemodiafiltration techniques.

HEMOFILTRATION

Hemofiltration is an extracorporeal technique in which solutes and electrolytes are removed from the patient by convective transport owing to large amounts of ultrafiltration. The fluid lost by ultrafiltration is then replaced with selected substitution fluids in a proportion adequate to maintain the desired fluid balance. Ultrafiltration was originally intended and used to control the patient's fluid overload during dialysis or in a separate session.[1] Subsequently, the introduction of a new highly permeable membrane led Henderson and co-workers in 1967 to use ultrafiltration to remove solutes, thus achieving blood purification.[2] A few years later Quellhorst et al.[3] in Germany reported a similar treatment based on high ultrafiltration rates and replacement with pyrogen-free solutions. The new treatment, named hemofiltration, was first used as a chronic renal replacement therapy only when reliable ultrafiltration control systems and fluid balancing machines were made commercially available by the industry.[4]

Multicenter studies demonstrated that this treatment is associated with high patient tolerance and cardiovascular stability as well as with higher clearances of medium and large molecules.[5,6] The real advantages of medium and large solute removal was never proved,[7] and interest in this technique rapidly decreased. The major problem was related to the high cost and the need for large amounts of commercially prepared substitution fluids. This problem was partially solved by the on-line production of sterile replacement solution from fresh dialysate,[8] but nevertheless the method did not achieve worldwide application, even though some patients are still treated by hemofiltration in Italy, France, and Germany.

Basic Principles

Solute removal (Js) is affected by convection and therefore will be proportional to the amount of ultrafiltration (UF) and the solute sieving coefficient (S)

$$Js = UF \times S \tag{1}$$

where S, the sieving coefficient, is defined as the ratio between the concentrations of the solute in the ultrafiltrate ([s]uf) and in plasma water ([s]pw).[9–13]

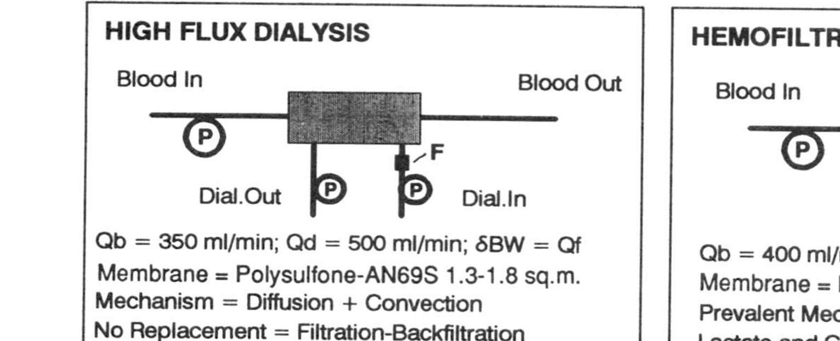

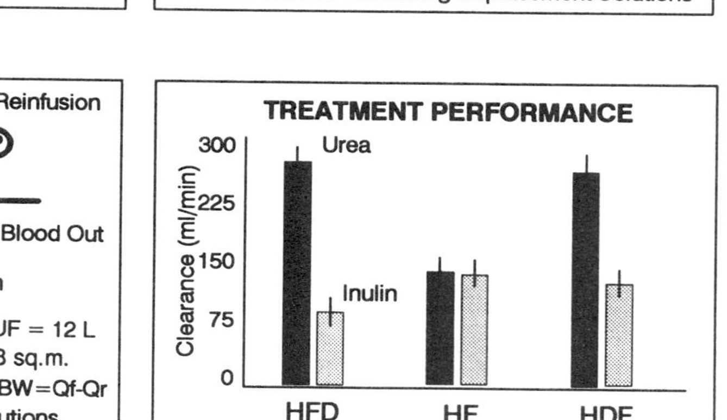

Fig. 9-2. Possible approaches to the use of highly permeable membranes are depicted schematically, with the standard characteristics of each technique. In high-flux dialysis urea clearance is as high as in hemodiafiltration, while inulin clearance is lower because of the lower amount of ultrafiltration and convection. In hemofiltration urea and inulin clearances are identical to ultrafiltration rate because of the completely convective nature of the technique.

It is evident that the solute clearance (C) will be proportional to the fractional ultrafiltration rate (Qf) and the sieving coefficient:

$$C = Qf \times S = Qf \times \frac{[s]uf}{[s]pw} \tag{2}$$

In the case of solutes freely crossing the membrane, the sieving coefficient will be unity and clearance will equal ultrafiltration rate. Solutes that are completely restrained by the membrane, such as proteins will have a sieving coefficient of zero, resulting in zero clearance. In Figure 9-3 the sieving coefficients for different membranes are plotted against solute molecular weight and Einstein-Stockes radius. It can be noted that while in cuprophane membranes the sieving coefficients dramatically decrease for solutes with a molecular weight larger than 200, in synthetic membranes they remain fairly high over a wide range of molecular weights up to the cutoff value of the membrane.

The rate of ultrafiltration is therefore the factor that strongly influences the efficiency of hemofiltration in terms of solute removal, since highly permeable membranes with high sieving coefficients are commonly used. Ultrafiltration rate is governed by the permeability coefficient of the membrane (Kf) and the transmembrane pressure (TMP). It should be noted, however, that protein concentration in the plasma water, hematocrit, and blood viscosity may strongly affect the rate of ultrafiltration. At low blood

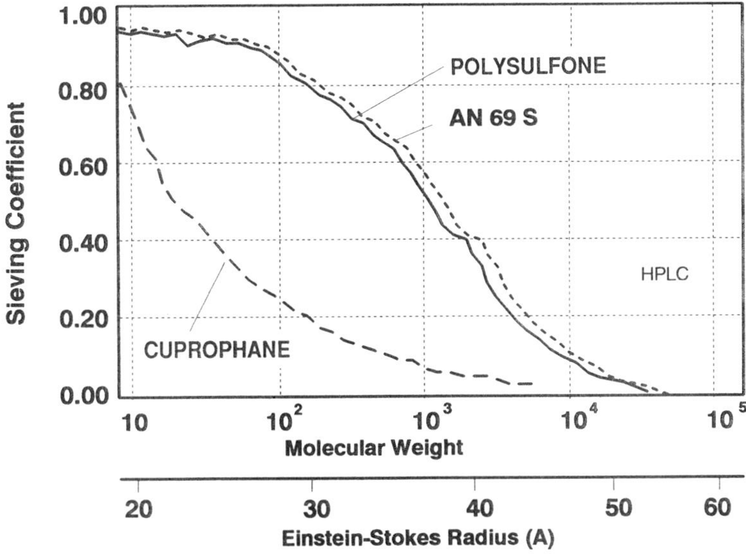

Fig. 9-3. Sieving coefficients of neutral dextrans of increasing molecular weight. It is evident that sieving values decrease early with cuprophane membranes, while they remain fairly stable over a wide range of molecular weights with synthetic membranes.

flows, the ratio between ultrafiltration rate and plasma flow (filtration fraction) may become higher than 20 to 30 percent. In this case the protein concentration increases dramatically in the blood compartment and an important oncotic pressure is generated against filtration. On the other hand, proteins may form a secondary layer on the inner surface of the membrane, thereby reducing significantly the effective permeability of the membrane (concentration polarization phenomenon). For all these reasons high blood flows (> 400 ml/min) must be used in hemofiltration; this will permit reduction of the filtration fraction and will increase the "washing" effect of the blood at the blood-membrane interface (high wall shear rate). In some cases the replacement solution can be administered in the predilution mode—in such instance the final effect will be relatively higher blood flow with lower hematocrit, viscosity, and plasma protein concentration. It should be noted, however, that since solute removal is proportional to solute concentration in the plasma water entering the filter, predilution may reduce this concentration and, despite higher filtration rates, may result in a reduced amount of solute removal removed during treatment. Most commercial hemofiltration machines have the built-in capability to perform pre- or postdilution hemofiltration according to the desired treatment schedule.

Techniques and Prescription

In postdilution hemofiltration, blood is circulated in the hemofilter, and the amount of ultrafiltration taking place is determined by both the positive hydraulic pressure in the blood compartment and the negative pressure exerted by the ultrafiltration pump on the other side of the membrane. The oncotic pressure generated by plasma proteins acts against filtration. Once water has been removed by ultrafiltration, blood leaves the filter and must be reconstituted at least in part in the venous line. The replacement solution is therefore infused in amounts adequate to achieve the desired patient weight loss. With large hemofilters, the initial ultrafiltration rate is generally 170 to 180 ml/min, but ultrafiltration capacity progressively decreases during treatment down to 100 to 120 ml/min. Therefore, an average ultrafiltration rate of 140 ml/min is the rule in hemofiltration. Accordingly, since clearance is equal to ultrafiltration rate, to achieve a Kt/V (where K is dialyzer clearance, t is dialysis time, and V is solute distribution volume) of 1 in a 70-kg patient with a V value of 42 L, 42 L of ultrafiltrate must be produced during treatment, and the treatment time will be 5 hours. There has been much debate on the prescription of hemofiltration,[14,15] and it has been suggested that owing to the peculiar characteristics of the treatment, Kt/V may not be the appropriate parameter to be used. It is a common observation, in fact, that most patients can have an adequate renal replacement therapy by exchanging 30 L per session, with an average duration of 215 minutes. Despite a Kt/V lower than 1 and a total clearance volume equal to 40 percent of the body weight, in hemofiltration uremic toxins are fairly well controlled and nutrition can be adequate.[16–18]

In patients with high hematocrit or blood viscosity, hemofiltration can only be performed in the predilution mode. This method is still used in some centers in Europe, and filtration rates up to 250 ml/min can be achieved. As a consequence of the reduction of solute concentration in the plasma water, the total amount of fluid exchanged per session must be significantly increased.

Clinical Tolerance

A remarkable hemodynamic stability and a reduction of the intradialytic symptomatology with hemofiltration were described as early as 1973 by Henderson et al.[19] The method was reported to be superior to bicarbonate hemodialysis in terms of vascular stability and tolerance in response to fluid withdrawal,[20] a feature that was confirmed in short sessions with relatively rapid patient weight loss.[21] The excellent hemodynamic response seems to be related to the patient's capacity to maintain sympathetic tone, thus adapting the vascular resistances to the reduced blood volume. Adequate blood pressure values are generally maintained in the presence of significant amounts of ultrafiltration, owing to a progressive rise in plasma noradrenalin concentration and hence in peripheral vascular resistance.[18] The acid-base status is generally satisfactory in patients undergoing chronic hemofiltration, and daily acid production is adequately compensated by the buffer contained in the replacement solution. For this purpose lactate has generally been used, since calcium ions and other electrolytes must also be present in the same bag. Recently bicarbonate-containing replacement solutions have been used experimentally, but in this case calcium must be added separately or empirically mixed in a few minutes prior to the session.

Hemofiltration was the treatment supposed to prove the middle molecule hypothesis, since large amounts of such molecules are removed by convection. Although it has proved to be a reliable form of renal replacement therapy, real advantages over hemodialysis were never demonstrated. Average levels of urea and creatinine were generally higher in patients treated with hemofiltration, even though this did not result in increased uremic symptoms. Since the expected advantages for treatment of uremic neuropathy and other uremic derangements as compared with hemodialysis were not demonstrated, interest in hemofiltration has been lost over the last few years. The technique is still used in Italy, France, and Germany but only for a few patients and in a limited number of centers. Its high cost and remarkable technical complexity, together with the need for large pools of replacement solutions, are the major drawbacks of the technique. Even with on-line production of replacement solutions, hemofiltration remains complex and expensive. For these reasons other methods of using highly permeable membranes, such as hemodiafiltration and high-flux dialysis, have generated more interest. The possibility of combining diffusion and convection in these treatments has been demonstrated, and increased number of patients are now undergoing these renal replacement therapies.

HEMODIAFILTRATION

The major drawback of hemofiltration is its comparatively low efficiency in the removal of small solutes. This problem is overcome in hemodiafiltration, in which diffusion and convection are combined. This method, first proposed in 1969 by Shinaberger,[22] was practically applied only in 1977 by Leber et al.[23] and by Kunitomo et al.[24] Because of its complexity and the need for specialized equipment and replacement solutions, hemodiafiltration was almost abandoned. Recently, however, new interest in this technique has been generated by its potential for greater efficiency and the possibility of reducing dialysis treatment time.

In hemodiafiltration small solutes are effectively removed by diffusion into a dialysate by a mechanism similar to that in standard hemodialysis, but ultrafiltration, achieved by a more permeable membrane (polysulfone or polyacrylonitrile), exceeds the needed amount of fluid withdrawal. The excess ultrafiltrate is replaced with a substitution fluid, 6 to 15 L of which is infused per session depending on the specific strategy and dialysis schedule. In fact, the term *hemodiafiltration* today includes a series of treatments called diafiltration, biofiltration, high-flux hemodiafiltration, and paired filtration dialysis. These treatments are briefly described later in this chapter.

Figure 9-4 shows the clearances obtained in hemodiafiltration at various blood flows, as well as the effects of membrane surface area and the volumes of exchanged fluid. It may be noted that urea clearances are remarkably high at blood flows above 300 ml/min. This may lead to a significant reduction of dialysis treatment time while maintaining a Kt/V index greater than 1. Meanwhile the clearances of inulin, taken as a marker for larger solutes, are significantly higher than those observed in hemodialysis at comparable blood flows.[25]

Equipment

Since large amounts of fluid are exchanged in hemodiafiltration, although not as large as in hemofiltration, an accurate system for ultrafiltration control is definitely required. Hemodiafiltration is performed with manual or automatic control. In manual control the ultrafiltrate achieved with the dialyze is balanced by manual regulation of the substitution fluid infusion pump in order to achieve the final net amount of ultrafiltration and fluid balance. The patient must be placed on a bed scale. Modern dialysis machines are equipped with an ultrafiltration control system connected to the substitution fluid infusion pump. It is sufficient to preset the treatment duration and

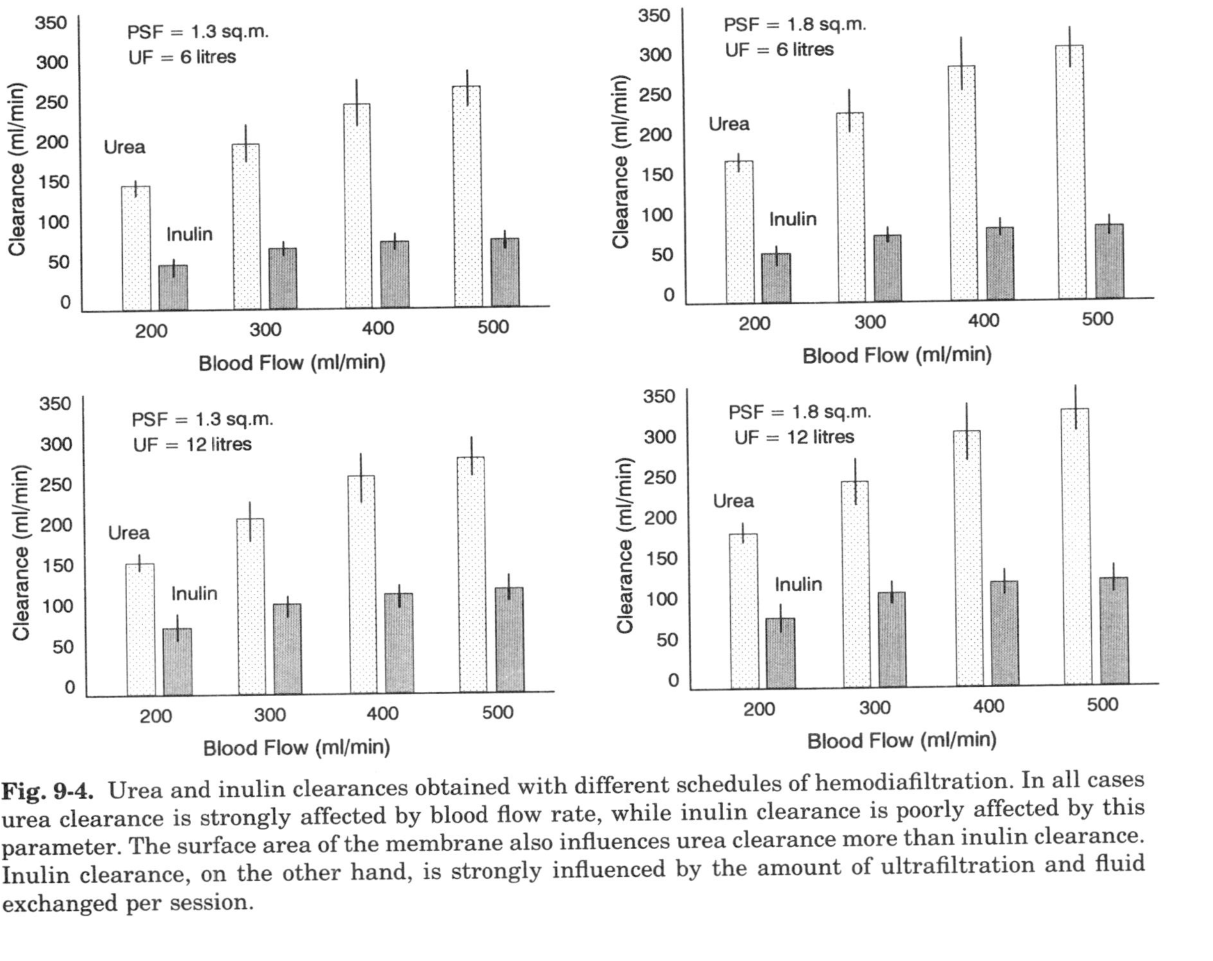

Fig. 9-4. Urea and inulin clearances obtained with different schedules of hemodiafiltration. In all cases urea clearance is strongly affected by blood flow rate, while inulin clearance is poorly affected by this parameter. The surface area of the membrane also influences urea clearance more than inulin clearance. Inulin clearance, on the other hand, is strongly influenced by the amount of ultrafiltration and fluid exchanged per session.

the volume of fluid to be infused, together with the desired patient weight loss, for the machine to automatically generate the transmembrane pressure to achieve the necessary ultrafiltration rate. The system is connected for safety to the blood module and ultrafiltration stops in case of sudden decreases in blood flow.

Systems for the on-line preparation of the replacement solution from fresh dialysate, such as that depicted in Figure 9-5, are today being used experimentally in order to reduce the cost and the complexity of the treatment. In this case the ultrafiltration control system operates as a dialysate flow equalizer and an auxiliary pump. Part of the fresh dialysate is withdrawn from the inlet line, filtered through a small polysulfone filter, and then infused into the venous line to compensate for the excess ultrafiltration volume achieved in the filter. A small pump extracts the net amount of ultrafiltrate corresponding to the patient's prescribed fluid loss.

Dialysate and Substitution Fluid Composition

The high mass transport and clearance values obtained in hemodiafiltration render the use of bicarbonate in the dialysate mandatory. With such high clearances, in fact, the mass transfer of acetate would exceed the metab-

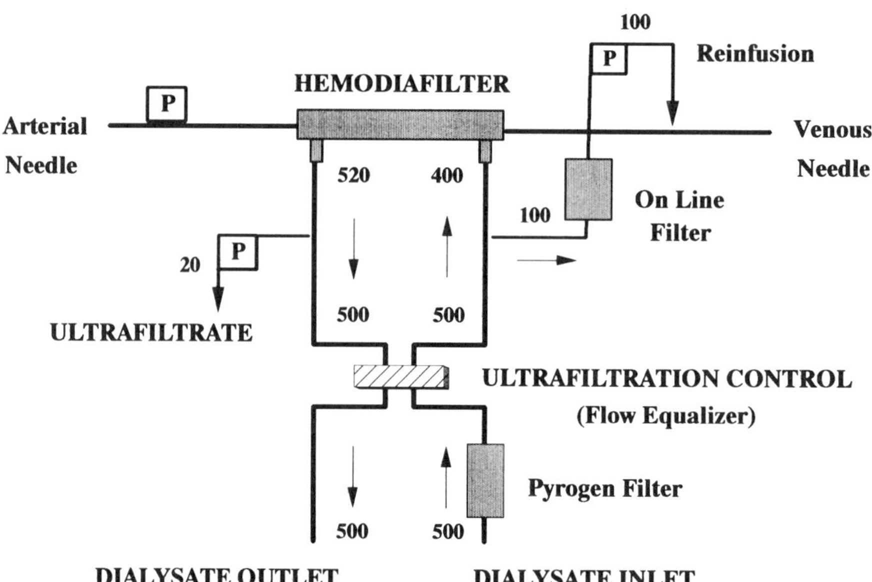

Fig. 9-5. Schematic representation of hemodiafiltration with on-line preparation of the reinfusion fluid. As the ultrafiltration controller acts as a flow equalizer, the amount of fresh dialysate withdrawn from the inlet line, filtered, and reinfused into the venous line must be replaced in the dialysate circuit by an equal amount of ultrafiltrate from the dialyzer. Net ultrafiltration is regulated by a small pump placed in the dialysate outlet line. The numbers in the figure represent a typical condition. A small polysulfone filter is generally used to filter the fresh dialysate and increase its quality.

olizing capacity (3 mmol/min) and would result in a series of side effects, including hypoxia, hypotension, depression of myocardiac contractility, and worsening acidosis. Furthermore, the different schedules of hemodiafiltration may require a wide variation in the sodium concentration of the dialysate. The commonly used dialysate sodium concentration is 138 mmol/L, even though variations over the range of 135 to 145 mmol/L have been reported.[26,27]

The quantity of replacement solution varies from 6 to 15 L per session. The fluid generally contains lactate (40 to 42 mmol/L) as a buffer so that calcium and magnesium can be added as well. However, in some cases calcium-free and bicarbonate-containing replacement solutions are used. In these circumstances the calcium concentration in the dialysate must be increased in order to avoid negative balances of this cation. However, the same result can be obtained by prescribing adequate oral calcium supplementation.

The sodium concentration of the substitution fluid varies typically between 138 and 145 mmol/L, and specific concentrations can be chosen according to the patient's clinical requirements.

Techniques

Classic Hemodiafiltration

As proposed by Leber et al.,[23] the original hemodiafiltration technique used acetate dialysate and lactate substitution fluid, lasted 180 minutes and exchanged 9 to 12 L of ultrafiltrate per session. The various current techniques of hemodiafiltration have some common aspects, which can be summarized as follows:

1. Blood flow is greater than 300 ml/min and generally ranges between 300 and 500 ml/min. A blood flow of 350 ml/min represents a good compromise and can be used in most patients.
2. Dialysate flow is between 500 and 800 ml/min with bicarbonate dialysate. Although most modern machines can accurately deliver dialysate flows of 800 ml/min, most treatments are still carried out at a dialysate flow of 500 ml/min.
3. The membranes used are polysulfone, polyacrylonitrile, polyamide, polymethylmethacrylate, cellulose acetate, or cellulose triacetate, with a surface area ranging between 1.3 and 1.8 m^2.
4. The average treatment time is between 180 and 210 minutes, even though treatment time must be individualized to achieve an adequate result for the particular patient.

Some other techniques of hemodiafiltration have recently been proposed, but their use is mostly confined to Europe.

Paired Filtration Dialysis (Two-Chamber Hemodiafiltration)

Paired filtration dialysis is a form of hemodiafiltration carried out with a special filter, in which a small hemofilter and a dialyzer are combined in series. Ultrafiltration and convection take place in the hemofilter, and substitution fluid is reinfused between the two units. Blood is then dialyzed in the second unit. In this technique diffusion and convection take place separately, and final clearances are comparable to those of classic hemodiafiltration. The main advantage is the fact that the ultrafiltrate is continuously available for on-line biochemical measurements and monitoring.[28]

Acetate-Free Biofiltration

Acetate-free biofiltration is a special form of hemodiafiltration in which the dialysate is completely buffer-free. The entire amount of buffer, sufficient to compensate for bicarbonate losses from the dialyzer during treatment and for interdialytic acid production, is infused with the substitution fluid. The apparent advantages are better vascular stability of the patient, an individualized acid-base correction, and the absolute sterility of the dialysate.[29]

High-Flux Hemodiafiltration (Double High-Flux)

High-flux hemodiafiltration was first described in 1984 by von Albertini et al.[30] In an innovative design, two large, highly permeable dialyzers are placed in series, and the ultrafiltrate removed in the first unit is automatically replaced by backfiltration of dialysate in the second unit, thereby alleviating the need for parenteral substitution fluid. High blood flows (500 to 600 ml/min) and dialysate flows (1,000 ml/min) are used, and efficiency is more than doubled as compared with conventional treatments. Although this technique allows reduction of dialysis treatment time to less than 6 hours per week, its use remains confined to only a few dialysis centers because of the complexity of the system.

Although the high filtration rates obtained in hemodiafiltration should be sufficient to avoid untoward effects due to backfiltration of contaminated dialysate, most dialysis machines today are equipped with a system for dialysate cleaning. These systems consist of a polysulfone or polyamide filter placed in the line of dialysate inlet, just ahead of the dialyzer. This generally ensures a high quality of dialysate and reduces the risk of pyrogenic reactions during treatment. Obviously, use of these cleaning systems is strongly advised in high-flux dialysis and double high-flux hemodiafiltration, in which backfiltration of dialysate is included in the system design.

CLINICAL IMPLICATIONS

The presence of convection associated with diffusion, together with more effective correction of metabolic acidosis, may partially explain the excellent observed clinical tolerance to hemodiafiltration and derived techniques. Significant reductions in hypotensive episodes and in the frequency of intradialytic symptoms as compared with hemodialysis have been demonstrated by several authors.[27,30–34] Removal of β_2-microglobulin is definitely higher in hemodiafiltration than in hemodialysis and is directly proportional to the amount of fluid exchanged per session.[35] Improved nerve conduction velocity has also been described and has been explained on the basis of the higher permeability of the membrane used.[36] Finally, use of synthetic membranes favors lower immunostimulation of the patient, owing to the better biocompatibility of the membrane material.

The necessity for relatively high blood flows and the possible complexity of hemodiafiltration techniques may present some limitations to their widespread, routine clinical use. However, it should be noted that these treatments represent a useful alternative to more conventional techniques in cases of unstable or critical patients, and they may represent a tentative further individualization of the dialysis treatment according to the specific clinical requirements. The possibility of individualizing the amount of fluid exchanged, the composition of the replacement solution, and the treatment efficiency represents definite advantages to be considered in the final cost-benefit evaluation.

REFERENCES

1. Malinow MR, Korzon W: An experimental method for obtaining an ultrafiltrate of the blood. J Lab Clin Med 32:461, 1947
2. Henderson L, Besarb A, Michaels A, Bluembe LW: Blood purification by ultrafiltration and fluid replacement (diafiltration). Trans Am Soc Artif Int Organs 16:216, 1967
3. Quellhorst E, Plaschues E: Ultrafiltration: Elimination harnpflichtiger Substanzen mit Hilfe neuartiger Membranen. p. 216. In Ditrich P, Skabal F (eds): Aktuelle Probleme der Dialyseverfahren und der Niereninsuffizienz. Bidernagel, Friedberg, 1971
4. Quellhorst E, Schuenmann B, Doth B: Hemofiltration—a new method for the treatment of chronic renal insufficiency. p. 96. In Frost TH (ed): Technical Aspects of Renal Dialysis. Pitman Medical, Kent, England, 1978
5. Quellhorst E, Rieger J, Doht B et al: Treatment of chronic uremia by an ultrafiltration kidney: first clinical experience. Nephrol Dial Transplant 13:314, 1976
6. Mackey BB: Proceedings of the Tenth Annual Contractors Conference of the Artificial Kidney Program of the National Institute of Arthritis, Metabolism and Digestive Diseases. Dept. Health and Human Services, Publication 77-1422, 1977
7. Schaffer K, von Herrat D: Impact of hemofiltration on various metabolic and endocrine disturbances of chronic uremia. p. 211. In Henderson LW, Quellhorst CA et al (eds): Hemofiltration. Springer-Verlag, Berlin 1986
8. Henderson LW, Beans E: Successful production of sterile pyrogen-free electrolyte solution by ultrafiltration. Kidney Int 522, 1978
9. Streicher E: Transport properties in filtration and dialysis membranes. Contrib Nephrol 14:522, 1982

10. Ofsthun NJ, Colton CK, Lysaght MJ: Determination of fluid and solute removal rates during hemofiltration. p. 18. In Henderson LW, Quellhorst CA et al (eds): Hemofiltration. Springer-Verlag, Berlin 1986
11. Henderson LW: Biophysics of ultrafiltration and hemofiltration. p. 300. In Maher F (ed): Replacement of Renal Function by Dialysis. 3rd ed. Kluwer, Boston, 1989
12. Colton CK, Henderson LW, Ford CA, Lysaght MJ: Kinetics of hemodiafiltration. I. In vitro transport characteristic of a hollow-fiber blood ultrafilter. J Lab Clin Med 85:355, 1975
13. Henderson LW, Colton CK, Ford CA: Kinetics of hemodiafiltration. II. Clinical characteristics of a new blood cleasing modality. J Lab Clin Med 85:372, 1975
14. Okazaki M, Yoshida F: Ultrafiltration of blood; effect of hematocrit on ultrafiltration rate. Ann Biomed Eng 4:138, 1976
15. Bosch JP, von Albertini B, Glabman S: Prescription for hemofiltration. Contrib Nephrol 32:137, 1982
16. Canaud B, Mayr H, Garred LJ et al: Urea kinetic model for hemofiltration, abstracted. Blood Purif 1:42, 1983
17. Canaud B, Mayr H, Araujo A et al: Protein catabolic changes induced by postdilution hemofiltration, abstracted. Blood Purif 1:42, 1983
18. Minetti C, Civati G, Guastoni C et al: Minimal standard for hemofiltration. Kidney Int, Suppl. 28:S116, 1985
19. Henderson LW, Livoti LG, Ford CA et al: Clinical experience with intermittent hemodiafiltration. Trans Am Soc Artif Intern Organs 19:119, 1973
20. Baldamus CA, Pollok M: Ultrafiltration and hemofiltration: practical applications. p. 327. In Maher F (ed): Replacement of Renal Function by Dialysis. 3rd ed. Kluwer, Boston, 1989
21. Shaldon S, Beau MC, Deshodt G, Mion C: Mixed hemofiltration (MHT): 18 months experience with ultrashort treatment time. Trans Am Soc Artif Intern Organs 27:610, 1981
22. Shinaberger JH, Miller JH, Rubini ME et al: Initial clinical evaluation of diafiltration. Trans Am Soc Artif Intern Organs Vol. 25, 1969
23. Leber WW, Wizemann V, Goubeaud G et al: Simultanous hemofiltration-hemodialysis: an effective alternative to hemofiltration and conventional hemodialysis in the treatment of uremic patients. Clin Nephrol 9:115, 1978
24. Kunitomo T, Lowrie EG, Kumazawo S et al: Controlled ultrafiltration (UF) with hemodialysis: analysis of coupling between convective and diffusive mass transfer in a new HD-UF system. Trans Am Soc Artif Intern Organs 23:234, 1977
25. Ronco C, Fabris A, Chiaramonte S et al: Comparison of four different short dialysis techniques. Int J Artif Organs 3:169, 1988
26. Cambi V, Buzio C, Arisi L et al: Vascular stability and middle molecules removal in hypertonic hemodiafiltration. Proc Eur Dial Transplant Assoc 18:681, 1981
27. Teo KK, Basile C, Ulan RA et al: Effects of hemodialysis and hypertonic hemodiafiltration on cardiac function compared. Kidney Int 5:226, 1987
28. Ghezzi PM, Frigato G, Fantini GF et al: Theoretical model and first clinical results of the paired filtration dialysis (PFD). Life Support Syst 1 (suppl 1):S271, 1983
29. Santoro A, Ferrari G, Spongano M et al: Acetate free biofiltration: a viable alternative to bicarbonate dialysis. Int J Soc Artif Organs 13:476, 1989
30. Von Albertini B, Miller JH, Gardner PW, Shinaberger J: High-flux hemodiafiltration: under six hours/week treatment. Trans Am Soc Artif Intern Organs 30:227, 1984

31. Basile C, Di Maggio A, Longo S: Sodium balance in hypertonic hemodiafiltration. Blood Purif 2:70, 1984
32. Basile C, Coates JE, Ulan RA: Plasma volume changes induced by hypertonic hemodiafiltration and standard hemodialysis. Am J Nephrol 7:264, 1987
33. Wizemann V, Rawer P, Schmidt H et al: Efficiency of hemodialysis, hemofiltration and hemodiafiltration. In Shutterle, Wizemann V, Seyffart (eds): Hemodiafiltration. Hygienplan, Oberursel 1982
34. Sprenger K, Bundschuh D, Figueroa P, Franz HE: Vergleich von Hämodiafiltration gegunüber Hämodialyse mit kontinuierlicher Ultrafiltration in einer ABA-Langzeitstudie. Nieren Hochdrucker 5:226, 1981
35. Gorevic PD, Casey TT, Stone WJ et al: Beta-2 microglobulin is an amyloidogenic protein in man. J Clin Invest 76:2425, 1985
36. Basile C, Di Maggio A, Ulan RA, Scatizzi A: Hypertonic hemodiafiltration: a preliminary report on a cross-over study. Kidney Int 33 (suppl 24):S132, 1988

10

Prescribing High-Efficiency Treatments

Juan P. Bosch

NEED FOR PRESCRIPTION

Despite the accomplishment of dialysis in preventing death from uremia, complete recovery of health is not always possible. Some of the limited success achieved may be due to factors such as the age of the patient, the cause of uremia, and socioeconomic issues. It is also conceivable that failure to attain full rehabilitation may result from insufficient correction of the uremic syndrome by dialysis. Clinical judgment alone may not permit assessment as to which of these factors is the most important. We cannot modify most of the patient-related variables, but we can at least define the role of dialysis. Therefore prescription of a standardized quantity of dialysis is an important requirement in the treatment of uremic patients.

The quantity of dialysis must be stated in terms that are easily conveyed to the dialysis personnel. The role of the treatment variables, such as type of dialyzer, blood and dialysate flow rates, and treatment time must be defined to allow the procedure to be standardized independently of the equipment used in the procedure.

ADEQUACY OF THERAPY

Definition

A renal replacement therapy must provide the quantity of dialysis necessary to allow patients to reach their potential for rehabilitation, eat a reasonable diet, and maintain near normal blood pressure and it must prevent the development or progression of neuropathy.[1]

Proposed Indices for Adequate Treatment

Over the years several studies have examined the issue of dialysis prescription.

Glomerular Filtration Rate

Teschan and co-workers[2] determined through a series of elegant experiments that approximately 10 percent of the normal glomerular filtration rate (GFR) was sufficient to prevent appearance of most uremic symptoms. In their view, for example, a 70-kg man would require 18 L/d of clearance or 126 L/wk. This number, expressed in terms of a normalized dialysis dose (Kt/V corresponds to the ratio of clearance [in liters] to total body water), would represent a weekly Kt/V of 3.0—in other words, each treatment on a three times per week schedule should provide a Kt/V of 1.0.

Time-Averaged Urea Concentration

The National Cooperative Dialysis Study (NCDS) was a comprehensive study undertaken by the National Institutes of Health in 1976. The partial results were published in 1981. The investigation evaluated the effects on clinical outcome of two treatment parameters: the time-averaged concentration of urea nitrogen (TAC urea in milligrams per deciliter) and the length of each dialysis treatment (Td, in hours or minutes). Protein intake was monitored carefully using the protein catabolic rate (PCR, in grams per day) and food records. The frequency of dialysis was fixed at three times per week, and the length of dialysis was at one of two levels allowed by the study protocol. The dialyzer model for treating each patient was selected before the patient was randomly assigned to an experimental group, which could not be changed. Blood urea nitrogen (BUN) concentration was then controlled by manipulating the dialyzer clearance of urea (Kd, in milliliter per minute) to achieve the desired TAC urea over the length of dialysis specified by the protocol.[3]

In the selection of the dialyzer urea clearance, certain characteristics of the patient were considered: the volume of urea distribution (V in liters), which closely approximates body water, the residual renal clearance of urea, and the PCR.

A total of 165 patients entered the experimental phase and were randomly assigned to four groups, as shown in Figure 10-1.[4] The experimental phase was 52 weeks long. The general approach of the analysis was to determine the clinical predictors of successful therapy. Each patient was classified as being a treatment failure or a success, using only those patients who had entered one of the four therapy groups. Failure was defined in two ways: any patient who died or withdrew for medical reasons at any time during the experimental phase was designated F1; any patient who died, withdrew for medical reasons, or was hospitalized prior to 24 weeks of the experimental phase was designated F2. Vascular access hospitalization was excluded as a cause of failure. All other patients were considered treatment successes.

Analysis of the results demonstrated that the probability of a patient suffering morbid events is strongly associated both with baseline attributes

		Group I	**Group II**	**Group III**	**Group IV**
Dialysis Length min	Control	274	274	278	275
	Exp.	271	268	200	190
TAC urea mg/dl	Control	52.0	51.4	50.8	52.0
	Exp.	51.1	87.8	54.7	93.6
Mid week BUN mg/dl	Control	74	75	72	75
	Exp.	76	108	77	115
Dialyzer Urea Clearance ml/min	Control	158	161	162	165
	Exp.	171	77	206	107

Fig. 10-1. Mean values in the different treatment groups in the National Cooperative Dialysis Study. (From Parker et al.,[4] with permission.)

of the patient (age, sex, etc.) and with the dialysis prescription. Hospitalizations during the control phase had significant predictive power, particularly for F2 patients. TAC urea and PCR estimates were the most powerful predictors of failure. The length of dialysis had also a significant impact on the probability of F2 failure, although this was small compared with TAC urea, PCR, and hospitalization during the control phase. Dialysis length had no impact on the F1 group.

The NDCS clearly established the importance of both the quantity of dialysis and protein intake in determining outcome. Patients in group I and III received 46 and 41 L of urea clearance per treatment, respectively. These groups were associated with good outcome. Patients in groups II and IV received 20.6 and 20.3 L, respectively, of urea clearance per treatment. These groups were associated with poor outcome. The study also proposed a systematic method for prescribing hemodialysis around a target BUN and an assumed protein intake of at least 1 g/kg/d (Fig. 10-2).

The study has been praised and criticized. Certainly it is the only large-scale clinical hemodialysis trial, and it is a valuable reference source. The main objection has been the use of BUN as a target for the treatment. Recent studies have suggested that protein intake is related to the quantity of dialysis.[5] If this is the case, it is unlikely that a target TAC urea can be reached if the amount of treatment is not also adjusted.

Quantity of Dialysis (Kt/V Value)

In 1985 Gotch and Sargent re-analyzed the NCDS data.[6] They suggested that patients with a PCR below 0.80 have a poor outcome and would not benefit from increased dialysis. Their analysis indicated that patients with a PCR below 0.80 received a greatly reduced quantity of dialysis (Kt/V <0.70); with these low Kt/V levels, there is a high probability of failure at all levels of PCR. When the probabilities of failure (*P*F1 and *P*F2) were analyzed as functions of Kt/V, it was found that there was a persistently high *P*F2 at Kt/V values of 0.4 to 0.8, which dropped to low levels when Kt/V values exceeded 0.9 (0.9 to 1.5). A step function relating morbidity to normalized treatment was suggested. These authors concluded that a fully adequate dialysis prescription is provided with a PCR of 1.0 and a Kt/V of 1.0. To prescribe higher levels of protein intake and Kt/V would be of no apparent clinical value with the cellulosic dialyzers in current use on a three times per week treatment schedule.

Keshaviah and Collins also reanalyzed the NCDS data and suggested that there was a continuous distribution between Kt/V and the probability of failure.[7] These authors suggested that the probability of failure is negligible at a Kt/V of 1.3.

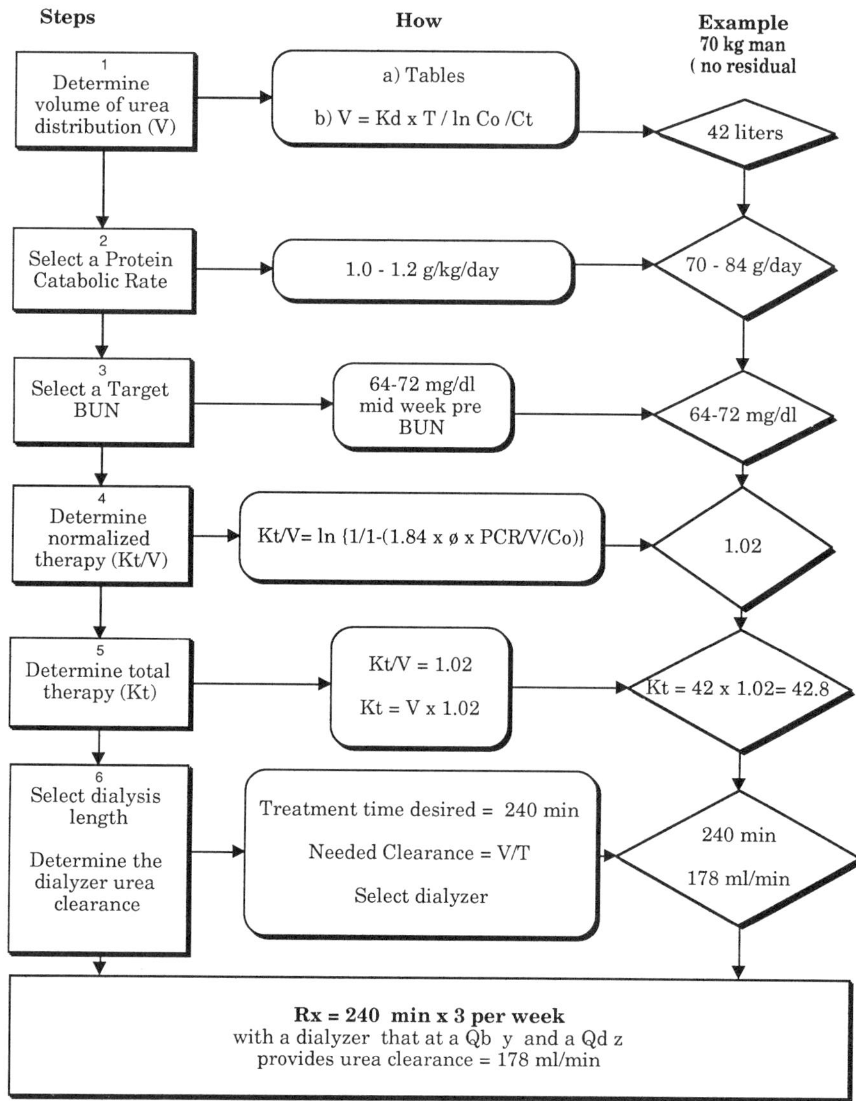

Fig. 10-2. Dialysis prescription as suggested by the National Cooperative Dialysis Study. V, total body water or urea space; Co, concentration at the end of the treatment; Ct, initial concentration; Kd, dialyzer clearance; ϕ, time interval between dialysis; PCR, protein catabolic rate. Concentrations and clearance refer to urea nitrogen. (From Lowrie et al.,[3] with permission.)

NUTRITIONAL PRESCRIPTION

It has been traditional to prescribe a protein intake of 1.0 to 1.2 g/kg/day to patients on maintenance dialysis. The NCDS showed the importance of PCR to the outcome and Gotch and Sargent have also recommended a PCR of 1.0 g/kg/day as needed to achieve a healthful outcome. In these studies protein intake was examined independently of the quantity of treatment administered. The relationship between renal function and dietary protein intake has been under close scrutiny because of the possible impact of diet on the progression of renal disease. It is now evident that these two variables are related.

1. In normal subjects, renal function as measured by 24 hour creatinine clearance was found by Lew and Bosch to be significantly related to protein intake.[5] The greater the protein intake, the higher the creatinine clearance observed. Conversely, the lower the protein intake, the lower the level of renal function. These authors suggested that GFR is not a fixed function but in normal subjects it is highly variable and dependent on dietary habits.
2. In patients with renal disease it is also possible to demonstrate a relationship between dietary protein intake and GFR. At low GFR (<15 ml/min) the relationship is also significant but has a steeper slope, suggesting a lower protein intake per level of GFR. This observation is supported by the clinical observation that patients with chronic renal failure and low GFR will develop malnutrition if dialysis is delayed.
3. There is considerable evidence to suggest that in dialysis patients PCR is dependent upon the amount of therapy (i.e., on Kt/V). This relationship has been demonstrated in hemodialysis patients[8] as well as in peritoneal dialysis patients.[9]

One of the functions of the kidney is to eliminate protein waste. The higher the dietary protein, the greater the GFR required. In patients with renal disease the relationship between protein intake and renal function is also apparent, but owing to the renal parenchymal injury, the internal environment is not preserved and plasma concentrations of BUN and other toxins are increased. There is a point, at a GFR of approximately 15 ml/min, at which appetite is markedly influenced by the uremic state and protein intake diminishes significantly. Intake will only be restored if renal function increases or is replaced by dialysis. Those treating dialysis patients should place emphasis on the quantity of therapy received by the patient rather than only on compliance with a dietary prescription.

In the follow-up of dialysis patients two easily measured parameters give powerful insight into their nutritional status, namely, albumin concentration and predialysis BUN. Low albumin levels are powerful predictors of poor outcome, and patients with such low levels should be examined carefully to detect causes of malnutrition. Delivery of prescribed dialysis must also be checked carefully. Low predialysis BUN (<40 mg/dl in patients with no residual kidney function) also is associated with poor outcome and should suggest a careful assessment of both quantity of dialysis delivered and protein intake.

DIALYSIS PRESCRIPTION

Goals of Therapy

The goals of hemodialysis therapy are (1) to remove during the treatment a certain quantity of uremic solutes so that the patient's plasma levels remain within acceptable minimal ranges; (2) to correct electrolyte imbalance, bone metabolism, and acid-base derrangements; and (3) to remove the interdialytic weight gain with the least morbidity for the patient. From the literature cited above it would appear that "adequate dialysis" is achieved if the total volume of urea clearance per treatment approximates the urea distribution space in patients who are receiving therapy three times per week and who have negligible residual renal function. This state is characterized by a Kt/V index of about 1, K being the average dialyzer urea clearance in milliliters per minute, t the treatment time in minutes, and V the distribution space or total body water. Dialysis prescribed on the basis of this index provides midweek pretreatment plasma urea nitrogen levels below 90 mg/dl in patients with adequate dietary protein intake. For a normal-size person (i.e., 70 kg) this requires about 42 L of total urea clearance or 126 L/week. This quantity represents approximately 10 percent of the normal glomerular filtrate volume for the same period. The total quantity of solutes removed at a Kt/V of 1 is approximately 60 to 65 percent of the predialysis urea nitrogen[7]

$$Kt/V = \ln \left(\frac{1/(1 - [BUN]_{post}}{[BUN]_{pre}} \right) \tag{1}$$

Figure 10-3 shows the relationship between urea reduction ratio (URR) and Kt/V. We have elected to depict this relationship as a curvilinear function; however, others have use a linear regression analysis to describe this relationship.[10] In both cases the fit is reasonably good and is useful in clinical practice.

$$URR\,\% = \left(\frac{1 - [BUN]_{post}}{[BUN]_{pre}} \right) \times 100 \tag{2}$$

The quantity of urea removed during dialysis is the product of the dialyzer clearance and the treatment time (Kt). To remove 60 to 65 percent of the predialysis urea in a given patient, a dialyzer with a low urea clearance will require a longer treatment time than a dialyzer with a high urea clearance. In this sense the dialysis prescription is independent of time.

In the NCDS short dialysis time was marginally associated with a high probability of failure, which suggests that time in itself is a factor in the outcome of dialysis therapy. The impact of treatment time on the outcome in the NCDS is clouded by the fact that in both "short" treatment groups (II

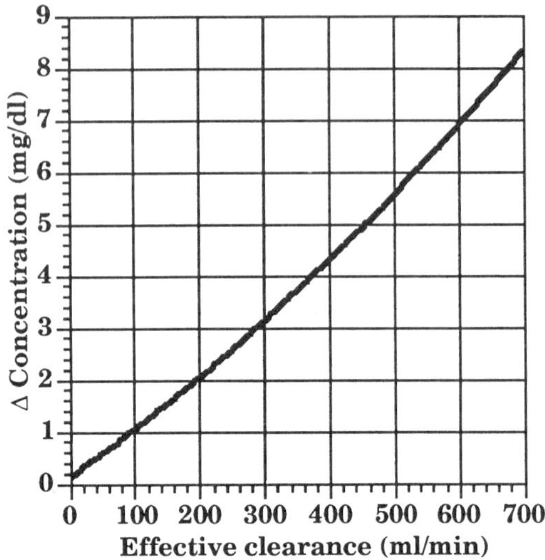

Fig. 10-3. Effect of effective clearance on urea gradient between a central and a peripheral compartment. Δ concentration refers to the difference between BUN in the peripheral compartment and in the central compartment, assuming a double pool model for urea distribution in high-efficiency treatments. (From Abramson et al.,[15] with permission.)

and IV), the total amount of therapy averaged a Kt/V of only 0.5 to 0.6. Lowrie and Lew compared a model based on the urea reduction rate as a predictor of outcome with the model used in the NCDS.[11] Patient outcome was found to be well predicted by the URR, which suggests the time independence of the dialysis prescription.

The statement that long and less efficient treatments are comparable with short and efficient treatments[12] appears to be justified by the evidence available. In high-efficiency treatments urea removal must be adjusted for the reduction in volume of urea observed during the treatment or the rebound observed after the treatment.

Translation of the Prescription into Dialysis Terms

Once the individual prescription has been determined (i.e., the number of liters per treatment) it must be translated into dialysis terms—dialyzer type, blood flow, and dialysate flow. The issue of ultrafiltration during dialysis requires the definition of dry body weight, which will have to be frequently adjusted in the early stages of therapy. Residual renal function is also important, but in general we tend to overlook residual function, since it will decrease with time. The loss in renal function will have to be compensated later on if residual function is initially added to the quantity of treatment received. This is clinically difficult since patients are always reluctant to increase dialysis time. Most patients who start hemodialysis with a residual function of approximately 5 ml/min will, within 2 years of starting therapy, have no more than 1 ml/min.[13]

As an example, we may consider a 70-kg man starting hemodialysis.

1. Total amount of treatment needed equals body weight (i.e., 70 kg) multiplied by urea space (60 percent of body weight), which equals 42 L per treatment.
2. The dialyzer type, available in the clinic with a KoA (area-mass transfer coefficient product) of 500 at a blood flow rate (Qb) of 300 ml/min and a dialysate flow rate (Qd) of 1,000 ml/min has a clearance of 230 ml/min (see Ch. 13).
3. Treatment time will be $\frac{42{,}000 \text{ ml}}{230 \text{ ml/min}}$, which equals 183 minutes
4. Knowing the Koa (calculated from the known clearance at a given Qb and Qd), it is possible to predict the performance of the dialyzer at different Qb and Qd values. In this example increasing Qb to 400 ml/min will increase clearance to 250 ml/min and reduce treatment time to 168 minutes.

The dialysis prescription should then be written as:

> Patient x to be dialyzed for 3 hours and 10 minutes three times weekly. Blood flow rate should be 300 ml/min from the start of the treatment. Dialysate flow should be 1,000 ml/min. Ultrafiltration should not exceed y.

All the other elements of the dialysis prescription should also be defined, namely, calcium, potassium, sodium, and bicarbonate concentration in the dialysate bath.

Delivered versus Prescription Therapy

The next step after prescribing a "dose" of dialysis is to assess whether the patient actually received the quantity of treatment assigned. The prescription of the treatment is calculated to provide a Kt/V of 1.0. Whether this amount of therapy was actually delivered to the patient can be determined readily by assessing the URR, the urea kinetics, or other indices. My colleagues and I have chosen to use URR as the primary indicator to monitor delivery of the prescribed treatment. Since a Kt/V of 1.0 corresponds to a URR of 60 to 65 percent we accept that the prescription was actually delivered to the patient when this URR is demonstrated at the end of the treatment. The post-treatment value, critical in the calculation, must be obtained with the patient disconnected from the machine before removal of the needles.

The use of kinetic modeling based on a set of clinical values, pre- and postdialysis BUN, and body weight depends on the specific model used by the computer program chosen. Different programs are available; some use a variable volume in which the patient's total body water changes during the treatment, while others use a fixed urea volume; and some models require three BUN determinations, while others require only two. Urea kinetic modeling permits computation of PCR, Kt/V, and volume of urea distribution. A number of investigators have used statistical techniques to calculate Kt/V rather than standard urea kinetics.[14]

Our preference is to use URR as a tool to assess the actual treatment delivered. Despite the fact that this method neglects convective solute losses (± 8 percent of total solutes removed during treatment), it is a simple method and does not require a computer. Urea kinetics provide a value not only for Kt/V but also for PCR. This is only an apparent advantage because, as stated earlier, if adequate treatment is provided, nutritional status should also be adequate. Albumin and predialysis BUN, when examined carefully, provide as much insight into nutrition as PCR. Complicated formulas used to estimate Kt/V are an extension of the predialysis/postdialysis BUN ratio and do not provide additional information.

SPECIAL ISSUES IN HIGH-EFFICIENCY TREATMENTS

In my experience a two-compartment model better describes the behavior of urea at the high clearances used in high-efficiency dialysis.[15] The intercompartmental resistance to urea transport become clinically apparent with extracorporeal urea clearances in excess of 200 ml/min (Fig. 10-3), and the intercompartmental concentration gradient is likely to increase with increasing treatment efficiency (Fig. 10-4). Therefore, during dialysis the urea nitrogen concentration in the extracellular compartment, reflected in the plasma concentration, will be the lowest in the body. The total volume of urea clearance (Kt product) must consequently be higher in order for high-efficiency treatments to provide equivalent solute removal. The concentration gradient between a small central and a larger peripheral compartment is eliminated after the treatment. This equilibration between compartments is the so-called urea rebound, which is proportional to the gradient between compartments.

Methods that rely on the post-treatment urea nitrogen concentration such as use of the URR, to estimate Kt/V will overestimate the treatment delivered. This error will increase proportionally with the efficiency of the treatment, as is clearly demonstrated in Figures 10-4 and 10-5. In order to provide the prescribed amount of solute removal, the goals of the methods used to assess treatment actually delivered must be changed. These goals for high-efficiency treatments are tabulated in Table 10-1 and depicted in Figure 10-6.

Table 10-1. Goals for High-Efficiency Treatments

	Treatment Length		
	240 min	180 min	120 min
URR	60–65%	65–70%	70–75%
Kt/V	1.0	1.05–1.10	1.2–1.35

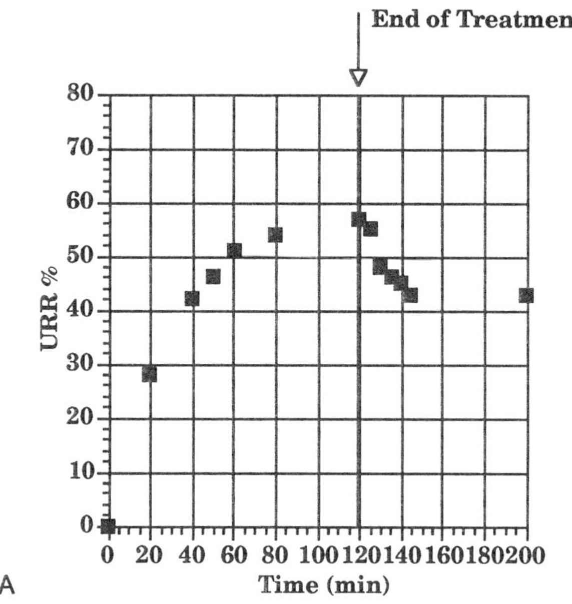

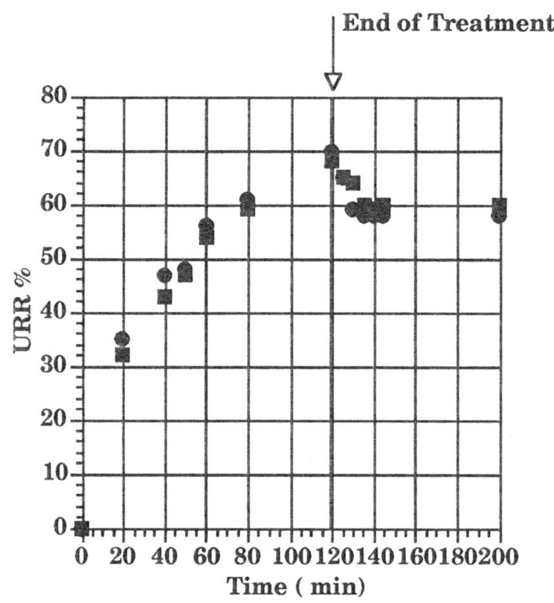

Fig. 10-4. Urea reduction ratio in high-flux hemodiafiltration (treatment time 120 minutes. Examples highlighting the importance of rebound in assessing the URR in high-efficiency treatments. (**A**) *Inadequate prescription delivered.* At the end of the treatment a URR of 58 percent was achieved; after the rebound UUR was only 41 percent. (**B**) *Adequate prescription delivered:* At the end of the treatment URR was 68 and 70 percent; after rebound, it was 59 to 60 percent, within the target range.

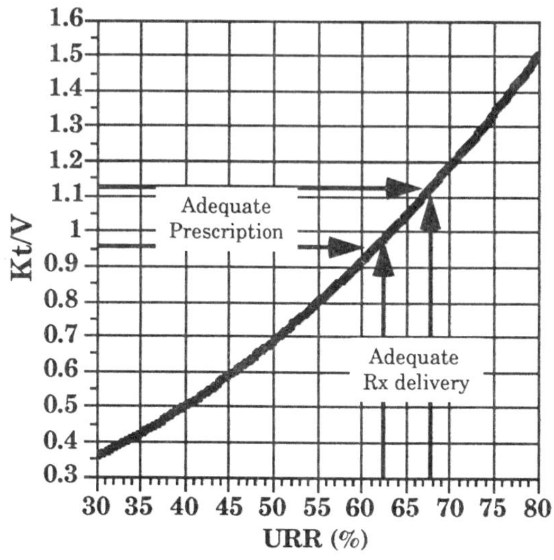

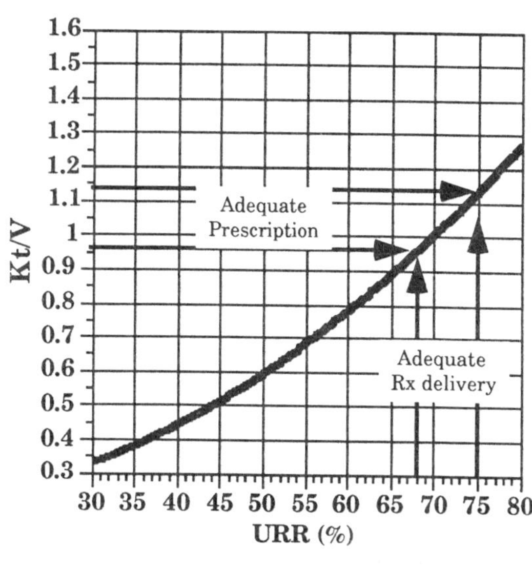

Fig. 10-5. URR targets in (**A**) conventional hemodialysis and (**B**) high-efficiency treatments. In conventional hemodialysis and high-efficiency treatments the prescription is the same, Kt/V 0.96 to 1.14. The URR targets are different because of the urea gradient generated at high urea clearances.

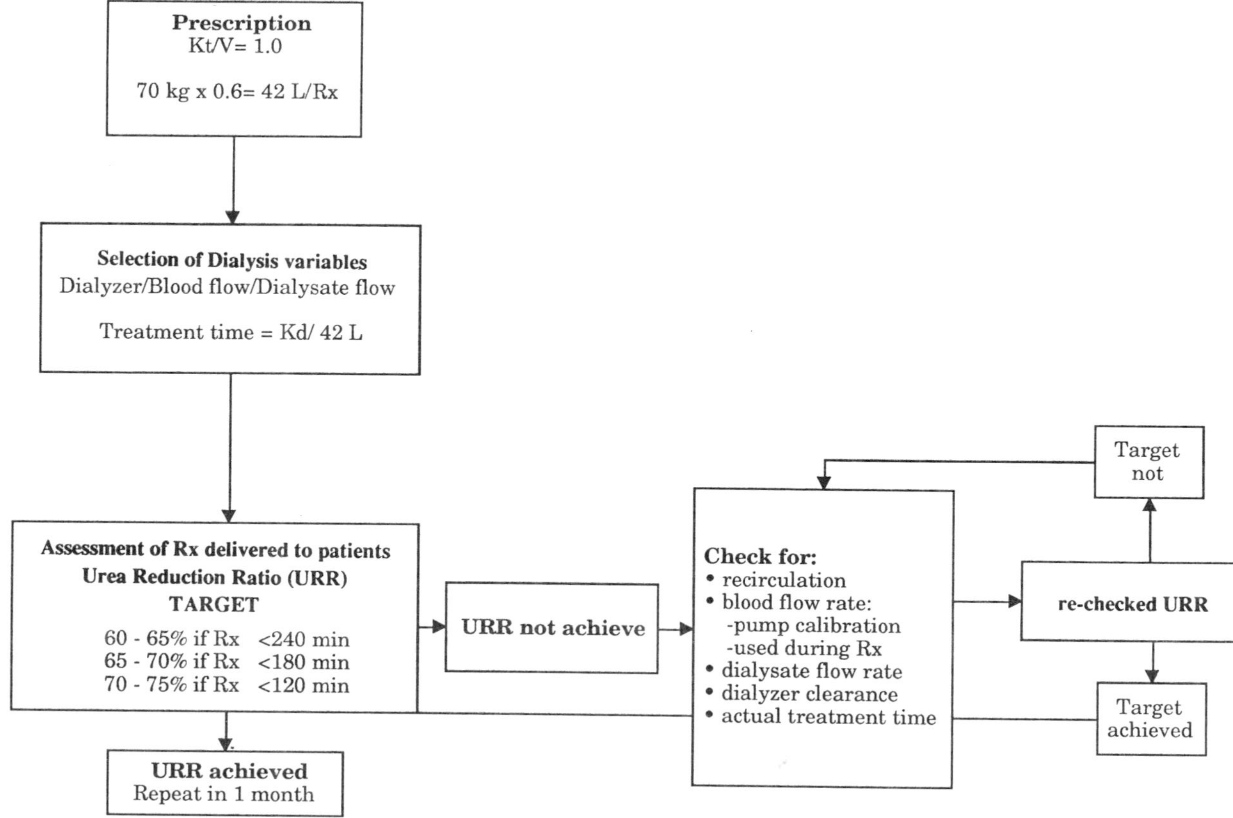

Fig. 10-6. Dialysis prescription in high-efficiency treatments.

FACTORS THAT MAY INTERFERE WITH THE ADMINISTRATION OF THE PRESCRIBED TREATMENT

A detailed discussion of problems encountered in the performance of high-efficiency treatments is included in Chapter 13. The following is a list of items to check if the target URR is not achieved during the treatment.

Factors affecting extracorporeal clearance

Extracorporeal blood flow rate: It is essential that over the entire treatment time (t) the blood flow be maintained at the level required to obtain the clearance used in the prescription (Kt). Calibration of the blood pump to deliver the flow rate shown by the blood flow indicator is also essential.

Dialysate flow rate: If dialysate flow rates in excess of 500 ml/min are used, care must be taken to ensure that the rate is constant throughout the treatment. High pressure in the dialysate path, adequate heating, degassing procedures, and adequate mixing with the concentrate are required.

Dialyzer clearance: The assumed dialyzer clearance may be less than anticipated. This is particularly important if the device is being reused.

Nursing factors

Actual treatment time may be less than time spent by the patient in the dialysis unit.

There may be a failure to prolong treatment to compensate for time lost by interruptions in blood flow or other events such as needle disconnections, bubble trap problems, or clotting of the dialyzer.

Prolonged episodes of hypotension that lead to reductions in blood flow must be compensated with extra treatment time.

Patient factors

Poor patient compliance with treatment time

Access recirculation

REFERENCES

1. DePalma JR: Adequate hemodialysis schedule. N Engl J Med 285:353, 1972
2. Teschan PE, Ginn HE, Bourne JR, Ward JW: Neurobehavioral probes for adequacy of dialysis. Trans Am Soc Artif Organs 23:556, 1977
3. Lowrie EG, Teehan BP: Principles of prescribing dialysis therapy: implementing recommendations from the National Cooperative Dialysis Study. Kidney Int 23(suppl 13):S113, 1983
4. Parker TF, Laird NM, Lowrie EG: Comparison of the study groups in the National Cooperative Dialysis Study and a description of morbidity, mortality, and patient withdrawal. Kidney Int 23(suppl 13):S42, 1983
5. Lew SQ, Bosch JP: Effect of diet on creatinine clearance and excretion in young and elderly subjects and in patients with renal disease. J Am Soc Nephrol 2:856, 1991

6. Gotch FA, Sargent JA: A mechanistic analysis of the National Cooperative Dialysis Study (NCDS). Kidney Int 28:526, 1985
7. Keshaviah P, Collins A: A re-appraisal of the National Cooperative Dialysis Study, abstracted. Kidney Int 33:227, 1988
8. Lindsay RM, Spanner E: A hypothesis: the protein catabolic rate is dependent upon the type and amount of treatment in dialyzed uremic patients. Am J Kidney Dis 13:382, 1989
9. Bergstrom J, Alvestrand A, Lindholm B, Tranaeus A: Relationship between Kt/V and protein catabolic rate (PCR) is different in continuous peritoneal dialysis (CAPD) and haemodialysis (HD) patients, abstracted. J Am Soc Nephrol 2:618, 1991
10. Daurgidas JT: The pre:post dialysis plasma urea nitrogen ratio to estimate Kt/V and NPCR: validation. Int J Artif Organs 12:420, 1989
11. Lowrie EG, Lew NL: The urea reduction rate (URR). A simple method for evaluating hemodialysis treatment. Contemp Dial Nephrol 12:11, 1991
12. Von Albertini B, Bosch JP: Short hemodialysis. Am J Nephrol 11:169, 1991
13. Lysaght MJ, Vonesh E, Gotch F et al: The influence of dialysis treatment modality on the decline of remaining renal function. ASAIO Trans 37:598, 1991
14. Ijelu G, Carrona M, Raje RM: Various methods for calculation of Kt/V: a clinical comparison. ASAIO Trans 36:364, 1990
15. Abramson F, Gibson S, Barlee V, Bosch JP: Urea kinetic modeling in hemodialysis at high urea clearance, abstracted. J Am Soc Nephrol 2:312, 1991

11

Erythropoietin and High-Efficiency Dialysis

Atef Wadie B. Morcos
Allen R. Nissenson

INTRODUCTION

The availability of recombinant human erythropoietin (r-HuEPO) as a treatment for the anemia of end-stage renal disease (ESRD) has led to a remarkable improvement in the quality of life of patients undergoing dialysis.[1,2] The enhancement of tissue oxygenation that occurs when anemia is corrected ameliorates many of the symptoms previously believed to be due to uremic toxins and inadequate dialysis.[3] Objective improvements in exercise performance, cardiovascular function, and brain electrophysiology have all been documented.[4–6]

Adequate dialysis is necessary to provide a healthy environment for red blood cell function and survival,[7,8] anemia generally being worse when dialysis is poor. This may in part be related to insufficient removal of high molecular weight inhibitors of erythropoietin (EPO) action on the bone marrow.[9–11] These substances are better removed by the more permeable peritoneal membrane, thus accounting for the higher hematocrit seen with peritoneal dialysis.[12] Newer hemodialysis techniques including high-efficiency and high-flux dialysis, which provide a high rate of solute and fluid removal, usually with a short treatment time, may also result in higher hematocrits[13] or in the need for lower r-HuEPO doses in part because of their solute clearance profiles.[14] However, hematocrits consistently above 30 percent, the generally used lower acceptable limit, are rarely achieved. Thus, even with high-efficiency dialysis, r-HuEPO will be needed for many patients.

Concern has been raised over the possible adverse impact of hematocrit elevation on high-efficiency dialysis. This includes effects on solute clearance and thus on dialysis adequacy, as well as on the physical characteristics of the dialyzer, including the possibility of backfiltration of dialysate into the bloodstream and consequent pyrogenic reactions, especially with the use of bicarbonate-containing dialysate as required for high-efficiency dialysis.[15]

Opinions based on theoretical analyses or small clinical studies are divided regarding the possible impact of higher hematocrits on high-efficiency dialysis, with some investigators supporting and others disagreeing with some or all of these concerns. Not only are there a variety of opinions and data among investigative groups, but differences have emerged between theoretical analyses and clinical data. Differences in methodology, including differences in the type of dialyzer used and in the mathematical and technical estimation of solute clearance, may in part explain these discrepancies. Much more in vitro and in vivo research, using well-designed and validated techniques, will be needed to clarify these important issues and therefore to avoid catastrophic problems in the future, particularly as the use of both r-HuEPO and high-efficiency dialysis increases.

IMPACT OF HEMATOCRIT ON DIALYZER SOLUTE CLEARANCE: THEORETICAL ANALYSIS

The mass transfer performance of any dialyzer may be viewed as the volumetric rate (volume per minute) at which whole blood is completely cleared of a solute. Mass transfer across a membrane is determined by the driving forces relative to the resistances to transfer:

$$\text{Mass transfer per unit area} = \frac{\text{driving forces}}{\text{resistances to transfer}} \tag{1}$$

A mathematical formula that describes mass transfer rate (MTR) at any point N of a dialyzer is

$$\mathrm{MTR(N)} = \frac{\mathrm{A}}{\mathrm{RO}} \Delta \mathrm{C} \tag{2}$$

where A is the membrane surface area, ΔC is the logarithmic concentration difference across the membrane, representing the mean driving force for solute transfer, and RO (in minutes per centimeter) is the overall mass transfer resistance, which is an index of the resistance encountered by a solute in moving from the center of the bloodstream to the center of the dialysate stream. RO is the sum of membrane-side resistance (R_m), dialysate-side resistance (R_d), and blood-side resistance (R_b):

$$\mathrm{RO} = R_m + R_d + R_b \tag{3}$$

The diffusivity of a solute across these resistances differs, an increase in hematocrit affecting only blood-side resistance.

Membrane-Side Resistance

Transfer of solute across a membrane is predominantly by diffusion and dependent on the concentration difference between the blood and the dialysate stream. Estimation of mass transfer resistance (R_m) for a particular membrane and solute requires knowledge about the effective diffusion coefficient of the solute through this membrane. This is proportional to the diffusivity of the solute in water as shown in equation 4

$$R_m = \frac{\Delta \mathrm{xm}}{\mathrm{Dm}} \tag{4}$$

where Δxm represents the wet membrane thickness (in centimeters), and Dm is the effective diffusion coefficient of a solute through the membrane. Hematocrit change has no influence on membrane resistance, which may, however, be decreased by making the membrane thinner, with larger pores, as in high-efficiency dialyzers.

Dialysate-Side Resistance

Hematocrit rise does not affect dialysate-side resistance, since the diffusivity of a solute in the dialysate is proportional to its diffusivity in water. This resistance can be expressed as

$$R_d = \frac{\Delta xd}{Dd} \tag{5}$$

where Δxd represents the thickness of the dialysate film and Dd is the diffusivity of a solute through the dialysate. Dialysate-side resistance can be minimized by making the dialysate fluid channels small and enhancing turbulence within the dialysate stream.

Blood-side Resistance

Diffusivity of a solute in blood is greatly dependent on the composition of the blood. The higher the red blood cell mass, the greater the resistance to solute transfer. Solute diffusion in plasma is not equal to that in water, higher values being seen with the latter. Estimation of blood-side resistance for a solute therefore requires consideration of the hematocrit value. According to the work of Zydney and Colton[16] on solute transport in concentrated suspensions, diffusivity of a solute in plasma is related to the hematocrit (Hct) as indicated by the equation

$$Db_{eff}(Hct) = DbHct \times K + D\ RBC\ (1 - Hct) \tag{6}$$

Here $Db_{eff}(Hct)$ is the effective diffusion coefficient of a solute in the blood as a function of hematocrit, D RBC is the diffusion coefficient in the red blood cell, and K is the overall solute equilibrium distribution coefficient calculated from the value of the hematocrit by the equation

$$K = 1 - Hct + Hct \times K_{eq} \tag{7}$$

where K_{eq} represents the solute equilibrium coefficient between red blood cell and plasma. K is found to be nearly unity for urea, 0.731 for creatinine, 0.5 for phosphorus, and zero for potassium. D RBC in equation 6 can be approximated from

$$D\ RBC = 0.03 \times a^2 \times y \tag{8}$$

where a is the red cell radius and y is the local shear rate. Blood-side resistance can then be estimated based on the blood film thickness (Δxb) and the effective diffusion coefficient of a solute in the blood at any hematocrit value [$Db_{eff}(Hct)$]:

$$R_b = \frac{\Delta xb}{Db_{eff}(Hct)} \tag{9}$$

From equation 9 it can be seen that R_b increases as $Db_{eff}(Hct)$ decreases with rising hematocrit. Consequently, the overall mass transfer resistance RO will increase as R_b increases (see equation 3), with a resultant decrease in the rate of solute mass transfer (equation 2). The theoretical effect of hematocrit on the blood diffusion coefficient, mass transfer resistance, and clearance for urea predicts that diffusion of urea will be reduced in whole blood relative to plasma.[17] Figure 11-1A represents this relationship, showing a 33 percent decrease in effective diffusion coefficient as hematocrit rises from 20 to 40 percent. This decrement in diffusion coefficient increases blood-side resistance by 50 percent (Fig. 11-1B) and has an impact on the overall resistance to solute transfer but not on membrane resistance or dialysate resistance, since these are independent of hematocrit. Figure 11-1C shows the whole blood urea clearance calculated from the overall resistance. In spite of the decrement in the latter, clearance is reduced only by 5 percent when hematocrit is increased from 20 to 40 percent; this is because of the nearly instantaneous and complete equilibrium of urea between red blood cells and plasma.[18,19] This minor decrease in clearance can be compensated by a slight increase in total blood flow through the dialyzer or in dialysis time or by use of a dialyzer with a higher permeability-surface area coefficient (KoA).[20] For solutes that have a slow red blood cell-plasma equilibrium, increasing blood flow alone will be effective only if a high-efficiency dialyzer is used because of the relation between dialyzer solute clearance, blood flow, and dialyzer KoA.[15]

Experimental models are in agreement with these theoretical results over the range of hematocrits tested, and in vivo studies by Schmidt and Ward[17] showed only a minor effect of hematocrit on urea clearance after EPO therapy. Similar results have been obtained by other groups,[21,22] who also were unable to find any influence of hematocrit on urea clearance either in vivo or in vitro.

Quantification of Dialyzer Solute Clearance

The mass transfer rate of a dialyzer can be estimated quantitatively from the measured solute concentrations at the blood side (Cb) and the dialysate side (Cd) by the formula

$$MTR(N) = Q_b(Cb_{in} - Cb_{out}) = Qd(Cd_{out} - Cd_{in}) \tag{10}$$

where Q_b and Q_d represent blood and dialysate flow rates, respectively. The equation considers the whole blood flow rate(Q_b) rather than the flow rate in the blood water (Q_{bw}) in which the solutes are distributed, but the latter is needed for accurate estimation of solute clearances. Solutes differ in their equilibrium distribution coefficient (K) between red blood cells and plasma. Blood water consists of a plasma water fraction (F_P) and a red cell water fraction (F_r), and the proportion of blood water flow of each can be estimated. F_p and F_r have been found to be 0.94 and 0.72 respectively.[20] The total blood water flow rate can be estimated as follows:

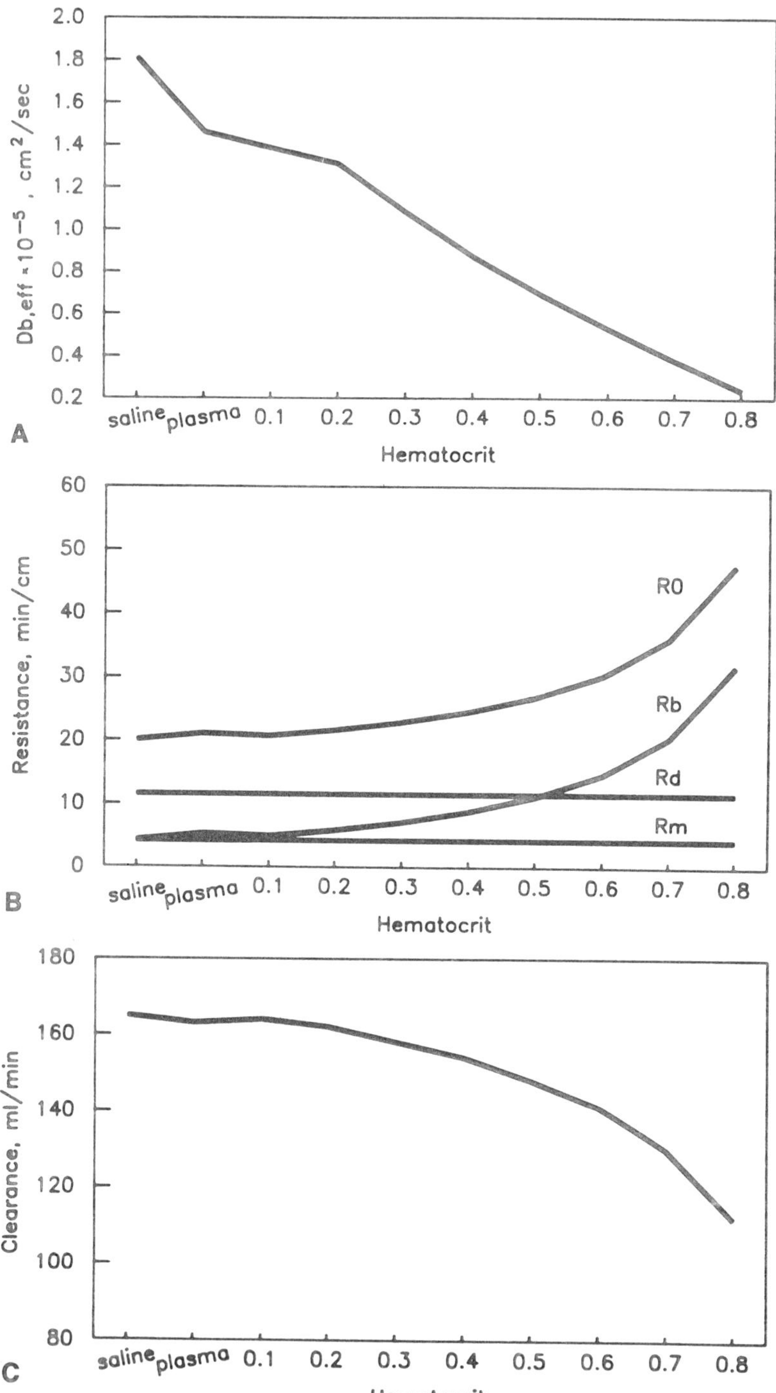

Fig. 11-1. Predicted transport parameters for urea plotted as a function of hematocrit: (**A**) whole blood diffusion coefficient (Db_{eff}); (**B**) mass transfer resistances (RO, overall resistance; R_b, blood-side resistance; R_d, dialysate side resistance; R_m, membrane resistance). (**C**) Urea clearance. (From Schmidt and Ward,[17] with permission.)

$$Q_{bw} = Q_b\{F_p - [(Hct/100) \times (F_p - F_r)]\} \tag{11}$$

Transfer of a solute out of the red blood cell should be modified by a factor of γ, which represents the fraction of red blood cell water that participates in solute transfer during a transit of the blood through the dialyzer. Equation 11 needs to be corrected for both K and γ to yield the effective blood flow rate (Q_e):

$$Q_E = Q_b[F_p - Hct/100\ (F_p - F_r K\gamma)] \tag{12}$$

Effective blood water flow can then be used instead of Qb to calculate the mass transfer rate for a dialyzer for any hematocrit value, and equation 10 can be modified to

$$MTR(N) = Q_e\ (Cb_{in} - Cb_{out}) \tag{13}$$

It can be concluded from equation 12 that effective blood flow rate and thus dialysate clearance is diminished if the hematocrit value is increased. The effect differs according to the values of γ and K for each solute. For a substance that has a K value nearly unity, such as urea, effective blood flow would decrease only slightly when hematocrit rises from 20 to 40 percent, and only a 5 percent increase in whole blood flow rate is needed to correct for effective blood water flow in this situation. Other solutes, (e.g., potassium and phosphorus salts) do not move out of red cells very rapidly or may not do so at all during transit through the dialyzer. Effective blood flow rates for these solutes may approach or equal the plasma flow rate and will be substantially reduced as the hematocrit rises. Accordingly, solute transfer calculations must be made on the basis of the effective blood flow rather than the whole blood flow, taking into account the solute's diffusivity from red blood cells to plasma (Table 11-1). This applies to high-efficiency as well as to conventional hemodialysis modalities.

Table 11–1. Solute-Specific Conversion of Whole Blood Flow to Effective Blood Water Flow[a]

Solute	k	α	Q_bH_2O
Urea	0.859	Instant	0.93 (1 − H + kH)Qb
Creatinine	0.731	4.4%/min	0.93 (1 − H + 0.02H)Qb
PO_4	0.5	Very slow	0.93 (1 − H)Qb
Inulin	0	None	0.93 (1 − H)Qb
Potassium	30	None	0.93 (1 − H)Qb

Abbreviations: k, red cell solute concentration as compared with plasma; α, rate of diffusion of solute from red blood cells to plasma; H, hematocrit expressed as a decimal fraction.

[a] Serum solid correction of 0.07 used.

(From Shinaberger et al.,[29] with permission.)

Table 11–2. Summary of Clinical Results on the Impact of Hematocrit on Dialysis Efficiency

Authors	Dialysis Modality	Hct Level (%)		Dialyzer Clearance Measurement	Changes in Dialyzer Solute Clearance				Changes in Predialysis Blood Chemistries	Kt/V
		Before EPO	After EPO		urea	Cr	K	PO_4		
Paginini et al.[23]	Conventional (n = 25)	23	34	Dialysate quant	↓ 3.7%	↓ 14%	n.c.	n.c.	↑ K, Cr and PO_4	↓
Kaupke et al.[24]	Conventional (n = 12)	22	33	Blood water	↓	↓	↓	↓	↑ urea, Cr, K	n.c.
Shinaberger et al.[29]	High-efficiency (n = 30)	20	40	Blood water	↓	↓	↑ 19.3%	↓ 10%	↑ K, PO_4	↓
Van Gleen et al.[32]	Conventional (n = 8) High-flux (n = 8)	20	28	Dialysate quant	↓	↓	↓	↓	↑ urea, Cr, K, PO_4	↓
Acchiardo et al.[34]	Conventional (n = 9) High-flux (n = 11)	19	34	Blood water	↓ 9% ↓ 7%	↓ 16% ↓ 15%	↓ 14% ↓ 15%	↓ 18% ↓ 14%	↑ urea, K, PO_4 ↑ urea, K, PO_4	↓ ↓

Acchiardo et al.[36]	High-flux (n = 20)	19	35	Blood water	↓ 9%	↓ 15%	↓ 15%	↓ 15%	↑ BUN, PO_4	↓
Collins et al[37]	High-efficiency (n = 11)	23	35	Blood water	↓	↓	↓	↓	↑ urea, Cr, K (some patients)	↓
Lim et al.[38]	High-efficiency (n = 5)	16	44	Whole blood	Minimal	↓	n.c.	n.c.		
				Blood water	↓ 5%	↓	↓ 8%	↓ 13%	↑ PO_4 only	No change
				Dialysate quant	↓	n.c	↓	↓		
Movilli et al.[46]	Conventional (n = 36)	16	46	Whole blood	↓ 5%	n.c.	n.c.	n.c.	n.c.	↓
Buur and Lundberg[49]	Conventional (n = 14)	21	34	Whole blood	↓ 5%	↓ 15%	n.c.	n.c.		
				Blood water	n.c.	n.c.	↓ 8.6%	↓ 16.5%		
				Dialysate quant	↓	↓	n.c.	n.c.		
				Dialysate side	↓	↓	n.c.	n.c.		

Abbreviation: n.c., no comment.

HEMATOCRIT AND HIGH-EFFICIENCY DIALYSIS: CLINICAL RESULTS

The impact of hematocrit rise on dialyzer solute clearance, the clinical significance of this effect for both the steady-state blood levels of these solutes, and the clinical outcomes of patients have been studied by many investigators (Table 11-2).

Reduced solute clearance due to hematocrit rise has been found by most investigators.[22–38] This has been confirmed following blood transfusion[37] as well as following administration of erythropoietin and is similar when either conventional or high-efficiency dialysis is used.[32,34,49] Most studies agree that reduction in clearance occurs when dialyzer clearance is calculated on the basis of blood water flow (see table 11-3) as opposed to whole blood clearances (for solutes other than urea). Figure 11-2 shows this effect on potassium and phosphate clearances. The same results are obtained when clearance is calculated from the dialysate side by the more accurate direct dialysate quantification method.[32,49] This effect on solute clearance occurs at the onset of dialysis[49]; this is important, since some have suggested that microclotting in the dialyzer secondary to high blood viscosity could be one possible explanation for the observed fall in dialysis efficacy. Most studies show that solute clearances are reduced by about 5 percent for urea, 10 to 15 percent for potassium and creatinine, and 15 to 18 percent for phosphorus when hematocrit is raised from 20 to 40 percent.

The clinical significance of reduced clearance on predialysis blood solute concentration is still being debated. Shinaberger et al.[29] suggest that elevation of steady-state predialysis blood levels of potassium and phosphorus occurs with higher hematocrits and that this effect is magnified when rapid dialysis is used. Predialysis hyperkalemia and hyperphosphatemia have been reported by many groups after correction of anemia with r-HuEPO.[30–32] Others, however, do not concur with these findings[33–38] despite the reported reduction in dialyzer clearances of these solutes when high-efficiency dialyzers are used. The observed rise in serum potassium and phosphorus has been debated by some authors, who attribute it to improved appetite and improved

Table 11–3. Impact of Hematocrit Rise on Measurements of Solute Clearances

		Before EPO	After EPO
Urea	K_b	149 ± 8	139 ± 9
	K_d	10 ± 12	146 ± 13
	K_c	139 ± 21	132 ± 1
Creatinine	K_b	119 ± 7	102 ± 10
	K_d	118 ± 11	101 ± 11
	K_c	103 ± 14	87 ± 11
Potassium	K_p	70 ± 10	64 ± 8
Phosphate	K_p	8 ± 9	71 ± 11

(From Buur and Lundberg,[49] with permission.)

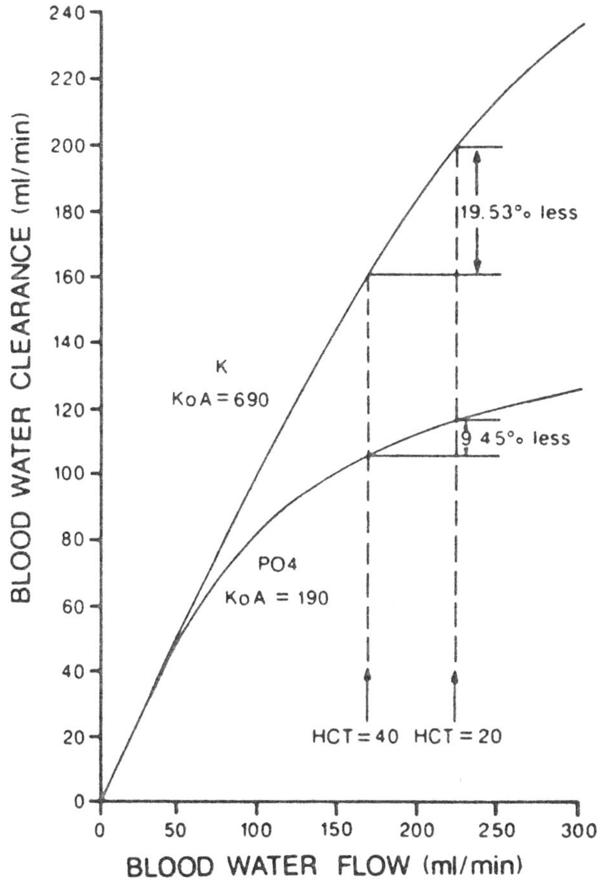

Fig. 11-2. The effect of increasing hematocrit from 20 to 40 percent on blood water flow and clearances of potassium and phosphate in high-efficiency dialysis. (From Shinaberger et al.,[29] with permission.)

dietary intake of these solutes rather than to changes in removal by dialysis.[24–28]

Gotch and Sargent[20] have shown, however, that regardless of the mechanism accounting for the rise of serum levels of these solutes, the blood levels can be controlled even with the use of high-flux dialysis and short treatment time. For phosphorus, an increase in a predialysis blood level of only 0.5 mg/dL is seen when the hematocrit is raised from 20 to 40 percent. This is because blood phosphorus level is mainly dependent on gut control of phorphorus absorption. An increase of phosphate binder dose by 3 percent can sufficiently control the serum phosphorus as hematocrit rises, as shown in Figure 11-3. For potassium, dietary intake restriction and use of low dialysate potassium can effectively control predialysis levels, but hyperkalemia may still occur in patients who are poorly compliant with potassium restriction, despite the use of a zero potassium dialysate, as shown in Figure 11-4.

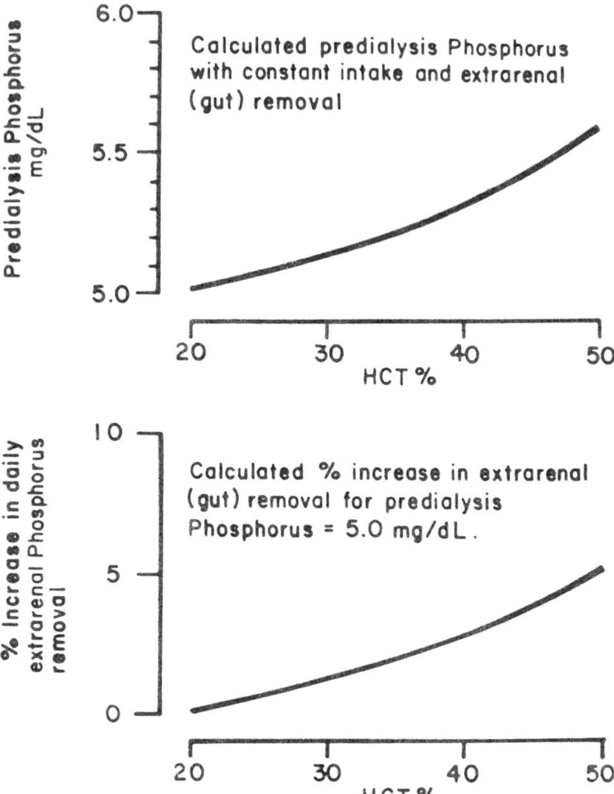

Fig. 11-3. Expected phorphorus levels and extrarenal removal requirements with increasing hematocrit. (From Sargent and Gotch,[20] with permission.)

The clinical outcomes of patients undergoing high-efficiency therapy who receive r-HuEPO suggest that changes in solute removal or predialysis blood levels are easily compensated for and of little clinical significance. Acchiardo and colleagues[34–36] and Collins et al.[37] have found no significant increase in morbidity or hospitalization before and after treatment with EPO in patients undergoing high-efficiency dialysis. Moreover, this was also the case for patients receiving EPO who were undergoing conventional dialytic therapy.

In summary, elevated hematocrit reduces solute mass transfer in general (for solutes other than urea) by reducing effective blood water flow through the dialyzer and also by interfering with solute movement within the flowing bloodstream in the dialyzer. Accurate estimation of solute clearance should be based on effective blood water flow rather than on whole blood flow. These effects on clearance have led to only minor changes in predialysis blood chemistries, although some alterations in the dialysis prescription or in

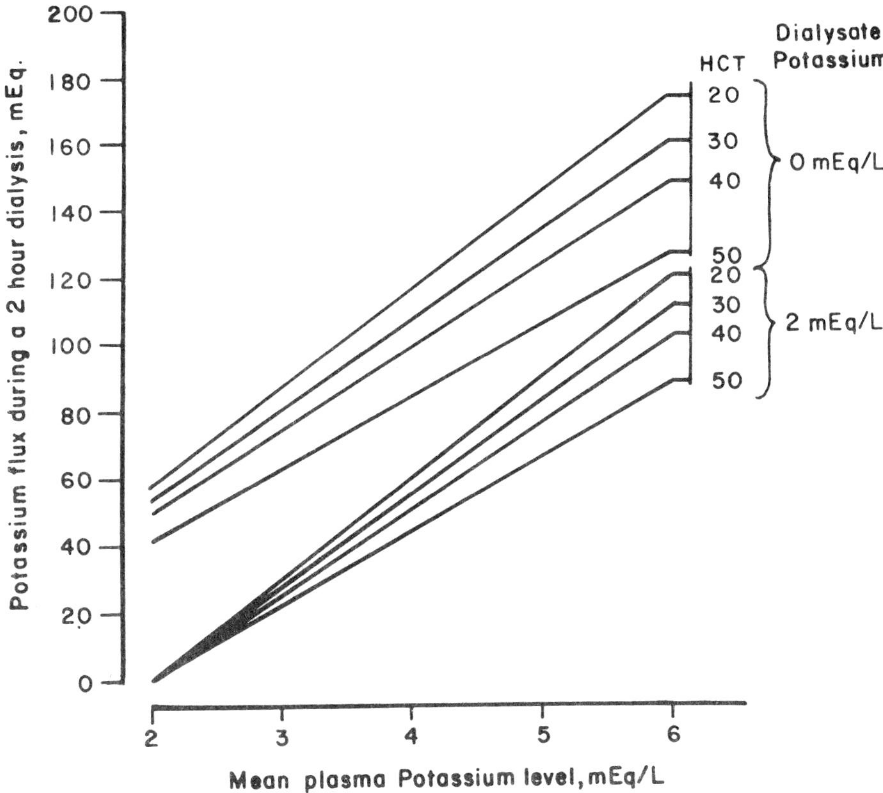

Fig. 11-4. The effect of hematocrit on potassium transport during dialysis. (From Sargent and Gotch,[20] with permission.)

medications have been required even when rapid high-efficiency therapy is used.

ERYTHROPOIETIN AND UREA KINETIC MODELNG (Kt/V) IN HIGH-EFFICIENCY DIALYSIS

Urea kinetic modeling is an effective tool for prescribing and monitoring dialysis therapy and nutritional status.[39] The mechanistic analysis by Gotch and Sargent[40] of the data from the National Cooperative Dialysis Study (NCDS) indicates that adequate dialysis will occur if the body distribution volume of urea is totally cleared in a single treatment (assuming appropriate protein intake). This can be expressed mathematically as Kt/V, where K is dialyzer urea clearance, t is treatment time, and V is urea distribution volume. When less urea is removed than that contained in the body urea

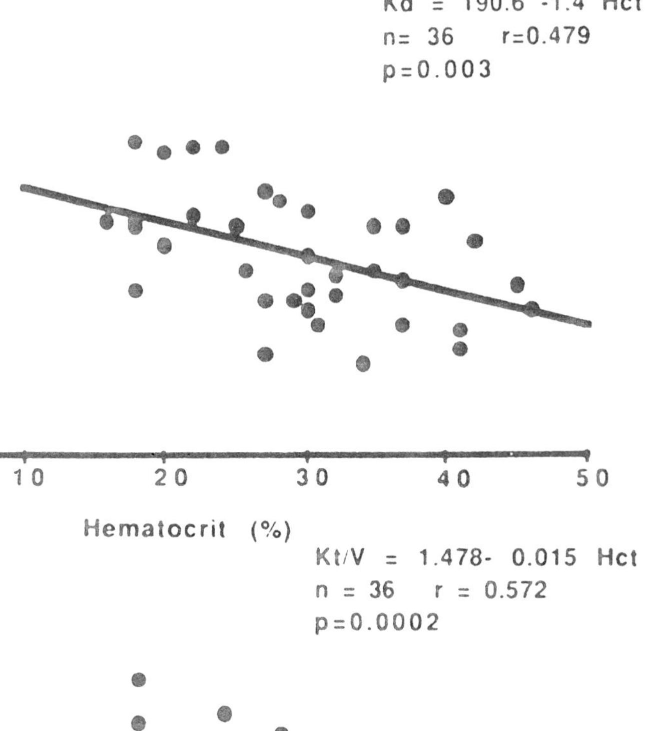

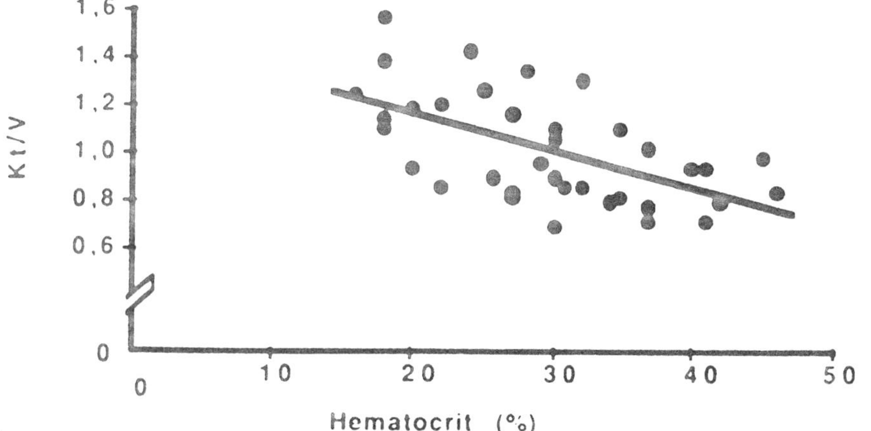

Fig. 11-5. Correlation between hematocrit and dialyzer clearance (**A**) and between hematocrit and Kt/V (**B**) during conventional dialysis. (From Movilli et al.,[46] with permission.)

space, morbidity rises. Accurate estimation of Kt/V requires measurement of dialyzer clearance and volume of urea distribution.

Questions have been raised regarding the possible impact of increased hematocrit on Kt/V measurement and thus on the adequacy of dialysis, especially with rapid high-efficiency dialysis.[29,30] The potential risks of inadequate removal of solutes of middle as well as those of small molecular size, resulting in underdialysis of patients, have been of concern as dialysis time is shortened.[29–32,41–45] The results of the NCDS mechanistic analysis are based on a particular relationship between the removal of urea (the surrogate uremic toxin) and other uremic toxins. The increase in hematocrit when EPO is given has a minimal effect on urea removal but a greater effect on the removal of other toxins. This may invalidate the urea kinetic targets established in anemic dialysis patients. This possibility requires further careful study. The fact that EPO can improve the patient's sense of well-being by correcting the anemia makes it more difficult to identify underdialyzed patients, which constitutes a real problem for the clinician.

Movilli et al.[46] have found an inverse correlation between hematocrit and dialyzer clearance (Kd) and Kt/V but no relation to the volume of urea distribution. These effects are shown in Figures 11-5 and 11-6, respectively, where the lowest Kt/V values were found in the group of patients with hematocrit above 37 percent. On the other hand, r-HuEPO has been reported to have a beneficial effect on the nutritional status in stable dialysis patients by stimulating appetite and dietary protein intake,[47,48] which may alter the kinetic parameters,[28–32] but this view is not supported by Buur and Lundberg,[49] who did not find any significant change in nutritional status after r-HuEPO administration. However, some suggest modifying the dialysis regimen to offset any potential decrease in delivered dialysis due to a higher hematocrit by increasing dialysis time or by using a higher blood flow rate or a larger dialyzer to improve dialyzer performance.[48]

Lim et al.[38] found conflicting results when clearances and Kt/V were studied. Their study showed that a rise in hematocrit did not affect urea kinetic parameters, including Kt/V and protein catabolic rate, when high-efficiency dialysis was used. Regression analysis of their results on the mass removal-to-whole blood clearance ratio versus hematocrit showed no effect on urea clearance when the hematocrit was raised from 16 to 44 percent. These results were confirmed by using the direct dialysate quantification technique. The clearance of both creatinine and phosphate was significantly reduced as hematocrit rose, however, and a 10 to 15 percent increase in dialysis prescription when hematocrit is raised to near 40 percent is recommended. The same technique of measuring dialysis adequacy was used by Van Gleen et al.[32] for both high-flux and conventional dialysis. They found that urea kinetic parameters, including Kt/V and protein catabolic rate, were decreased as hematocrit rose. It is worth noting that the range of hematocrit in this study was 20 to 30 percent and that the results of conventional and high-flux dialysis were similar.

If Kt/V is to be used to prescribe adequate dialysis, dialyzer urea clearance should be corrected for effective blood water clearance or measured directly. Furthermore, the target Kt/V values for urea should be increased as dialysis

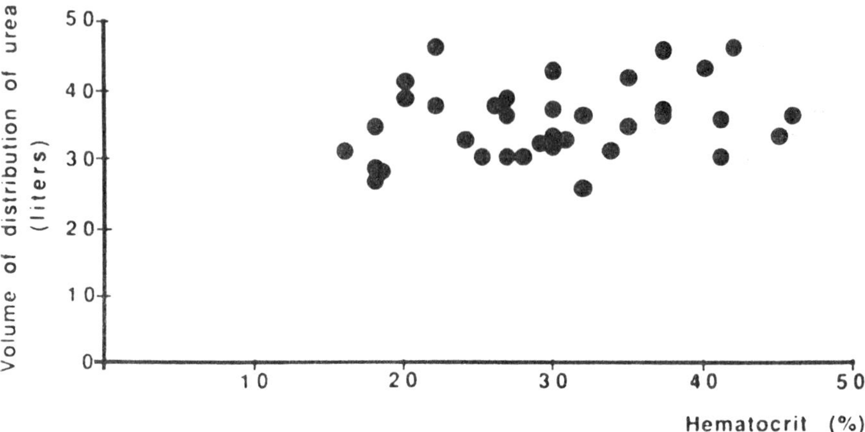

Fig. 11-6. Correlation between hematocrit and volume of distribution of urea. (From Movilli et al.,[46] with permission.)

time shortens and hematocrit rises to ensure adequate mass removal of solutes other than urea.

IMPACT OF HEMATOCRIT ON BACKFILTRATION OF THE DIALYZER WITH HIGHLY PERMEABLE MEMBRANES

Controversy continues over the effect of hematocrit on the physical characteristics of the dialyzer and dialysate delivery systems. Shinaberger et al.[29] and Stiller et al.[50] studied the forces present on the dialysate side of the membrane when highly permeable membranes are used in patients with high hematocrits. These studies showed that the operational capabilities of the dialysate delivery system can be exceeded owing to increased dialysate pressure in response to an increase in blood compartment pressure, which in turn is due to higher viscosity caused by the hematocrit and ongong ultrafiltration. This may result in imprecision of the ultrafiltration balancing system, which may exceed the alarm limits and/or may lead to backfiltration of dialysate into the blood (Fig. 11-7). When bicarbonate dialysate is used, as is required with high-efficiency dialysis, the risk of pyrogenic reactions becomes higher.[15,16] These concepts have been confirmed by Robertson and Curtin.[51]

The effect of increased hematocrit on the rate of backfiltration when a high-flux dialyzer is used is shown in Figure 11-8. The rate of backfiltration is increased from 10.1 ml/min at a hematocrit of 20 percent to 15.7 ml/min at a hematocrit of 33 percent. This means that the patient may gain "obligatory" dialysate of about 2.4 L/wk in the model used. Also, the rate of blood flow has an impact on backfiltration, which increases with higher

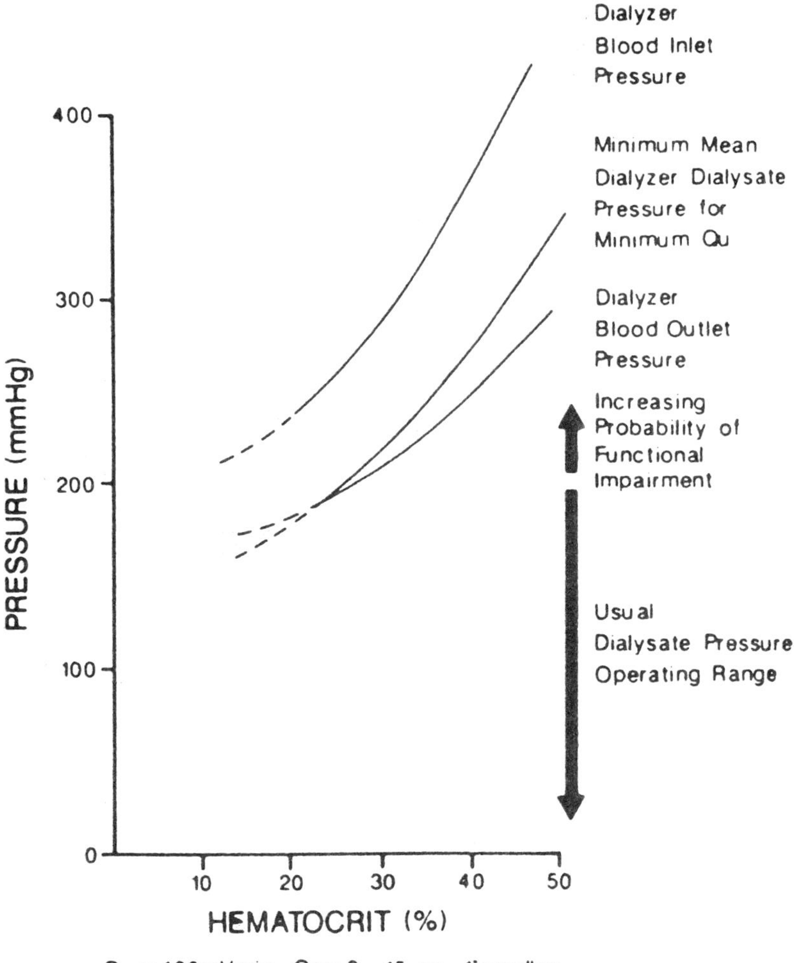

Fig. 11-7. Effect of increasing hematocrit on blood and dialysate compartment pressures. The probability of functional impairment of some dialysate delivery systems begins when dialysate pressures more than 200 mmHg above ambient are required. (From Shinaberger et al.,[29] with permission.)

hematocrit (Fig. 11-9) and is significant at the high blood flows used with high-efficiency dialysis. As ultrafiltration increases, the amount of back filtration decreases until the minimum obligatory ultrafiltration (ultrafiltration at which there is no backfiltration)[55] is reached, as shown in Figure 11-10.

A possible remedy for this problem would be to increase the inside diameter of the dialyzer fiber or to decrease the fiber length, with subsequent addition of more fibers to compensate for the decrease in surface area. The resultant shorter, wider dialyzer would abolish backfiltration due to increased hemato-

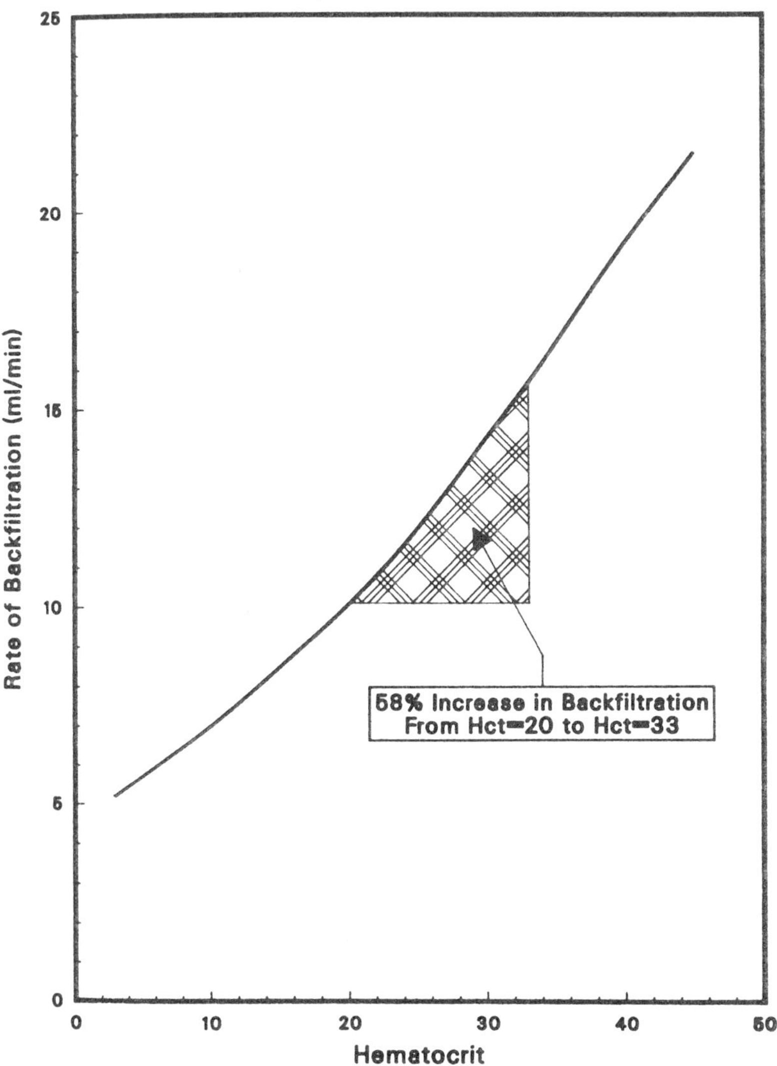

Fig. 11-8. Model predictions for the effect of hematocrit on back filtration in a typical high-flux dialyzer. (From Robertson and Curtin,[51] with permission.)

crit, but the impact of these modifications on solute clearances needs careful study.

These theoretical concerns were not confirmed in clinical practice by Lim et al.[38] when a volumetric fluid controller was used. These investigators found no pyrogenic reactions at higher hematocrits, which suggests but does not prove that backfiltration was not taking place when a dialyzer with an ultrafiltration coefficient of 15 ml/h/mmHg was used. They cautioned, however, about the possibility of backfiltration with the use of more porous, high-flux membranes.

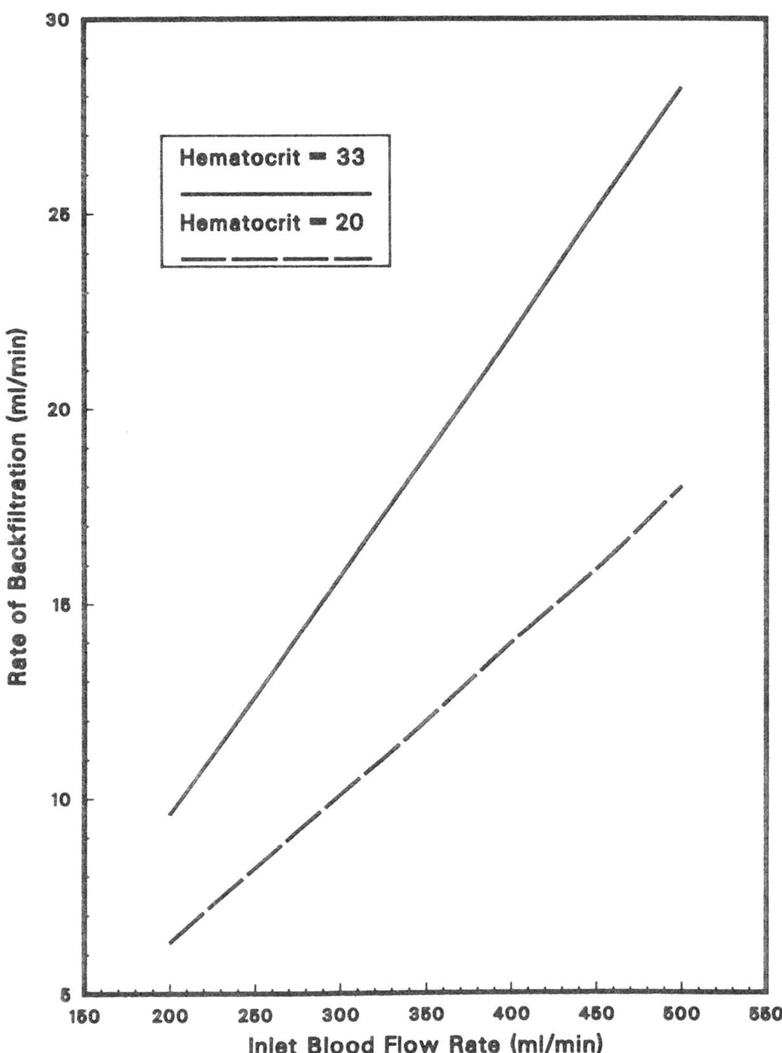

Fig. 11-9. Effect of inlet blood flow rate on back filtration under conditions of high-flux dialysis. Dashed curve is for a hematocrit of 20 percent and solid curve for a hematocrit of 33 percent. (From Robertson and Curtin,[51] with permission.)

SUMMARY AND CONCLUSIONS

In conclusion, use of EPO and the resultant increase in hematocrit may affect the process of high-efficiency dialysis if high hematocrits (>35 percent) are reached. The impact on solute clearance may be explained by the difference between solute clearance calculated according to blood water flow and that based on whole blood flow. For urea, the effect of increased hematocrit has little impact on overall mass transfer, at least at hematocrits less than

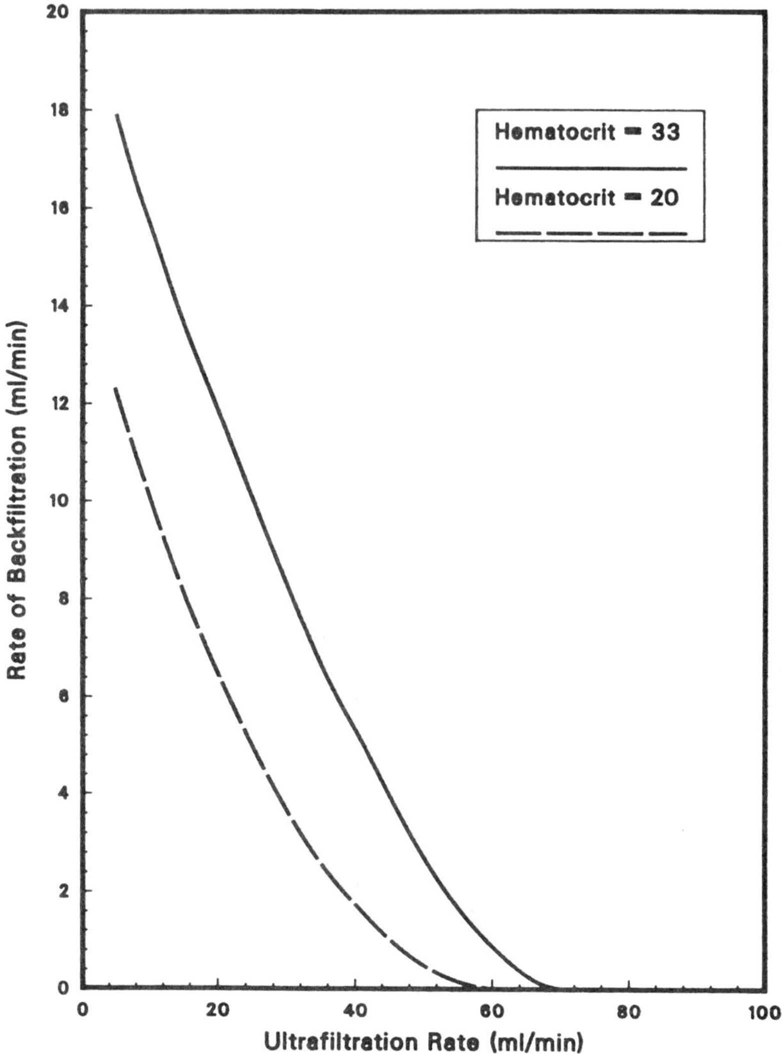

Fig. 11-10. Effect of net ultrafiltration rate (UFR) on back filtration. Minimum obligatory UFR is approximately 60 ml/min for a 20 percent hematocrit (dashed curve) and 70 ml/min for a 33 percent hematocrit (solid curve). (From Robertson and Curtin,[51] with permission.)

37 percent. For other solutes such as potassium and phosphate ions, there may be a clinically significant reduction in mass transfer, which needs to be considered. Appropriate changes in dialysate potassium or ingestion of phosphate binders may be needed to avoid predialysis hyperkalemia or hyperphosphatemia. This effect may be aggravated by the increased appetite and dietary intake seen when hematocrit rises.

Reduced clearance of other uremic toxins, including creatinine and solutes of middle molecular weight, will occur as hematocrit rises. Whether adverse clinical effects will be seen remains to be determined. The effect of hematocrit rise on solute removal occurs with conventional as well as with high-efficiency dialysis. Although clinical data are lacking, theoretical considerations would suggest that the impact will be greater with the latter than with the former. In addition, the use of urea as a surrogate for other uremic toxins and in the mathematical assessment of dialysis adequacy needs to be reexamined for patients with higher hematocrits. Finally, backfiltration is a serious concern with highly permeable membranes in high-hematocrit patients. This area requires further study, with redesign of dialyzers indicated if significant backfiltration is documented. At the present state of knowledge, it appears that high-efficiency dialysis is compatible with higher hematocrits. Close clinical observation and well-designed research studies are needed to better define and resolve any remaining problems or incompatibilities.

REFERENCES

1. Eschbach J, Adamson J: Recombinant human erythropoietin: implications for Nephrology. Am J Kidney Dis 11:203, 1988
2. Gibilaro S, Delano B, Quinn R et al: Improved quality of life while receiving erythropoietin, abstracted. Kidney Int 35:247A, 1989
3. Nonnast-Daniel B, Creutzig A, Kuhn K et al: Effects of treatment with recombinant human erythropoietin on peripheral hemodynamics and oxygenation. Contrib Nephrol 66:185, 1988
4. Nissenson A, Himer S, Wolcott D: Recombinant human erythropoietin and renal anemia: molecular biology, clinical efficacy, and nervous system effects. Ann Intern Med 114:402, 1991
5. Tzutzui M, Suzuki M, Hirasawa Y: Renewed cardiovascular dynamics induced by recombinant human erythropoietin administration. Nephrol Dial Transplant 4:146, 1989
6. Nissenson A, Marsh J, Brown W et al: rHuEPO treatment improves brain and cognitive functions of anemic dialysis patients. Kidney Int 39:155, 1991
7. Von Hartitzsch B, Carr D, Kjellstrand CM et al: Normal red cell survival in well dialyzed patients. Trans Am Soc Artif Intern Organs 19:471, 1973
8. Santiago G, Rao TK, Laird N: Effects of dialysis therapy on the hematocrit system: the National Cooperative Dialysis Study. Kidney Int (suppl 23):S95, 1983
9. Wallner SF, Vautrim RM: Evidence that inhibition of erythropoietin is important in the anemia of chronic renal failure. J Lab Clin Med 97:170, 1981
10. Eschbach JW, Adamson JW, Cook JW: Disorders of red blood cell production in uremia. Arch Intern Med 126:812, 1970
11. Nathan DG, Chess L, Hillmann DG et al: Human erythropoid-burst forming unit: T-cell requirement for proliferation in vitro. J Exp Med 14:195, 1978
12. Zappacosta A, Caro J, Erslev A: Normalization of hematocrit in patient with end stage renal disease on continuous ambulatory peritoneal dialysis. Am J Med 72:53, 1982
13. Mastrangelo F, Rizzelli S, Alfonso L: Anemia in high-efficiency dialysis. Nephrol Dial Transplant 116(suppl 2):S:127, 1991

14. Depner T, Rizwan S, James L: Effectiveness of low dose erythropoietin: a possible advantage of high flux hemodialysis. ASAIO Trans 36:M223, 1990
15. Collins A, Keshaviah P: High efficiency therapies for clinical dialysis therapy. p. 687. In Nissenson A, Fine R, Gentile D (eds): Clinical Dialysis. Appleton-Century Crofts, East Norwalk, CT, 1990
16. Zydney A, Colton C: Augmented solute transport in the shear flow of a concentrated suspension. J Colloid Interface Sci (submitted), 1992
17. Schmidt B, Ward R: The impact of erythropoietin on hemodialyzer design and performance. Artif Organs 13:35, 1989
18. Colton C, Smith K, Merril E, Reece J: Diffusion of organic solutes in stagnant plasma and red cell suspension. Chem Eng Progr Symp Ser 99:66, 1970
19. Cheung A, Alford M, Wilson M, et al: Urea movement across erythrocyte membrane during artificial kidney treatment. Kidney Int 23:866, 1983
20. Sargent J, Gotch F: Principles and biophysics of dialysis. p. 59. In Maher JF (ed): Replacement of Renal Function by Dialysis. 3rd ed. Kluwer, Boston, 1989
21. Delano B, Lundin A, Galonsky R et al: Dialyzer urea and creatinine clearance are not significantly altered in erythropoietin treated maintenance hemodialysis. ASAIO Trans 36:36, 1990
22. Besarb A, Anzalone J: Effect of erythropoietin (EPO) induced changes in hematocrit on dialysis solute clearance (cl), abstracted. Kidney Int 35:240, 1989
23. Paganini EP, Abdulhadi MH, Garcia J, Magnusson MO: Recombinant human erythropoietin correction of anemia. Dialysis efficiency, waste retention and chronic dose variables. ASAIO-Trans 35:513, 1989
24. Kaupke C, Vaziri N, Sampson J, Atkins L: Effect of erythropoietin therapy on diet and dialysis clearance in hemodialysis patients. Int J Artif Organs 13:218, 1990
25. Grutzmacher P, Bergmann M, Weinreich T et al: Benefits and adverse effects of correction of anemia by recombinant human EPO in patients on maintenance hemodialysis. Contrib Nephrol 66:104, 1988
26. Fernandez E, Betriu MA, Sorribas A, Montioliu J: Influence of increase in hematocrit induced by recombinant human erythropoietin on dialysis efficiency. Nefrologia (Spain) 11:66, 1991
27. Eschabach J, Egrie J, Downing M et al: Correction of the anemia of end stage renal diseases with recombinant human EPO. N Engl J Med 316:73, 1987
28. Casati S, Passerini P, Campise M et al: Benefits and risks of protracted treatment with human recombinant EPO in patient during hemodialysis. Br Med J 295:1017, 1987
29. Shinaberger J, Miller J, Gardner P: Erythropoietin alert: risks of high hematocrit hemodialysis. ASAIO Trans 34:179, 1988
30. Von Albertini B: Effect of hematocrit on solute removal during hemodialysis abstracted. Am Soc Artif Intern Organs Abstracts 17:62, 1988
31. Walczyk M, Gopler T: Letter to the editor: N Engl J Med 314:250, 1978
32. Van Gleen J, Nube M, Zuurbier P: Influence of erythropoietin treatment on urea kinetic parameters in hemodialysis patients. Clin Nephrol 35:156, 1991
33. Mohini R, Michaels R, Troste C et al: Comparison of effects of recombinant human erythropoietin EPO in patients on high flux (HF) vs conventional (C) hemodialysis, abstracted. Kidney Int 35:256, 1989
34. Acchiardo S, Quinn B, Burk L: Are high flux dialysis and erythropoietin in a collision course?ASAIO Trans 35:308, 1989
35. Acchiardo S, Moore L, Miles D et al: Does erythropoietin (EPO) treatment change hemodialysis (HD) requirement? (abstracted). Kidney Int 35:237A, 1989

36. Acchiardo S, Quinn P, Moore L et al: Evaluation of hemodialysis patients treated with erythropoietin. Am J Kidney Dis 17:290, 1991
37. Collins A, Keshaviah P, Berkseth R et al: Impact of erythropoietin therapy on rapid high efficiency hemodialysis, abstracted. Kidney Int 35:243A, 1989
38. Lim S, Flanigan M, Fangman J: Effect of hematocrit on solute removal during high efficiency hemodialysis. Kidney Int 37:1557, 1990
39. Laird NM, Berkey CS, Lowrie EC: Modeling success or failure of dialysis therapy: the National Cooperative Dialysis Study (NCDS). Kidney Int (suppl 23):S101, 1983
40. Gotch F, Sargent J: A mechanistic analysis of the National Cooperative Dialysis Study (NCDS). Kidney Int 28:526, 1985
41. Keshaviah P, Collins A: Hemodialysis: how much is enough? Semin Dial 1:3, 1988
42. Bosl R, Shideman JR, Mayer RM et al: Effects and complication of high efficiency dialysis. Nephron 15:151, 1975
43. Held P, Levin N, Bovbjerg R et al: Mortality and duration of hemodialysis treatment. JAMA 265:871, 1991
44. Nolph KD: Short dialysis, middle molecule and uremia. Ann Intern Med 86:99, 1977
45. Bergstrom J, Furst P: Uremic middle molecule. Clin Nephrol 5:143, 1976
46. Movilli E, Cancarini G, Mobelloni S et al: The role of hematocrit in efficiency of dialysis. Blood Purif 8:183, 1990
47. Zehnter E, Pollok M, Ziegenhager D et al: Urea kinetics in patients on regular dialysis treatment before and after treatment with recombinant human EPO. Contrib Nephrol 66:149, 1988
48. Canaud B, Boulox C, Rivory J et al: Erythropoietin induced changes in protein nutrition: quantitative assessment by urea kinetic modeling analysis. Blood Purif 8:301, 1990
49. Buur T, Lundberg M: Secondary effects of erythropoietin on metabolism and dialysis efficiency in stable hemodialysis patients. Clin Nephrol 34:230, 1990
50. Stiller S, Mann H, Brunner H: Backfiltration in hemodialysis with highly permeable membranes. Contrib Nephrol 46:23, 1985
51. Robertson B, Curtin C: Effects of EPO therapy on backfiltration of dialysate in high flux dialysis. ASAIO Trans 36:M447, 1990

12

Drug Removal During High-Efficiency and High-Flux Hemodialysis

Thomas A. Golper Hieronymus H. Vincent
John R. Gleason Margreet C. Vos

INTRODUCTION

Drug removal and dosing recommendations associated with either high-flux or high-efficiency dialysis have been grossly understudied, in view of their importance in the management of patients treated by these technical innovations. In this chapter we describe the principles and concepts that affect drug removal by these treatment modalities and apply those principles to devise a mathematical model for predicting drug removal behavior from certain manufacturer's data. Conventional dialysis and ultrafiltration (prototype continuous arteriovenous hemofiltration) have provided a framework for these concepts and applications.[1,2] However, specific studies are needed. In their absence our goal is to elucidate the issues involved and encourage a standardized approach for future studies of this topic.

HIGH-EFFICIENCY AND HIGH-FLUX HEMODIALYSIS VERSUS CONVENTIONAL DIALYSIS

The differences among high-efficiency hemodialysis, high-flux hemodialysis, and conventional hemodialysis are based upon membrane porosity, surface area, and the flow rates of blood and dialysate used with each technique. Table 12-1 summarizes these functional differences.

Table 12-1. High-Efficiency and High-Flux Hemodialysis

High-efficiency hemodialysis
Qb > 400
Qd > 700
T = "short"
Membranes tight
High-flux hemodialysis
Qb > 400
Qd > 700
T = "short"
Membranes open
Dialysate moves backwards (backfiltration) into patient

High-efficiency hemodialysis uses dialysis membranes with a large surface area and high blood and dialysate flow rates to improve clearance of low molecular weight substances. Thus, the duration of dialysis can be reduced without jeopardizing small solute clearances. However, high-efficiency dialysis techniques employ conventional dialysis membranes, which generate average or poor clearances of species of middle and large molecular size. With conventional membranes the clearance of these middle and larger size molecules is very dependent upon the duration of the dialysis.

In high-flux hemodialysis membranes with greater porosity allow substantial diffusive clearance of molecules in the middle to large molecular size range. In addition, because of the high hydraulic permeability of these membranes, greater ultrafiltration rates are used (intentionally or otherwise) to achieve maximum convective solute removal of middle and large molecules. If ultrafiltration rates are not high, dialysis with highly permeable membranes allows constant water and solute exchange (filtration/backfiltration) across the blood/dialysate membrane barrier.[3–5] On the other hand, high ultrafiltration rates cause unidirectional flow toward the dialysate side (filtration) and generally hinder backfiltration.

The backfiltration in high-flux hemodialysis is not unlike the technique of hemodiafiltration, which incorporates two filters in series, one for diffusion and one for convection. The goal of this procedure is to optimize the clearance of middle size and large molecules by maximizing diffusion and convection. The high ultrafiltration rates used with this technique require pre-or postfilter replacement fluids. Under certain conditions high-flux dialysis may operate in a similar fashion with a single filter-dialyzer; the backfiltration of dialysate in the distal end of the device then acts in the same manner as the replacement fluids of hemodiafiltration.

Modification of clearances across a broad spectrum of molecular sizes is of particular interest to a discussion of drug clearance, since most drugs fall in the low to middle molecular weight category. The adjustments made with high-efficiency dialysis suggest that drug clearance may not vary from that in conventional dialysis, but there may be significant differences in drug removal with high-flux dialysis, depending on the molecular size of the drug. These concepts are expanded further in the following sections.

PRINCIPLES OF DRUG DIALYSIS

Virtually all studies of drug removal during dialysis have been performed with conventional hemodialysis techniques. Specific data describing drug removal with highly permeable membranes are scarce and often based on continuous arteriovenous hemofiltration (CAVH) or continuous arteriovenous hemodiafiltration (CAVHD) techniques rather than on high-flux or high-efficiency hemodialysis. Current information must therefore be extrapolated from those drugs that have been tested and from clearance data on middle molecular weight markers such as vitamin B_{12} and inulin. To this

Table 12-2. Drug Properties that Affect Dialytic Clearance

Molecular weight
Protein binding
Volume of distribution
Charge
Water or lipid solubility
Membrane binding
Alternative excretory pathway

end drugs are considered solutes of variable water solubility, to which the principles for dialytic clearance apply. Table 12-2 summarizes the unique properties of drugs that affect their removal by dialysis.

Drug Properties that Affect Dialyzability

Molecular Weight

One of the most reliable predictors of the dialyzability of a drug is its molecular weight.[6,7] Drugs of molecular weight above 1,000 depend less upon diffusion and more upon convection for dialytic clearance.[7] Hemodiafiltration does not differ from conventional dialysis with respect to clearance of small solute (those with molecular weights < 500). However, the hemodiafiltration clearance of middle molecular weight molecules (500 to 5,000) exceeds that in conventional dialysis by 10 percent, and large molecular clearance (>5,000) in hemodialfiltration is increased by 24 percent over that in conventional hemodialysis.[8]

Molecular volume is determined by the weight, shape, and charge of the species in question. If a drug cannot fit through a dialysis membrane pore because of its geometric proportions, it is reflected and cannot be cleared by the dialyzer. The term *molecular size* is used to indicate the relationship of molecular weight, volume, shape, charge, and steric hindrance to the ability of a molecular species to permeate a membrane pore.

There is an inverse semilogarithmic relationship between dialysis clearance and molecular weight.[9] This inverse relationship has been mathematically applied to continuous hemodiafiltration, with creatinine clearance used as the reference valve.[6] The shortcomings of this mathematical expression limit its clinical application, since the estimates do not consider the dialytic effect of steric hindrance, molecular and membrane charge, protein binding, and lipid solubility. However, the same mathematical model could be applied to predict drug clearance during intermittent high-flux hemodialysis (see below).

Protein Binding

The binding of drugs to circulating plasma proteins is another reliable predictor of a drug's dialyzability. Most drugs bind to plasma proteins to a variable extent. Protein binding renders the drug pharmacologically inactive by preventing it from reaching its site of action and slows its metabolism for the same reason. The forces that affect protein binding include opposite charge attraction, pH, hydrophobic or hydrophilic environment, and van der Waals forces.

The bound and unbound fractions of the total drug are in constant equilibrium. If the drug is tightly protein-bound, then the flux between bound and unbound drug occurs more slowly. Unbound drug is the pharmacologically active form, for it can be freely distributed to targeted tissue receptor sites, metabolic inactivating sites (e.g., the liver), or excretory sites (e.g., the kidneys or dialyzer).

Certain conditions of uremia may inhibit or enhance protein binding. Malnutrition and proteinuria lower serum protein levels, thereby increasing the free fraction of drug owing to saturation of the reduced number of available protein binding sites.[10] Consequently, dialyzer clearance increases and the possibility of drug toxicity is enhanced, particularly if the drug has a narrow therapeutic window.

Accumulation of uremic toxins decreases the affinity of albumin for drugs such as penicillins, digitoxin, phenobarbital, phenytoin, warfarin, morphine, primidone, salicylates, theophylline, and sulfonamides.[11–13] Acidic drugs, (e.g., cephalosporins, imipenem, vancomycin, and ciprofloxacin) have a higher free fraction than do basic drugs such as tobramycin because of the chronic organic acidemia that accompanies renal failure.[14] Organic acids compete with acidic drugs for certain protein binding sites.

On the other hand, uncomplicated uremia causes few alterations in the protein binding of basic drugs. Basic drugs bind more avidly to nonalbumin serum proteins[14] than to albumin.[15] The protein binding of basic drugs is often increased owing to elevated levels of the acute-phase reactant α_1 acid glycoprotein, to which these drugs readily bind.[14,16] These basic drugs may bind still more avidly to these nonalbumin proteins during catastrophic illnesses. As a result, less unbound drug is available for dialytic clearance or for pharmacologic activity. However, since metabolism is slowed by the enhanced protein binding, drug presence may also be prolonged.

Heparin use during hemodialysis stimulates the activity of lipoprotein lipases, which break down triglycerides into free fatty acids.[15,17,18] Elevated levels of plasma free fatty acids compete with drugs such as tryptophan, sulfonamides, salicylates, phenylbutazone, phenytoin, thiopentone, and valproic acid for protein binding sites, causing an increase in the free fraction during and after the duration of the heparin effect. To illustrate the complexity of drug-protein interactions, free fatty acid may displace cefamandole but may enhance the binding of other cephalosporins such as cephalothin or cefoxitin.[19] Golper and associates[20] have shown that the addition of free fatty acids increases the free fraction of phenytoin, a highly protein bound drug. Thus, any perturbation in the serum free fatty acid concentration may alter drug-protein binding and ultimately drug clearance.

Volume of Distribution

The apparent volume of distribution (Vd) is a mathematical concept primarily based on protein and/or tissue binding. Avid protein or tissue binding "expands" the apparent Vd. Thus, Vd does not refer to actual fluid volumes for most drugs. It may coincidentally represent an actual volume as in the case of aminoglycosides, whose apparent Vd is the extracellular water or sodium space.

Drug clearance can be mathematically quantified in units of time with use of the iterative definition of elimination half-life:

$$T_{1/2} = \frac{0.693 \times Vd}{C1} \tag{1}$$

where $T_{1/2}$ is the elimination half-life, Vd is the apparent volume of distribution, and Cl is clearance. Thus, for a given clearance, $T_{1/2}$ is directly proportional to Vd. When the Vd is large, drug availability to the circulation is minimal and the half-life is long.[15] Drugs with Vd values below 1L/kg are more likely to be dialyzable[15]; those with Vd between 1 and 2 L/kg have marginal dialytic clearances; and drug removal is unlikely if Vd is greater than 2 L/kg.

The above simplified discussion ignores the effect of molecular size on dialytic clearance. Diffusive clearance is minimal under conditions of conventional dialysis if the molecular weight of the drug is greater than 1,000. It will be greater for membranes with greater porosity. Therefore, a middle molecular weight drug such as vancomycin, with a molecular weight of 1,448 and a Vd of 0.7 L/kg, has a better clearance (85 ml/min) with a high-flux polysulfone F-80 hemodialyzer than it does with a cuprophane dialyzer (9.6 ml/min).[21]

Despite rapid extracellular clearances with any type of short-time dialysis, intracellular equilibration with extracellular fluid can be slow, especially with middle to large molecular weight solutes.[22] This is probably related to the lipid solubility of the drug and to tissue compartmentalization. Quantitatively, postdialysis intracellular concentrations may vary by only 1 to 2 percent,[8] and as a result, there is a drug concentration gradient between intracellular and extracellular fluid. There may be a posthemodialysis rebound of 10 to 25 percent with intercompartmental equilibration.[23] Higher ultrafiltration rates, as with short-time high-flux hemodiafiltration, can aggravate this rebound phenomenon. Matzke et al.[24] found that for vancomycin the rebound level was 50 percent higher than the initial postdialysis drug concentration. The maximum posthemodiafiltration rebound time, defined as the time at which the maximum drug plasma concentration occurred postdialysis, was highly variable for vancomycin, ranging from 2.8 to 45.8 hours. Therefore it would be difficult to predict this phenomenon for a specific patient, and because of the significant interpatient variability in rebound time, it is advised to follow drug levels closely.

Drug Binding to Red Blood Cells

Related to tissue compartmentalization is the phenomenon of drug partitioning into red blood cells (RBCs). Marbury and associates[25] first raised this concern because ultrafiltration during dialysis raises hematocrit and complicates the determination of intradialytic drug clearance. The question is whether the whole blood concentration or the plasma concentration is the proper reference value; this is particularly relevant to the clearance of ethambutol, a drug known to partition into the RBCs.[26] Drugs that have a partition coefficient (whole blood to plasma concentration ratio) exceeding unity (e.g., procainamide, glutethimide, and acetaminophen) may have decreased clearances due to hemoconcentration at the end of dialysis.[15] Thus, for drugs that partition into RBCs, total dialytic clearance may be reduced in these hemoconcentrated states. Furthermore, the issue of rapid reequilibration between RBC drug and plasma drug becomes more important. This is discussed further below in connection with mathematical modeling.

These observations were made prior to the routine use of erythropoietin. Hematocrits are now higher than they were in the pre-erythropoietin era. Higher predialysis hematocrits will result in greater RBC partitioning and in less free drug, with the potential consequences described above.[27] Even for a drug with low RBC partitioning, clearance may be decreased in the setting of higher hematocrits because, as with all plasma solutes, dialytic clearance is dependent on delivery of plasma to the dialyzer. With higher hematocrits more red cell mass and less plasma are delivered to the dialyzer.

Elimination

The primary organs of drug elimination are the liver and kidneys, with the skin, gastrointestinal tract, and the lungs also involved to an appreciable degree. Dialysis may play a significant role in drug elimination for the individual with end-stage renal failure. If alternate routes of elimination are not available for drug clearance, the parent drug and its metabolites accumulate. Thus, the quantity of drug administered and/or the frequency of dosing must be considered.

Metabolic biotransformation is the chemical conversion of a drug to another form. This process, occurring mainly in the liver, results in a more polar, less lipid-soluble, and more extractable metabolite, which often differs from the parent drug in its pharmacologic effects. Most metabolites are pharmacologically inert, although some may possess pharmacologic activity and/or toxicity (e.g., *N*-acetylprocainamide).

Hepatic metabolism of most drugs is usually normal or accelerated with uremia.[15] This may be related to an increased availability of free drug because of decreased protein binding. Cytochrome P450 metabolism of phenytoin is accelerated in uremia, probably as a result of enzyme induction due to the increased free fraction. The metabolism of peptides (e.g., insulin) and procaine is reduced secondary to inhibition of ester hydrolysis, while hepatic acetylation (e.g., isoniazid) and glucuronide (e.g., acetaminophen) and sulfate conjugate hydrolysis (e.g., sulfa compounds) are usually normal.[28]

Drugs and metabolites that have a small molecular size, small volume of distribution, and high water solubility are more likely to be eliminated by dialysis. A dialytic clearance that increases plasma clearance by more than 30 percent is considered significant.[29,30]

Bioavailability

Bioavailability is defined as the fraction of administered drug that reaches the bloodstream. It is dependent on the completeness of and rate of absorption. The technique of administration will determine how much drug is bioavailable. A drug's absorption is affected by the character of the membranes it must cross to reach the circulation, the blood flow at the site of absorption, the absorptive surface area, and the contact time between the drug and the absorptive area. In addition, physicochemical drug properties such as molecular size and lipid solubility affect drug absorption, particularly after oral administration.

Routes of drug administration include the gastrointestinal tract and injection into subcutaneous tissue, muscle, and the bloodstream. Since maximum absorption is obtained with intravenous administration, this is the standard with which all other forms of administration are compared.

Interstitial edema can retard absorption after subcutaneous or intramuscular injection. If a dialysis patient has large interdialytic fluid gains, one would expect erratic or delayed absorption of drugs administered by either of these routes. A dosing regimen may be erroneously presumed to be stable under these conditions of volume overload. However, there is the potential for increase in either pharmacologic or toxic effect when the patient approaches dry weight and absorbs the drug properly.

In the uremic patient three factors affect gastric absorption: gastric pH, gastric motility, and mucosal integrity. An increase in gastric pH as a result of urea breakdown to ammonia greatly reduces absorption. Aluminum hydroxide, used as a phosphate binder, further raises gastric pH, delays gastric emptying, and forms poorly absorbed complexes with drugs. Drugs such as digoxin, tetracycline, and probably ciprofloxacin may form nonabsorbable chelation products with aluminum hydroxide. H_2-blockers and proton inhibitors may also raise gastric pH without concomitant motility effects. Mucosal edema delays absorption in the same manner as interstitial edema delays absorption after intramuscular and subcutaneous injection.

Bioavailability is closely related to hepatic metabolism owing to the first-pass effect of the enterohepatic circulation, which the drug enters following enteral absorption. The liver can metabolize and inactivate drugs before they reach the systemic circulation. Drugs may never reach their intended site of action due to this first-pass effect. One cannot consistently predict how uremia will affect hepatic metabolism.

Hemodialysis can indirectly alter absorption or bioavailability. It can reduce edema in the bowel, muscles, and skin as described above. Dialysis can lower urea levels and can slightly reduce the need for phosphate binders, which may improve absorption of some drugs. On the other hand, hypotension associated with dialysis can impair mesenteric blood flow and may contribute to malabsorption. Removal of uremic toxins may result in more available protein binding sites, thus increasing the fraction of drug bound to protein, and this in turn may affect drug metabolism by reducing the amount of free drug available for hepatic metabolism or removal by dialysis.

Properties of Dialysis that Affect Drug Clearance

Dialysis characteristics that affect drug clearance can be divided into three categories: properties of the dialyzer, properties of the dialysate, and technique of dialysis. These items are summarized in Table 12-3.

Membrane Materials

Hemodiafiltration membranes are fabricated from a variety of natural and synthetic polymers, including cellulose, cellulose acetate, polysulfone, polyamide, polyacrylonitrile (PAN) (e.g., AN69), and polymethylmethacrylate (PMMA). Concern over the possible importance of higher molecular weight toxins has led to the development of membranes with a wide range of solute permeabilities. This development has accelerated in recent years with the availability of dialysis equipment capable of controlling fluid removal.

With polysulfone membranes, trace quantities of albumin can appear in the dialysate.[31] Clearances of vancomycin vary with different membranes[21,23,32,33]. AN69 and polysulfone membranes have the greatest clearance, while cuprophane has minimal clearance of this drug under similar hemodialysis conditions.[21,33]

Table 12-3. Dialysis Properties that Affect Drug Clearance

Hemodialyzer properties
Pore size
Blood flow rate
Surface area
Membrane binding
Dialysate Properties
Dialysate flow rate
Solute concentration
pH
Temperature
Convection

Surface Area

The removal of small solutes is dependent upon the concentration gradient between blood and dialysate. This gradient can be maximized by increasing flow rates and/or by increasing surface area, thus dispersing the undialyzed blood to areas of fresh dialysate. Both these principles apply to either high-flux or high-efficiency dialysis. As molecular size increases and diffusivity is increasingly limited by membrane pore size, molecular clearance becomes more dependent upon convection. The hydraulic permeability of high-flux membranes exceeds that of conventional membranes, thus enhancing convective clearances of these larger molecules. When hydraulic permeability limits are achieved, larger surface area becomes the factor most influencing the total rate of convective clearance. Jindal and associates[34] have shown that for PAN, PMMA, and polysulfone dialyzers, surface area and ultrafiltration have a great effect on the clearances of B_2-microglobulin and phosphate, two poorly diffusible species.

This, of course, is not a new concept. Increasing surface area has been the mainstay of a variety of techniques to enhance clearances. Inulin clearances exceeding 150 ml/min were generated by von Albertini et al.[35] by increasing surface area, blood flow, ultrafiltration rate, dialysate flow rate, and needle size in high-flux hemodiafiltration. This was confirmed by Surian et al.,[36] who noted that with increasing surface area, blood flow, and ultrafiltration rate the clearances of all solutes, but especially of large molecules, increased.[35] Again, this demonstrates the importance of convection in the clearance of larger molecules. Surface area is a major determinant of the ultrafiltration rate in dialyzers with membranes of high hydraulic permeability. A clinical example of this phenomenon is a report that the amount of vancomycin removed by high-flux dialysis was correlated with membrane surface area.[21]

Drug-Membrane Charge Interaction and Membrane Binding

The negative charge of the PAN membrane repels anionic solutes such as gentamicin and doxycycline.[37] In one study theoretical estimates of gentamicin clearance did not to correlate well with clinical observations during continuous arteriovenous hemodiafiltration with PAN filters.[6] It was suggested that the negative charge of the membrane retarded gentamicin clearance.

Other possibilities for decreased gentamicin clearance could be drug adsorption on the dialysis membrane. Rumpf and associates[38] first proposed that drugs may bind to dialysis membranes. Kraft and Lode[39] noted membrane binding of gentamicin to an RP-6 hemofilter, while Kronfol et al.[40] described both tobramycin and amikacin binding to AN69 filters. Drug-membrane binding has also been demonstrated in the absence of proteins during experimental conditions of continuous arteriovenous hemofiltration.[20,41–43]

Diffusion

Hemodialysis membrane pores act as cylinders of uniform diameter. As the molecular volume (weight and ionic drag) increases, a drug's diffusivity will decrease. For a given drug or solute, there is a negative linear relationship between the logarithm of dialysance and the logarithm of molecular weight.[44] Henderson and associates have demonstrated that convection removes larger molecules more readily than does diffusion.[45–47] Diffusive clearance through conventional dialysis membranes is negligible for molecules with a molecular weight larger than 1,000.

Maneuvers that augment the concentration gradient between the blood and the dialysate make diffusion more efficient. Countercurrent flow combined with high blood and dialysate flow reduce the blood-dialysate contact time, thereby maximizing the concentration gradient. This is particularly important for low molecular weight species and for drugs in the lower range of middle molecular weights (e.g., aminoglycosides of 600). Clearances increase considerably as dialysate and blood flow increase. Under these conditions the solute removal rate is predominantly flow rate-limited.[10] For larger molecules, since their size limits the rate of diffusion through the membrane pores, the concentration gradient from blood to dialysate remains high, and flow rates have less influence for diffusion. However, the surface area and hydraulic permeability become important, allowing convective removal (see below). While convective removal occurs, the use of high ultrafiltration rates during high-flux hemodialysis causes admixture of the ultrafiltrate and the dialysate, which diminishes the concentration gradient and, as a result, the diffusive clearance of solutes.[14]

Nolph and associates demonstrated in coils and parallel-plate dialyzers that the diffusion of higher molecular weight species decreased with an increase in ultrafiltration rate. However, in hollow-fiber artificial kidneys there was an additive effect of ultrafiltration and diffusion upon clearance of high molecular weight solutes.[48–50] These observations were attributed to a widening of the blood pathway due to the increased transmembrane pressure (TMP) necessary to produce the ultrafiltration. The wider blood pathway increases the distance for diffusion and thus decreases the diffusion rate, and in plates it causes the membrane to abut against the support mesh, which decreases the functional surface area. Furthermore, ultrafiltration brings convectively transported solute into the dialysate, decreasing the concentration gradient from blood to dialysate. Compliant dialyzers such as coils and plates are vulnerable to these effects. Hollow-fiber dialyzers presumably maintain the integrity of their fiber pathways for blood under conditions of high TMP.

Convection

Convection is defined as bulk flow, or ultrafiltration, from the blood side to the dialysate side of the membrane. Negative TMP induces bulk flow of water and solute from the blood to the dialysate. Convection is unlimited until the permeability of the membrane is reached, when the negative TMP causes collapse of the dialysate compartment or the membrane ruptures. Ultrafiltration affects all sizes of molecules, but its effect is more evident with large molecules because these species are not diffusible. With cellulosic dialysis membranes, removal of solutes with molecular weights larger than 1,000 generally requires ultrafiltration. Depending on the type of membrane, even during ultrafiltration, molecules with a molecular weight larger than 2,000 are partially reflected by the membrane due to restrictions of porosity.[51]

Jaffrin et al.[51] and Vincent and colleagues[6,14,52] have separately attempted to quantify the contribution of convection to solute removal with PAN membranes under conditions of hemodiafiltration and continuous hemodiafiltration, respectively. Jaffrin et al.[51] concluded that diffusion dominates convection in most cases of solute removal. This is especially noted for solutes of small molecular size and less so for middle and large molecules. The clearance of middle-size and large molecules is dependent on convection. Using vitamin B_{12} as a marker for middle-size molecule clearance and myoglobin for large molecule clearance, Jaffrin and associates illustrated the dependence of middle-size and large molecule clearance on ultrafiltration. Furthermore, improvement in clearance of these markers with increased blood flow was minimal.[51]

Membrane-protein binding can adversely affect ultrafiltration. Vincent et al.[52] have shown predictable deterioration of ultrafiltration secondary to protein binding to the membrane. This is probably related to alteration in the porosity of the membrane by protein binding or to reduction in the surface area. Protein layering against the dialysis membrane (protein concentration polarization) creates a physical barrier has the effect of "widening" the membrane. Protein at the membrane surface results in increased osmotic and oncotic activity on the blood side, which ultimately retards convection.

In addition, protein concentration polarization, a direct consequence of high ultrafiltration rates, could negatively affect clearance of small solutes by creating another diffusion barrier. However, Bosch et al.[53] noticed no decline in creatinine clearance and only a slight decline in inulin clearance under these conditions. Therefore, protein accumulation at or on the membrane probably has its greatest impact on ultrafiltration.

Effect of Dialyzer Reuse

Dialyzer reuse was first described in 1964 by Shaldon et al.[54] Despite its long history, there is no mention in the literature of the possible effects of dialyzer reuse on drug clearance and scant mention of any effect on solute clearance in general. Adverse effects of reuse on drug clearance have not been clearly identified, which is partly related to the fact that several methods of reuse are currently employed. Despite this handicap, one may make inferences about drug removal from small and large solute clearance studies.

Reuse may affect clearance by reduction of fiber bundle volume (loss of surface area), by alteration in the diffusive property of the membrane, or by the loss of hydraulic permeability, which decreases convective clearances. Regarding the loss of hydraulic permeability, observations during continuous hemodiafiltration suggest a predictable decline in ultrafiltration with time due to either fibrin or protein adherence to the membrane.[55] This deterioration of ultrafiltration has been considered when predicting the clearance of several drugs.[52] Wetzelberger and Lucker[56] have described a time-dependent decrease in theophylline clearance during conventional dialysis. They suggested that increased membrane resistance due to clotting was responsible, but protein adsorption onto the dialysis membrane may also account for their findings. Consistent with this are the observations of Teehan et al.,[57] who suggested that there is deterioration in ultrafiltration due to protein adsorption associated with frequent reuse.

Reuse techniques using bleach remove much of the adsorbed protein, restoring the membrane properties lost by the protein layer effects. On the other hand, use of formaldehyde alone does not remove adsorbed protein, and multiple uses may result in a loss of membrane permeability. The Renatron system uses reverse ultrafiltration, followed by treatment with peracetic acid as a rinsing and sterilizing agent. Reverse ultrafiltration should remove adsorbed protein. Garred et al.[58] using the Renatron system, found no change in the clearance of small solutes with an average of 14 reuses of a polysulfone dialyzer. Ultrafiltration failure was not discussed, nor were the clearances of larger molecules evaluated.

Few researchers have undertaken the study of middle-size and large molecule clearance with the newer dialysis techniques. Teehan and associates[57] demonstrated in early studies that the diffusive clearance of vitamin B_{12} was not affected by membrane reuse, whereas its convection was reduced. Data obtained by conventional dialysis techniques have suggested that vitamin B_{12} clearance remains stable up to the twentieth reuse but drops off considerably after that.[59] Long-range studies such as these have not been applied to high-flux dialyzers. Petersen et al.[60] have reported the longest reuse experience with high-flux hemodialysis. Plasma B_2-microglobulin levels have been reported to decline by 57 percent after the first treatment and by 62 percent after the sixth reuse. The results of this study imply that B_2-microglobulin clearance is adequate after six reprocessing treatments when hypochlorite is used as the cleansing agent. These data suggest that there is no untoward affect of reuse upon the clearance of most drugs with molecular weights lower than that of B_2-microglobulin (11,900).

A small reduction in ultrafiltration has been demonstrated with peracetic acid and the Renatron system after the sixth reuse of cuprophane dialyzers.[61] Whether or not this applies to bleach or formaldehyde reprocessing techniques is not certain. It is also uncertain whether the data apply to other dialyzer materials.

In summary, it is difficult to draw conclusions about the effects of reprocessing upon drug clearance. Protein deposition on the dialyzer significantly reduces ultrafiltration and possibly middle-size and large molecule clearance. Despite these observations, the role of reuse in membrane deposition of protein has not been elucidated adequately, and its effect on drug clearance is also uncertain. On the basis of current data, if polysulfone and other high-flux dialyzer membranes are used more than six times, neither predictable drug clearance nor predictable membrane behavior can be ensured.

MATHEMATICAL MODELING OF DRUG REMOVAL

Mechanisms of Solute Removal by Diffusion and Convection

The total amount of a drug (or any solute) removed during dialysis is the sum of the amounts removed by diffusion and by convection. The mechanisms of solute removal by these two processes are entirely different. The rate of diffusion depends on the difference between the concentrations in blood and in dialysate and on the diffusive mass transfer coefficient, the value of which depends on the solute, the dialyzer, and the operating conditions. In hemofiltration and to some extent in hemodiafiltration and high-flux dialysis, solutes are removed by convection (i.e., plasma water is removed together with all dissolved molecules that are able to pass through the membrane pores). In convection the driving force is the TMP difference. In hemodiafiltration and high-flux dialysis convection and diffusion occur simultaneously and have an influence on one another.[8,48–50,62] Filtration delivers convectively derived solute to the dialysate, thereby decreasing the concentration gradient between blood and dialysate and decreasing the diffusion rate. Diffusive solute removal lowers the solute concentration in plasma water and thereby decreases the amount of solute that is removed by filtration. A detailed description of the mechanisms of solute removal by combined convection and diffusion is best given in mathematical terms.

A Model of Combined Convection and Diffusion

What follows is a simple mathematical model of solute transport from plasma water to dialysate. The model equations can easily be implemented in any spreadsheet computer program. By doing so, the reader may study the influence of the determinants of solute transport for a variety of compounds. This may be particularly applicable to the clearance of drugs when actual in vivo data are not available.

Input variables are blood flow rate at the dialyzer inlet (Qbi), hematocrit (Hct), plasma protein concentration (Cprot), dialysate flow rate at the dialysate inlet (Qdi), ultrafiltration rate (Qf), infusion rate of predilution fluid (Qpred) (applicable in hemodiafiltration or hemofiltration), and solute concentration in the arterial blood plasma (Cpi). The solute concentration of the dialysate at the dialysate inlet (Cdi) is taken to be zero. To calculate solute transport one also needs total membrane surface area (A) and solute mass transfer coefficient for diffusion (Ko). From these one first calculates the flow rate of plasma water at the blood inlet (Qwi) according to

$$\text{Qwi} = \text{Qbi} \times (1 - \text{Hct}) + \text{Qbi} \times \text{Hct} \times \text{f} + \text{Qpred} \tag{2}$$

where f is the fractional solute distribution in red blood cells. For urea, f is 0.8; for many other solutes, it may be taken to zero. However, as discussed in the section on drug binding to red blood cells, some drugs compartmentalize into red blood cells, and this effect, when known, must be included in the calculations. One next calculates the solute concentration in plasma water at the inlet of the dialyzer (Cwi) according to

$$\text{Cwi} = \frac{\text{Cpi}}{(1 - 0.00107 \cdot \text{Cprot})} \times \frac{(\text{Qwi} - \text{Qpred})}{\text{Qwi}} \tag{3}$$

From this formula it is clear that the concentration in plasma water is some 7 percent higher than that in plasma owing to the volume of plasma proteins if no predilution is used. The plasma water flow rate at the blood outlet (Qwo) is calculated by

$$\text{Qwo} = \text{Qwi} - \text{Qf} \tag{4}$$

and the dialysate flow rate at the dialysate outlet (Qdo) is

$$\text{Qdo} = \text{Qdi} + \text{Qf} \tag{5}$$

For simplicity, one first assumes that the volume flux (Jv) is constant along the length of the membrane. The value of Jv is given by

$$\text{Jv} = \frac{\text{Qf}}{\text{A}} \tag{6}$$

Solute flux (Js) through the membrane at a point occurs by convection and diffusion

$$\text{Js} = \text{Jv} \times \text{Cw} + \text{Ko} \times (\text{Cw} - \text{Cd}) \tag{7}$$

It should be noted that according to equation 7, diffusion results from the difference between blood and dialysate solute concentrations. Possible concentration gradients in the radial direction are not taken into account. In reality, owing to the axial flow profile and to the "stagnant" layers near the membrane, solute concentrations near the membrane differ from those in the middle of the stream. These differences may have an influence on the true driving force for diffusion and thereby on the calculated value of Ko.

Therefore, any possible influence of blood and dialysate flow rates on Ko should be investigated before the model can be used to extrapolate to different blood and dialysate flow rates.[54] For the calculation of total solute transport, equation 7 must be integrated in a stepwise manner. At each step dx one should define Qwx, Qdx, total solute mass (i.e., Qwx × Cwx and Qdx × Cdx), Cwx, Cdx, and Jsx. In order to avoid circular calculations, an approximation procedure must be used to find the input value of the dialysate outlet concentration (Cdo) at which the value of Cdi becomes zero. The model may be used to calculate the change in plasma water and dialysate solute concentrations along the length of the dialyzer. Figures 12-1 to 12-4 show the effects of blood flow rate (Qb) and dialysate flow rate (Qd) on changes in urea concentration along the dialyzer. They demonstrate that in the case of a very low dialysate flow rate, as with CAVHD, most diffusion will take place along a small part of the length of the fibers (to the right in Figs. 12-1 and 12-2). Furthermore, the dialysate is virtually saturated with solute during these conditions of low Qdi. Figure 12-3 represents the conditions seen during conventional dialysis, while Figure 12-4 represents some exaggerated conditions seen in high-efficiency dialysis.

It is customary to present dialyzer clearance rates as a function of Qb. Figures 12-5 and 12-6 show the influences of Qb, membrane surface area, and Ko on clearance rate. If Ko is constant, clearance rates are proportional to membrane surface area.[21]

Equation 7 has been solved analytically, primarily to obtain an expression for Ko as a function of Cdo and the other input variables,[52] but the solution

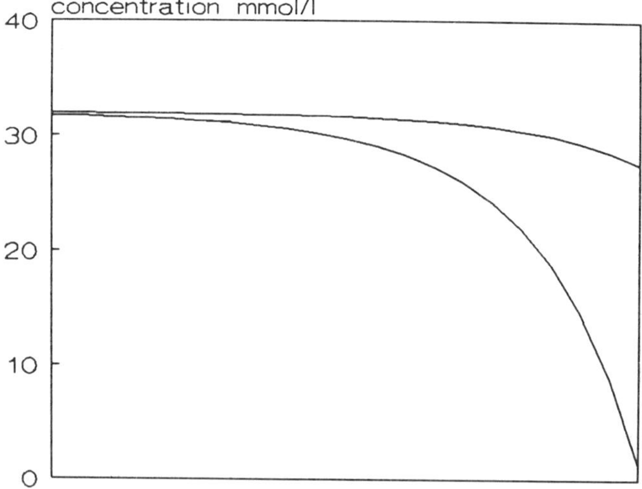

Fig. 12-1. Concentration profile of urea in plasma water (upper curve) and in dialysate (lower curve) under typical conditions of continuous hemodiafiltration (Qd, 1 L/h; Qb, 150 ml/min; Cl, 30 ml/min).

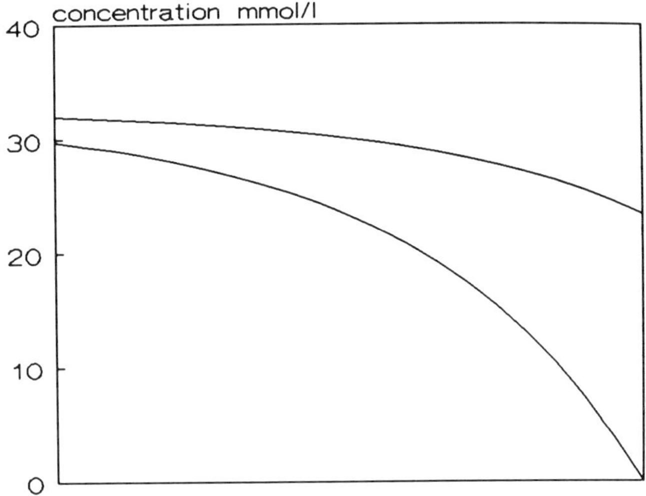

Fig. 12-2. Concentration profile of urea in plasma water (upper curve) and in dialysate (lower curve) under conditions of continuous hemodiafiltration with high dialysate flow (Qd, 2 L/h; Qb, 150 ml/min; Cl, 43 ml/min).

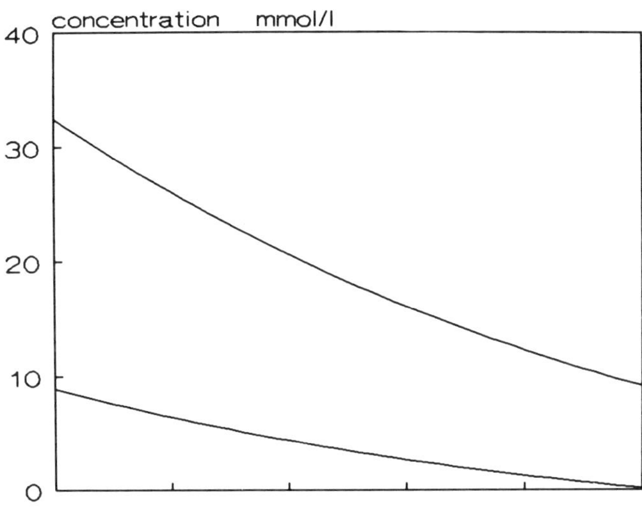

Fig. 12-3. Concentration profile of urea in plasma water (upper curve) and in dialysate (lower curve) under conditions of conventional hemodialysis (Qd, 500 ml/min; Qb, 200 ml/min; Cl, 152 ml/min; surface area, 1.1 m^2).

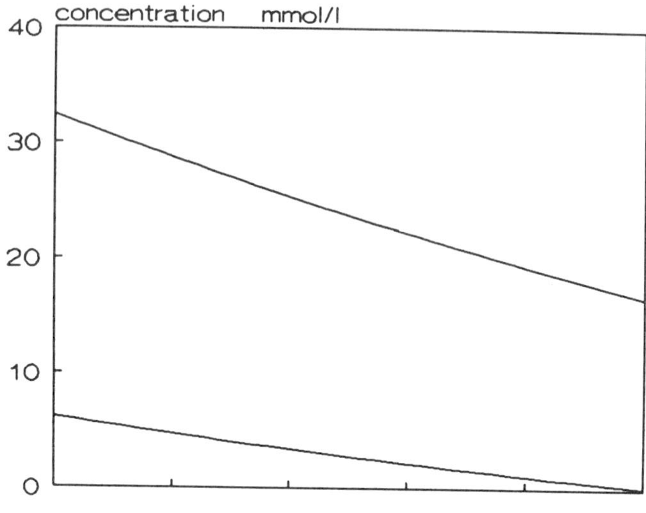

Fig. 12-4. Concentration profile of urea in plasma water (upper curve) and in dialysate (lower curve) under conditions of high-efficiency or high-flux hemodialysis (Qd, 1,000 ml/min, Qb, 400 ml/min; Cl, 207 ml/min; surface area, 1.1 m^2).

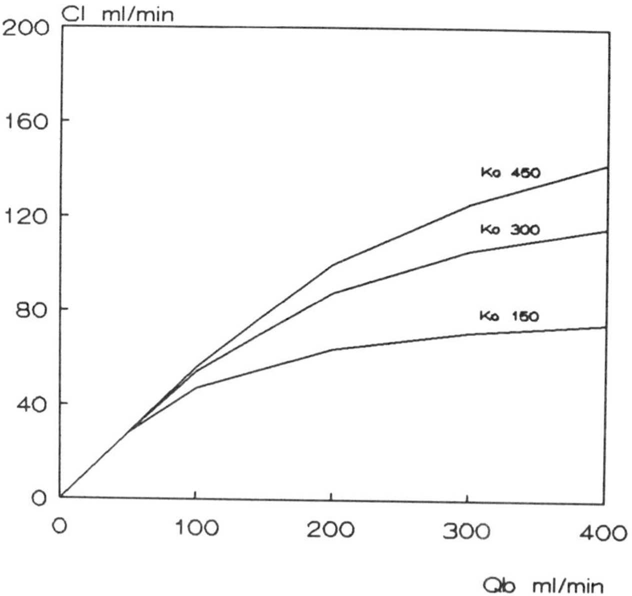

Fig. 12-5. Clearance rate versus blood flow at different Ko values (surface area, 0.75 m^2; Qf, 10 ml/min; α, 0.75).

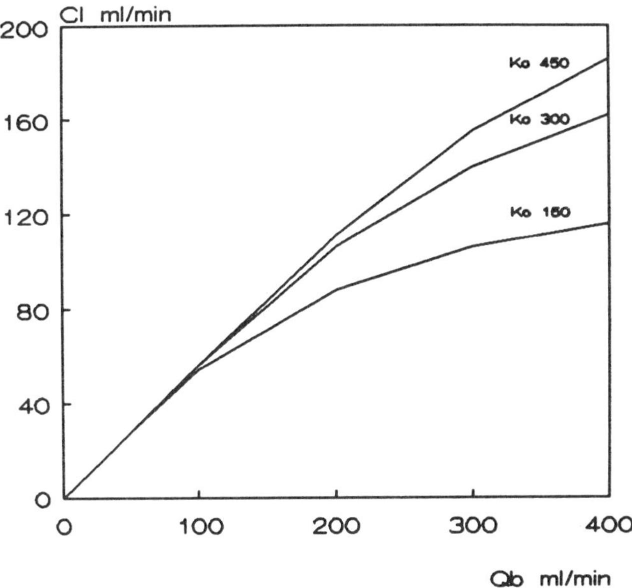

Fig. 12-6. Clearance rate versus blood flow at different Ko values (surface area, 1.5 m^2; Qf, 10 ml/min; α, 0.75).

may also be used to express Cdo as a function of Ko and the other input variables.[6] Thus the use of the numerical approach, as explained above, is obviated. It should be noted, however, that the analytical solution is valid only if the solute is not bound to proteins and the sieving coefficient is 1.0 (see below).

Protein Binding and Sieving

In the model described above it is assumed that the solute can freely pass through the dialyzer membrane. In the case of drugs, usually a fraction of the solute's total plasma concentration is bound to proteins and only the free fraction α is available for convection and diffusion. To take the effect of protein binding into account, in equation 7 the value of Cwx must be replaced with Cwx $\cdot$ α. A solute molecule may itself be so large that in the process of convection a portion of the solute is retained. The absolute sieving coefficient of the solute (s) is defined as the fraction of unbound solute that passes through the membrane during ultrafiltration. The values of α and s determine the ratio of drug concentration in ultrafiltrate (Cf) to that in plasma:

$$\text{Cf} = \text{Cw} \times \alpha \times \text{s} \qquad (8)$$

It is customary to define the *apparent* sieving coefficient of a solute as the ratio of the concentration in filtrate to that in plasma or plasma water. One should realize that the apparent sieving coefficient, thus defined, is the product of α and s. In the case of most drugs and small to medium-sized solutes, the apparent sieving coefficient in reality represents the free fraction, and the absolute sieving coefficient of the solute is unity.

In the model one may assume either that during passage through the dialyzer no reequilibration between bound and unbound drug takes place or that reequilibration takes place instantaneously. In the first case, Cwi should be substituted by Cwi $\cdot$ α and equation 3 replaced with

$$\text{Cwi} = \frac{\text{Cpi}}{(1 - 0.00107 \times \text{Cprot})} \times \frac{(\text{Qwi} - \text{Qpred})}{\text{Qwi}} \times \alpha \qquad (9)$$

Solute transport is then calculated by integration of equation 7. In the second case equation 3 is used without modification and equation 7 is replaced with equation 10:

$$\text{Js} = \text{Jv} \times \text{Cw} \times \alpha + \text{Ko} \times (\text{Cw} \times \alpha - \text{Cd}) \qquad (10)$$

Figure 12-7 shows the effect of reequilibration on the fall in concentration across the dialyzer. With immediate reequilibration (condition B in Fig. 12-7), the outlet concentration in blood (Cbo) is slightly lower than without equilibration, which reflects the additional removal of that small amount of drug freed from protein binding sites during passage through the dialyzer

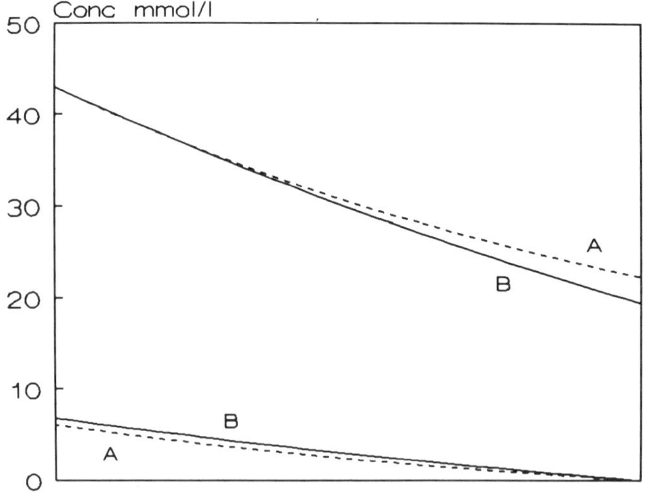

Fig. 12-7. Drug concentration profiles in plasma water (upper two curves) and in dialysate (lower two curves). Condition A is no reequilibration between bound and unbound fractions of the drug. Condition B is immediate reequilibration. Dialysis conditions are conventional.

blood pathway. With high rates of diffusion, reequilibration contributes to drug removal. Generally, however, this effect is small, and in the case of CAVHD the contribution of reequilibration may be neglected. It is probably not negligible in high-clearance procedures such as high-flux or high-efficiency dialysis, especially with changes in blood pH during transit through the dialyzer.

As a rule, drug clearance rate by dialysis and hemofiltration may be taken to be linearly related to its free fraction (Fig. 12-8). The value of the free fraction is a function of plasma protein concentration and intrinsic properties of the drug (see above discussion of protein binding). Accordingly, it may be appropriate to define Cprotx as a function of Cprot, Qwi, and Qwx and to define αx as a function of α, Cprot, and Cprotx. Generally, however, this will have little effect on the calculated results.

Influence of Transmembrane Pressure and Back Transport

If a high-flux dialyzer is used with a large membrane surface area, only a small TMP difference is needed to obtain a high rate of ultrafiltration. Indeed, in order to achieve zero net ultrafiltration, the dialysate pressure must exceed the blood pressure at the blood outlet of the dialyzer. In such a case ultrafiltrate is formed within the dialyzer at the blood inlet side and is reabsorbed at the blood outlet side (so-called backfiltration). Backfiltration is a potential problem because it may lead to movement of dialysate contaminants into the blood. On the other hand, as the concentration of uremic

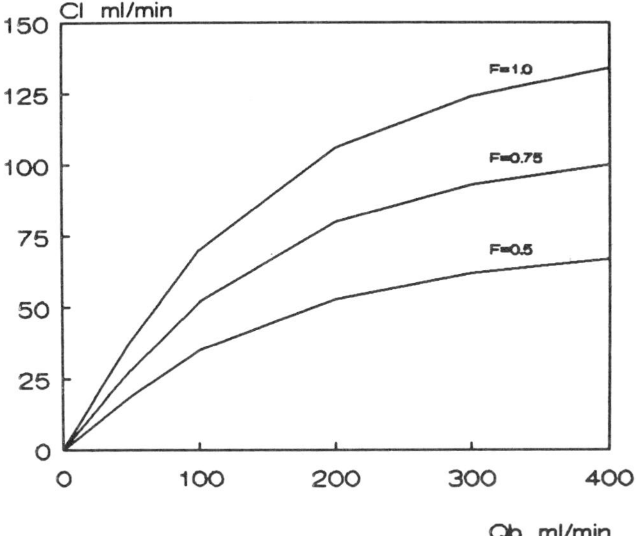

Fig. 12-8. Clearance rate versus blood flow at different values of F (free fraction, α in text) under conditions of conventional dialysis.

solutes will be higher in blood at the inlet than at the outlet, backfiltration will cause a net solute flux from blood to dialysate. It has been reasoned, therefore, that backfiltration may usefully contribute to clearance. In order to investigate this, we have modified the model as to take into account that volume flux (Jvx) is a linear function of TMPx. The value of TMPx is calculated from the blood- and dialysate-side pressures (Pbx and Pdx) and the oncotic pressure in blood (π) according to

$$\mathrm{TMP} = \mathrm{Pb} - \mathrm{Pd} - \pi \tag{11}$$

Here Pbx is taken to decrease as a linear function of x from the arterial to the venous pressure value. Pdx shows a similar but smaller decrease in the opposite direction. The value of π may be estimated from the blood protein concentration by the Landis-Pappenheimer equation.[63]

For most practical purposes, however, if the net ultrafiltration rate is known, this further sophistication of the model is not necessary. This is demonstrated in Figures 12-9 and 12-10, which show the contribution of convection and diffusion to the overall transport of deferoxamine (DFO), a molecule with a molecular weight of 657. Convective solute transport is closely related to net ultrafiltration. At zero net ultrafiltration, the convective contribution to solute clearance is negligible (Fig. 12-10).

Input Values of the Model

For the application of the above model the needed input values are the sieving coefficient s, the free fraction α, and Ko.

With high-flux dialyzers, data on sieving coefficients are provided by the manufacturer. Usually these data have been obtained in vitro. In clinical

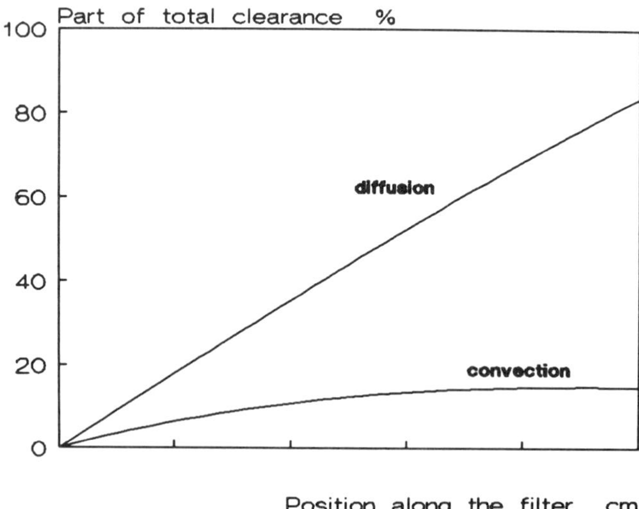

Fig. 12-9. Contributions of diffusion and convection to total dialytic clearance of DFO under conditions of standard dialysis with moderate ultrafiltration rates.

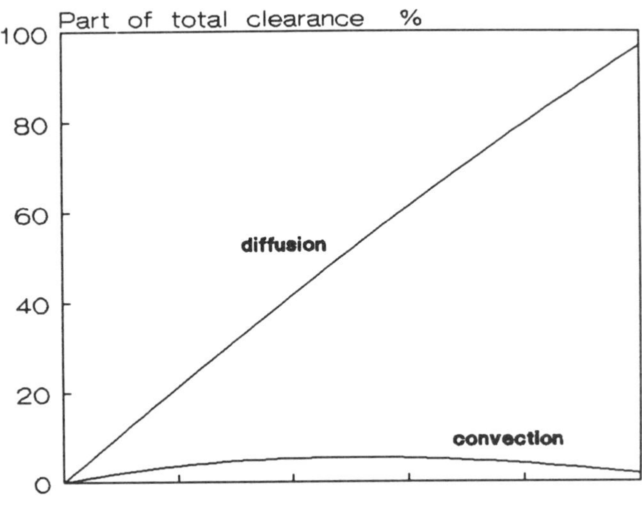

Fig. 12-10. Contributions of diffusion and convection to total dialytic clearance of DFO under conditions of standard dialysis with zero net ultrafiltration.

use, sieving coefficients will be lower because of protein adsorption on the membrane and, in case of high ultrafiltration rates, because of protein boundary layer formation. During CAVHD, using an AN69 dialyzer, we found that for drugs with a molecular weight of up to at least 1,500 the real sieving coefficient is unity, the apparent sieving coefficient thus reflecting the free fraction of the drug. The AN69 membrane has a pore size of 30 Å. It would seem reasonable to assume that for other high-flux dialyzers with pore sizes of about 30 Å or greater, the apparent sieving coefficient is equal to the free fraction.

There is a wealth of published data on apparent sieving coefficients of drugs. These data have been obtained with different dialyzers and at different operating conditions. For the reason given above, they may be taken to be applicable to different dialyzers; however, they are not readily applicable to different patients, since protein binding is affected by the condition of the patient. The binding of acidic drugs may be decreased because of uremia, low levels of albumin, or high levels of bilirubin and free fatty acids, and it may be altered by competition with other drugs. The binding of basic drugs may be increased by increased levels of acute phase proteins. Thus, we found that in intensive care patients the apparent sieving coefficient of cephalosporins was much higher than in normal subjects, whereas that of tobramycin was lower[2,64] (Table 12-4).

In conclusion, if the clinical condition of the patient is taken into account, literature data may be used to obtain a reliable estimation of the values of α and s. Accordingly, the rate of drug clearance (Cl) by

Table 12-4. Drug Protein Binding and Sieving Coefficient

Drug	Free Fraction in Normal subjects[a]	Apparent Sieving Coefficient in ICU Patients
Cefotaxime	0.60	0.80
Cefuroxime	0.67	0.85
Ceftazidime	0.83	0.99
Imipenem	0.80	1.05
Ciprofloxacin	0.75	1.07
Vancomycin	0.45	0.72
Tobramycin	1.00	0.89

[a] Data of protein binding in normal subjects were taken from literature.
(From Golper,[64] with permission.)

either intermittent or continuous hemofiltration may easily be calculated according to the equation

$$Cl = Qf \times s \times \alpha \tag{12}$$

which represents the result of the integration of equation 7 for Ko = 0.

Unfortunately, hemodialysis and hemodiafiltration are rather more complicated than hemofiltration. In addition to the values of α and s, one needs an input value of Ko. The value of Ko is determined by the resistance to diffusion of the blood side, the membrane, and the dialysate side of the dialyzer, which in turn depend on the solute, on membrane pore size and density, and on dialyzer geometry and operating conditions. Let us first consider the influence of solute. Figure 12-11 shows the relationship between

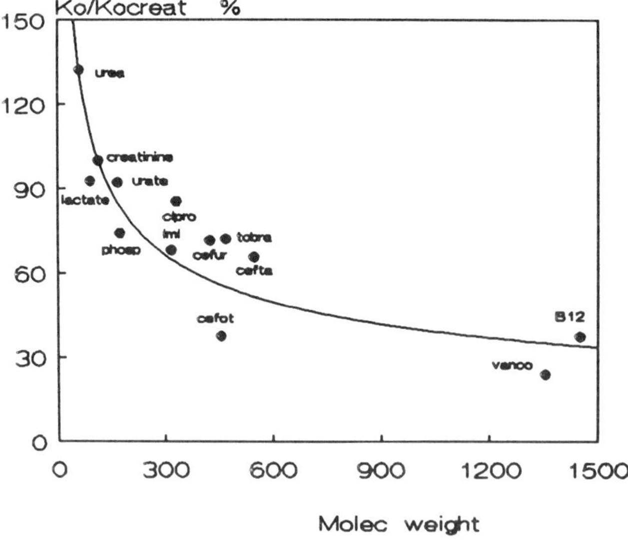

Fig. 12-11. Relation of diffusive mass transfer coefficient (Ko) to solute molecular weight.

Ko and solute molecular weight (MW),[65] which may be described by the equation

$$\frac{Ko}{KoCr} = \left(\frac{113}{MW}\right)^{w} \tag{13}$$

where KoCr is Ko of creatinine, 113 is the molecular weight of creatinine, and the exponent w depends on the membrane and its contribution to diffusion resistance.

To solve equation 10, one needs the Ko value of creatinine for the particular dialyzer and operating conditions. Unfortunately, Ko values are seldom provided by dialyzer manufacturers. In our experience, in the case of conventional hemodialysis typical values for Ko of creatinine are 100 μm/min for cuprophane dialyzers and 140 to 160 μm/min for more permeable membranes such as AN69 and cellulose triacetate. Using AN69 dialyzers in CAVHD, Vincent and colleagues[6,52] found Ko values to vary two- to threefold, depending on the membrane condition as reflected by the rate of ultrafiltration and on dialysate flow rate. An average value of the Ko of creatinine for AN69 dialyzers at a dialysate flow rate of 1 L/h is 120 μm/min. Although these values can seldom be found in the literature, they may be calculated from published data on creatinine clearance by using the analytical solution of equation 13.

The value of the exponent w in equation 13 depends on the membrane and on its relative contribution to the total resistance to diffusion. It may be calculated that *w* takes a value between 0.7 and 0.9 with conventional cellulosic membranes (e.g., cuprophane), and between 0.4 and 0.5 with high-flux membranes. For most practical purposes, more precise determination of w is not important.

Calculation of Drug Removal and Dose Adaptation

Drug elimination from plasma may be conceptualized as the sum of regional clearances, where "regions" may be hepatic metabolism/elimination, renal metabolism/elimination, other organ metabolism/elimination, and dialysis/hemofiltration. In order to calculate total drug removal one must take all these regions into account. At a certain total clearance rate, the plasma concentration half-life depends on the volume of distribution, as discussed earlier. The necessary dose adaptation is not only determined by the predicted plasma concentration but may also depend on the mode of action of the drug. For instance, in the case of an antibiotic that causes dose-dependent killing of bacteria, one aims for a certain peak level of the drug. If the action of the drug is time-dependent rather than dose-dependent, the minimum effective drug level must be maintained for a certain time period.

A simple model of the pharmacokinetics is based on the assumption that a single compartment contains the drug. This implies that removal of a certain amount of drug immediately results in a proportional decrease in the drug concentration. The fall in drug concentration over time is given by the formula

$$C_t = C_0 \times e^{\left(-\frac{Cl}{Vd} \times t\right)} \tag{14}$$

where Cl is the total drug clearance, which is the sum of the regional clearances, and Vd is the volume of distribution of the drug. Figure 12-12 shows the concentration in time of imipenem and cilastatin after starting treatment by CAVHD. During the untreated period, the concentration of cilastatin had increased due to its low clearance rate in renal failure. The contribution of the clearance by CAVHD to the total clearance rate is much higher in the case of cilastatin than in that of imipenem.

From equation 14 one may derive the formula for the calculation of the half-life of the drug:

$$T_{1/2} = \frac{0.693 \times Vd}{C1} \tag{15}$$

For steady-state conditions, dosage adaptations may be made either by changing the dose itself or by changing the dose interval according to the calculated drug half-life.[1] The impact of intermittent dialysis treatment may best be expressed in terms of the percentage of drug removal. If, for instance,

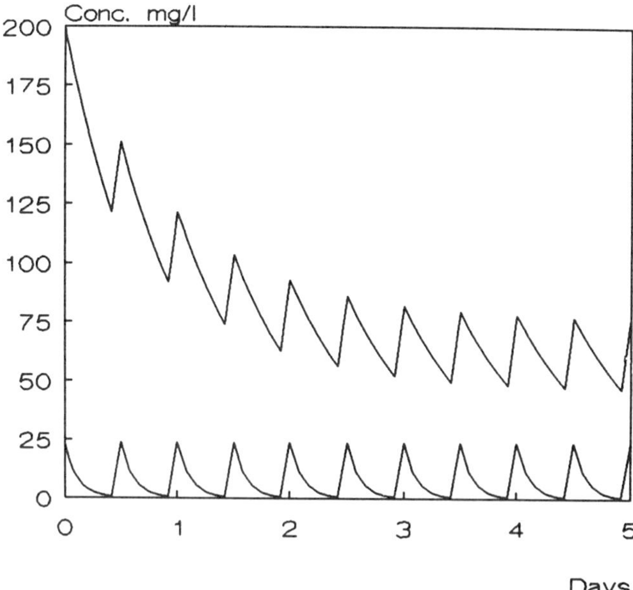

Fig. 12-12. Plasma concentration-time profiles of cilastatin (upper curve) and imipenem (lower curve).

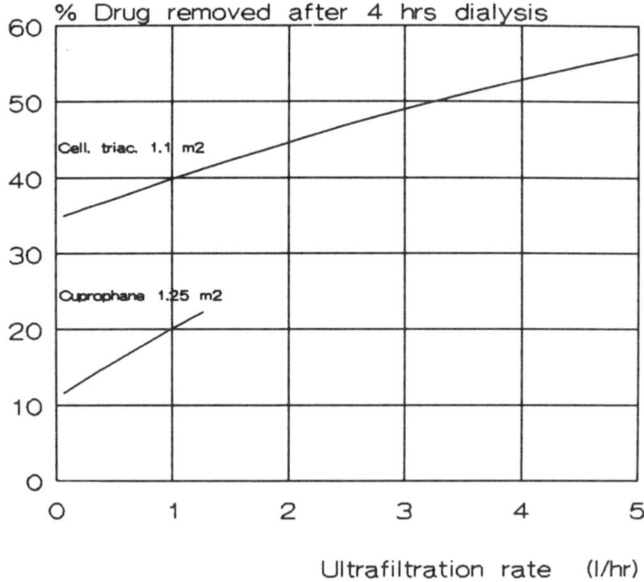

Fig. 12-13. Removal of vancomycin using a conventional cuprophane membrane dialyzer and a high-efficiency cellulose triacetate dialyzer.

half of the total amount of drug is removed by one dialysis session, one may administer half of the normal loading dose immediately after dialysis. The percentage of the drug that is removed by dialysis or hemofiltration may be calculated by equations 10 and 13. As an example, Figure 12-13 shows the percentage removal of vancomycin during hemodialysis/hemodiafiltration using a 1.25-m^2 cuprophane dialyzer or a 1.1-m^2 cellulose triacetate dialyzer. With both dialyzers, urea clearance is 140 ml/min at zero ultrafiltration and the corresponding urea reduction is 75 percent. Urea clearance may be increased to 180 ml/min and urea reduction to 83 percent by hemodiafiltration at an ultrafiltration rate of 5 L/hr. With vancomycin, very little is removed during conventional cuprophane hemodialysis, whereas one-third of the drug is removed by the high-efficiency cellulose triacetate dialyzer.[32] Drug removal may be further increased by hemodiafiltration. (See discussion of vancomycin below.)

CLINICAL APPLICATIONS

Vancomycin

Bastani et al.[32] first compared vancomycin and urea clearances through dialyzers of different membrane material. Employing conventional flow rates and dialyzer surface areas, they found that vancomycin clearance was highest with AN69 membranes, intermediate with cellulose acetate, and lowest with cuprophane. The exact opposite was noted for urea clearance. Barth et al.[33] reported similar findings and quantitated a threefold increase in vancomycin clearance with use of an AN69 membrane over that obtained with compared to a cellulosic membrane of comparable size. Torras et al.[66] demonstrated similar results and further showed that by increasing blood flow rates from 250 to 350 ml/min through an AN69 dialyzer, vancomycin clearance increased by another 50 percent. Up to 200 mg of vancomycin could be removed during a high-flux hemodialysis session. De Bock et al.[23] removed at least that much using a cellulose acetate dialyzer under standard operating conditions. With this particular membrane, Bastani et al.[32] found intermediate vancomycin clearances.

Lanese et al.[21] applied the principles described in detail above and examined the relationship among membrane surface area, ultrafiltration coefficient (hydraulic permeability), vitamin B_{12} clearance, and the removal of vancomycin. They demonstrated a strict linear relationship between vitamin B_{12} clearance and vancomycin clearance (Fig. 12-14). Lanese and Molitoris[67] concluded that the correlation between the clearance of vitamin B_{12} and the percentage of vancomycin removal may be the best available data in the absence of specific dialyzer vancomycin removal rates. Mathematically, they derived the following expression for vancomycin removal during dialysis:

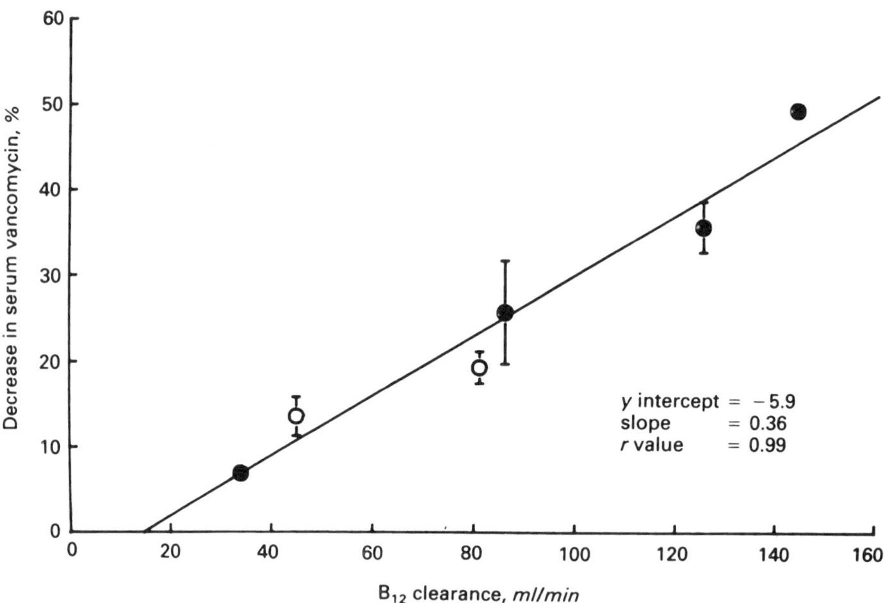

Fig. 12-14. The correlation between percentage decrease in plasma vancomycin levels and manufacturer's vitamin B_{12} clearance of individual dialyzers. For all data points Qb was 250 ml/min and duration of dialysis 4 hours. The solid symbols are from Lanese et al.[21] and form the basis for the linear regression. The open symbols represent the data of Bastani et al.[32] with cellulose acetate and AN69. (From Lanese et al.,[21] with permission.)

$$\text{Percent vancomycin removal during dialysis} = (0.09 \times Cl_{B_{12}} - 1.5) \times (0.75 + 0.001 \times Q_B) \times (\text{time, hours}) \quad (15)$$

where $Cl_{B_{12}}$ is the manufacturer's reported vitamin B_{12} clearance, Q_B is dialyzer blood flow, and "time, hours" is duration of dialysis.[21] This very clever analysis is an extrapolation of the principles described in this chapter. Such an approach is possible for many of the medications that we frequently use.

Deferoxamine

Deferoxamine (DFO) is a poorly protein-bound 657-dalton molecule, which is used to chelate body aluminum so that it can be removed by dialysis. Using a Q_b of 250 ml/min and a Q_d of 500 ml/min, Molitoris et al.[68] showed that total plasma aluminum clearance was four times greater with polysulfone dialyzers than with cuprophane dialyzers. Muirhead et al.[69] were not able to demonstrate such an advantage for AN69 dialyzers. Minimal ultrafiltration occurred during the study with the AN69 membrane, and Molitoris et al.[68] excluded ultrafiltration from their polysulfone calculations. However, the plasma clearance was calculated from arteriovenous differences. Convective losses may be masked by this calculation because the arterial and venous concentrations differ so little during hemofiltration. Since hemofiltration has been shown to be superior to dialysis in removing aluminum with DFO,[70,71] it is possible that the clearance noted by Molitoris et al.[68] is from combined convection and diffusion. Even with minimal net ultrafiltration, substantial convection and backfiltration can occur, contributing to the removal of relatively large solutes. Studies are currently in progress to determine the mode of solute transfer under these conditions.

CONCLUSIONS

There is a curious paucity of data regarding drug removal during high-efficiency or high-flux dialysis. Several explanations are plausible. First and foremost is that there are only a few centers performing these techniques whose medical staff interested in or experienced with such studies. Most published reports addressing these dialytic strategies emphasize control of uremia, metabolism in general, or survival. We are now just entering the next level of research in these technologies, which will include drug handling. Therefore, temporarily we must extrapolate from the conventional dialysis and CAVH data and the mathematical modeling described above.

Certain generalizations can be safely suggested. High-efficiency dialysis uses what are considered tight membranes. Urea clearance is high because flow rates and surface areas are increased above those seen in conventional dialysis. These adjustments allow for shortened dialysis time while overall dialysis delivery is probably unchanged from that of conventional dialysis. Therefore, drug dosing recommendations for conventional dialysis will probably apply reliably to high-efficiency dialysis.[1] This will need to be confirmed in clinical trials but is a reasonable assumption at present.

High-flux dialysis involves several variables that make generalizations more difficult and predictions risky. For example, while the open membranes used in this technique may demonstrate greater diffusivity and convectivity (and thus clearance) for middle molecular weight species, the shortened dialysis time may reduce overall clearance. The larger the molecule, the longer it takes to remove it, no matter what membrane is used. Even though most drugs are either small molecules with molecular weights less than 500 or are in the lowest ranges of middle molecular weight, this principle of time and clearance applies. In addition, any technique that uses shortened dialysis times jeopardizes the clearance of molecules that are bound to tissue or deposited intracellularly to a substantial degree. Unbound or extracellular drug that is rapidly removed by dialysis cannot be replaced quickly from protein-bound, tissue-bound, or intracellular stores. Therefore, the openness of the membrane and the shortening of dialysis time may counteract each other regarding overall drug clearance. Some membranes, particular AN69, bind drugs more readily than other high-flux membranes. Therefore, until actual studies are performed to define drug removal during high-flux dialysis, we must remain cautious.

ACKNOWLEDGMENTS

The authors extend their gratitude to Norma Thompson for her secretarial efforts and to Richard A. Ward, Ph.D., for his general advice.

REFERENCES

1. Bennett WM, Aronoff GR, Golper TA et al: Drug Prescribing in Renal Failure: Dosing Guidelines for Adults. 2nd Ed. Am College Physicians, Philadelphia, 1991
2. Golper TA: Drug handling during continuous therapies. p. 145. In Paganini EP (ed): Acute Continuous Renal Replacement Therapy. Martinus Nijhoff, Boston, 1993
3. Ronco C: Backfiltration in clinical dialysis: nature of the phenomenon, mechanisms, and possible solutions. Int J Artif Org 13:11, 1990
4. Leypoldt JK, Schmidt B, Gurland HJ: Measurement of backfiltration rates during hemodialysis with highly permeable membranes. Blood Purif 9:74, 1991
5. Leypoldt JK, Schmidt B, Gurland HJ: Net ultrafiltration may not eliminate backfiltration during hemodialysis with highly permeable membranes. Artif Organs 15:160, 1991

6. Vincent HH, Vos MC, Akcahuseyin E et al: Blood flow, ultrafiltration and solute transport rate in CAVHD: the AN69 flat plate haemofilter. Nephrol Dial Transplant 7:29, 1992
7. Keller F, Wilms H, Schultze G et al: Effect of plasma protein binding, volume of distribution, and molecular weight on the fraction of drugs eliminated by hemodialysis. Clin Nephrol 19:201, 1983
8. Sprenger KGB, Stephan H, Kratz W et al: Optimizing of hemodiafiltration with modern membranes? Contrib Nephrol 46:43, 1985
9. Lasrich M, Maher JM, Hirszel P, Maher JF: Correlation of peritoneal transport rates with molecular weight: a method of predicting clearances. ASAIO 2:107, 1979
10. Maher JF: Principles of dialysis and dialysis of drugs. Am J Med 62:475, 1977
11. Gulyassy PF, Depner TA: Impaired binding of drugs and endogenous ligands in renal disease. Am J Kidney Dis 98:730, 1983
12. McNamara PJ, Lalka D, Gibaldi M: Endogenous accumulation products and serum protein binding in uremia. J Lab Clin Med 98:730, 1981
13. Golper TA, Bennett WM. Drug usage in dialysis patients. In p. 608. Clinical Dialysis. 2nd Ed., Nissenson A, Fine R, Gentile D (eds): Appleton-Century-Crofts, Norwalk, CT, 1988
14. Vos MC, Vincent HH, Mouton JW et al: Drug clearance by continuous hemodiafiltration (CAVHD). Results with the AN-69 capillary hemofilter and recommended dose adjustments. (submitted for publication)
15. Lee CC, Marbury TC: Drug therapy in patients undergoing haemodialysis. Clin Pharmacokinet 9:42–66, 1984
16. Piafsky KM. Disease-induced changes in the plasma binding of basic drugs. Clin Pharmacokinet 5:246, 1980
17. Dromgoole SH: The effect of hemodialysis on the binding capacity of albumin. Clin Chim Acta 46:469, 1973
18. Rustein DD, Catelli WP, Nickerson RJ: Heparin and human lipid metabolism. Lancet 2:1003, 1969
19. Suh B, Craig WA, England AC, Elliot RL: Effect of free fatty acids on protein binding of antimicrobial agents. J Infect Dis 143:609, 1981
20. Golper TA, Saad AMA, Morris CD: Gentamicin and phenytoin sieving through hollow-fiber polysulfone hemofilters. Kidney Int 30:937, 1986
21. Lanese DM, Alfrey PS, Molitoris BA: Markedly increased clearance of vancomycin during hemodialysis using polysulfone dialyzers. Kidney Int 35:1409, 1989
22. Fabris A, La Greca G, Chiaramonte S et al: Total solute extraction versus clearance in the evaluations of standard and short hemodialysis. ASAIO Trans 34:627, 1988
23. De Bock V, Verbeelen D, Naes V, Sennesael J: Pharmacokinetics of vancomycin in patients undergoing hemodialysis and hemofiltration. Nephrol Dial Transplant 4:635, 1989
24. Matzke GR, O'Connell MB, Collins AJ, Keshaviah PR: Disposition of vancomycin during hemofiltration. Clin Pharmacol Ther 40:425, 1986
25. Marbury TC, Lee CC, Perchalski RJ, Wilder BJ: Hemodialysis clearance of ethosuximide in patients with chronic renal disease. Am J Hosp Pharm 38:1757, 1981
26. Lee CS, Marbury TC, Benet LZ: Clearance calculations in hemodialysis: application to blood, plasma, and dialysate measurements for ethambutol. J Pharmacokinet Biopharm 8:69, 1980

27. Buur T, Lundberg M: Secondary effects of erythropoietin treatment on metabolism and dialysis efficiency in stable hemodialysis patients. Clin Nephrol 34:230, 1990
28. Reidenberg MM: The biotransformation of drugs in renal failure. Am J Med 62:482, 1977
29. Levy G: Pharmacokinetics in renal disease. Am J Med 62:461, 1977
30. Gibson TP: Problems in designing hemodialysis drug studies. Pharmacotherapy 5:23, 1985
31. Brunner H, Mann H, Stiller S, Sieberth H-G: Permeability for middle and higher molecular weight substances. Contrib Nephrol 46:33, 1985
32. Bastani R, Spyker SA, Minocha A et al: In vivo comparison of three different hemodialysis membranes for vancomycin clearance: cuprophane, cellulose acetate, and polyacrylonitrile. Dial Transplant 17:527, 1988
33. Barth RH, DeVincenzo N, Zara AC, Berlyne GM: Vancomycin pharmacokinetics in high-flux hemodialysis. Am Soc Nephrol Abstracts and Program, 348, 1990
34. Jindal K, McDougall J, Goldstein M: High-flux dialyzers: impact of ultrafiltration and surface area on clearance of small and large molecular weight substances, abstracted. Natl Kidney Found. Annu Mtg Abstr: A10, 1987
35. Von Albertini B, Miller JH, Gardner PW, Shinaberger JH: Performance characteristics of high-flux haemodiafiltration. Proc Eur Dial Transplant 21:447, 1984
36. Surian M, Malberti F, Corradi B et al: Adequacy of haemodiafiltration. Nephrol Dial Transplant 4:32, 1989
37. Rumpf KW, Rieger J, Dohl B et al: Drug elimination by hemofiltration. J Dial 1:677, 1977
38. Rumpf KW, Rieger J, Ansorg R et al: Binding of antibiotics by dialysis membranes and its clinical relevance. Proc Eur Dial Transplant 14:607, 1978
39. Kraft D, Lode H: Elimination of ampicillin and gentamicin by hemofiltration. Klin Wochenschr 57:195, 1979
40. Kronfol NO, Lau AH, Barakat MM: Aminoglycoside binding to polyacrylonitrile hemofilter membranes during continuous hemofiltration. ASAIO Trans 33:300, 1987
41. Kronfol N, Lau AH, Colon-Rivera J, Libertin CL: Effect of CAVH membrane types on drug sieving coefficients and clearances. ASAIO Trans 32:85, 1986
42. Lau A, Kronfol N, Jaber N, Libertin C: Determinants of drug removal by continuous arteriovenous hemofiltration. Drug Intell Clin Pharm 20:467, 1986
43. Kronfol N Lau A, Jaber N, Libertin C: Effect of membrane properties on drug clearances by CAVH, abstracted. Natl Kidney Found Annu Mtg Abstr: A10, 1986
44. Henderson LW: Hemodialysis: rationale and physical principles. p. 1643. In Brenner BM, Rector FC (eds): The Kidney. 1st Ed. WB Sanders, Philadelphia, 1976
45. Henderson LW, Silverstein ME, Ford CA, Lysaght MJ: Clinical response to maintenance hemodiafiltration. Kidney Int, suppl. 2:S58, 1975
46. Hamilton R, Ford C, Colton C et al: Blood cleansing by diafiltration in uremic dog and man. Trans Am Soc Artif Intern Organs 17:259, 1971
47. Henderson LW, Ford C, Colton CK, et al: Uremic blood cleansing by diafiltration using hollow-filter ultrafilter. Trans Am Soc Artif Intern Organs 16:107, 1970
48. Husted FC, Nolph KD, Vitale FC, Maher JF: Detrimental effects of ultrafiltration on diffusion in coils. J Lab Clin Med 87:435, 1976

49. Nolph KD, Hopkins C, Van Stone J: Effects of ultrafiltration on solute clearances in parallel plate dialyzers. Clin Nephrol 8:453, 1977
50. Nolph KD, New DL: Effects of ultrafiltration on solute clearances in hollow fiber artificial kidneys. J Lab Clin Med 88:593, 1976
51. Jaffrin MY, Ding L, Laurent JM: Simultaneous convective and diffusive mass transfers in a hemodialyzer. J Biomech Eng 112:212, 1990
52. Vincent HH, van Ittersum FJ, Akcahuseyin E et al: Solute transport in continuous arteriovenous hemodiafiltration: a new mathematical model applied to clinical data. Blood Purif 8:149, 1990
53. Bosch T, Schmidt B, Samtleben W, Garland HJ: Effect of protein adsorption on diffusive and convective transport through polysulfone membranes. Contrib Nephrol 46:14, 1985
54. Shaldon SH, Silva H, Rosen M: Technique for refrigerated coil preservation haemodialysis with femoral vein catheterization. Br Med J 2:411, 1964
55. Vincent HH, Akcahuseyin E, Vos MC et al: Determinants of blood flow and ultrafiltration in continuous arteriovenous haemodiafiltration: theoretical predictions and laboratory and clinical observations. Nephrol Dial Transplant 5:1031, 1990
56. Wetzelberger N, Lucker PW: Simple method for prediction and estimation of hemodialyzability of incorporated drugs. Methods Find Exp Clin Pharmacol 7:217, 1985
57. Teehan BP, Smith LJ, Hartigan MF et al: Functional and morphological changes in reused Gambro-Lundia Nova dialyzers. Proc Dial Transplant Forum 5:51, 1975
58. Garred LJ, Canaud B, Flavier JL et al: Effect of reuse on dialyzer efficacy. Artif Organs 14:80, 1990
59. Gagnon RF, Kaye M: Dialyzer performance over prolonged reuse. Clin Nephrol 24:21, 1985
60. Petersen J, Roscoe MM, Kaczmarek RG et al: The effects of reprocessing cuprophane and polysulfone dialyzers on β_2-microglobulin removal from hemodialysis patients. Am J Kidney Dis 17:174, 1991
61. Fleming SJ, Foreman K, Stanley K et al: Dialyzer reprocessing with Renalin. Am J Nephrol 11:28, 1991
62. Golper TA, Cigarran-Guldris S, Jenkins RD, Brier ME: The role of convection during simulated continuous arteriovenous hemodialysis. Contrib Nephrol 93:146, 1991
63. Landis EM, Pappenheimer JR: Exchange of substances through the capillary wall. p. 962. In Handbook of Physiology. American Physiological Society Washington, 1963
64. Golper TA: Drug removal during continuous hemofiltration or hemodialysis. Contrib Nephrol 93:110, 1991
65. Vincent HH, Vos MC, Akcahuseyin E et al: Drug clearance by continuous haemodiafiltration (CAVHD). Analysis of sieving coefficient and mass transfer coefficients of diffusion. Blood Purif (in press)
66. Torras J, Cao C, Rivas MC et al: Pharmacokinetics of vancomycin in patients undergoing hemodialysis with polyacrylonitrile. Clin Nephrol 36:35, 1991
67. Lanese D, Molitoris BA: Removal of vancomycin by hemodialysis: a significant and overlooked consideration. Semin Dial 2:73, 1989
68. Molitoris BA, Alfrey AC, Alfrey PS, Miller NL: Rapid removal of DFO-chelated aluminum during hemodialysis using polysulfone dialyzers. Kidney Int 34:98, 1988

69. Muirhead N, Hollomby DJ, Leung FY et al: Removal of aluminum during hemodialysis: effect of different dialyzer membranes. Am J Kidney Dis 8:51, 1986
70. Weiss LG, Danielson BG, Fellstrom B, Wikstrom B: Aluminum removal with hemodialysis, hemofiltration, and charcoal hemoperfusion in uremic patients after deferoxamine infusion: a comparison of efficacy. Nephron 51:325, 1989
71. Sulkova S, Laurincova Z, Valek A: Haemofiltration or haemodialysis in aluminum elimination? Nephrol Dial Transplant, suppl. 3:S3, 1991

13

High-Efficiency Treatments: Risks and Common Problems Encountered in Clinical Application

Juan P. Bosch
Claudio Ronco

PATIENT COMPLIANCE
HEPARINIZATION
MACHINE MAINTENANCE
DIALYZER REUSE

INTRODUCTION

The clinical application of high-efficiency treatments demands a greater level of technical skills than those required in the practice of conventional hemodialysis. The reduction of treatment time that can be achieved with the use of these newer techniques must not be associated with a reduction in the total quantity of treatment delivered to the patient. This fundamental goal cannot be met unless the dialysis team—nephrologists, nurses, dialysis technicians and dietitians—works together and all members of the staff understand their respective roles in the delivery of the treatment. In high-efficiency treatments the safety margins are greatly reduced as compared with conventional hemodialysis. The dialysis personnel must be alert, have the knowledge required to identify the problems that may appear, understand these problems and execute the necessary changes.

RECIRCULATION

Recirculation in the vascular access has been known since the early years of hemodialysis.[1] The impact of recirculation on the efficiency of conventional hemodialysis was small, and thus it was not emphasized.[2] In high-efficiency treatments, recirculation is an important variable and must always be considered as a potential source of discrepancy between prescribed and delivered treatment. Figure 13-1 depicts schematically a vascular access for hemodialysis. In Figure 13-1A there is no recirculation; the blood from the systemic circulation is "pulled" by the blood pump and "pushed" toward the dialyzer, and the dialyzed blood returns to the systemic circulation through the venous line. Figure 13-1B depicts the same vascular access but this time a distal venous obstruction is assumed. If a high blood flow is used during the treatment, a significant fraction of the access blood is pulled to the extracorporeal circuit by the blood pump, and a negative pressure inside the vascular access is thus created. This newly generated negative pressure may increase even further the blood flow to the region where the vascular access is located. On the venous side of the vascular access, the blood returning from the dialyzer has a higher viscosity and because of this together with an increased volume of flow through the access, the forward flow may find a greater distal resistance and favor recirculation. This hypothesis may explain why recirculation

No recirculation - Conventional Hemodialysis

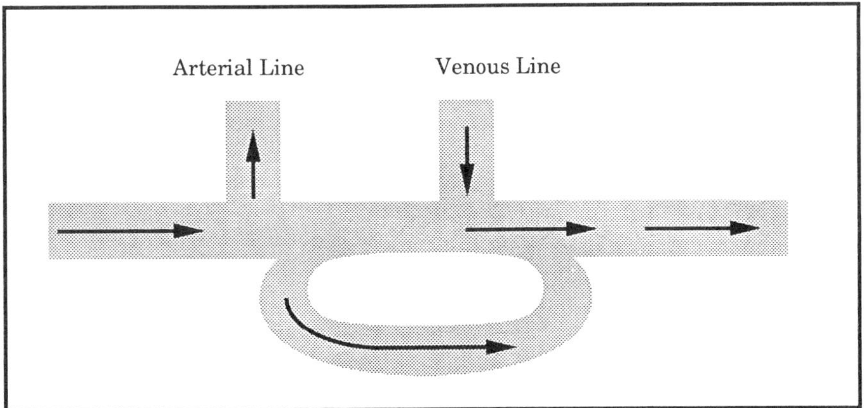

Recirculation - High-Efficiency Treatment

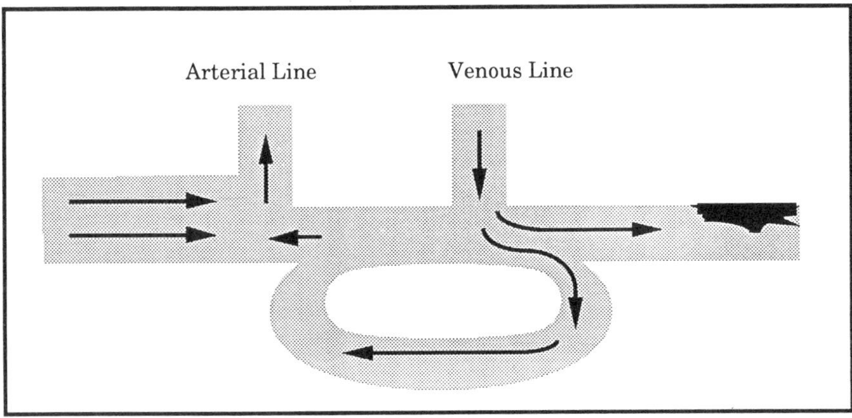

Fig. 13-1. Schematic drawings of a vascular access, (**A**) without and (**B**) with recirculation.

is likely to increase during treatment as well as why recirculation may occur in the vascular access at rest with blood flows over 800 ml/min.

Definition

Recirculation (R) during hemodialysis represents the fraction of the blood flow entering the dialyzer in the arterial line (Qbi) that derives from the blood exiting the dialyzer (Qr) rather than from the systemic circulation (equation 1). When the blood entering the dialyzer originates in its entirety from the systemic circulation, there is no recirculation. At the blood flows rates used in high-efficiency treatments, recirculation is always present to a greater or lesser extent during treatment.

$$R = \frac{Qr}{Qbi} \qquad (1)$$

Measurement

Recirculation can be calculated from the systemic concentration (Cs), the concentration at the dialyzer inlet (Ci), and the concentration at the dialyzer outlet (Cv) of urea nitrogen or other solute. Blood urea nitrogen (BUN) has been traditionally used for this calculation due to the ease of measurement and the large concentration gradients that exit between the inlet and outlet concentration (see equation 2, below).

Blood flow (Qb) dialyzer inlet	=	Qb from systemic circulation	+	Qb from venous outlet
Qbi	=	(Qbi − Qr)	+	(Qr)
Solute at dialyzer inlet	=	solute in the systemic blood	+	solute in recirculated blood
$Qbi \times Ci$	=	$(Qbi - Qr) \times Cs$	+	$Qr \times Cv$
and				
$Qbi \times Ci$	=	$Qbi \times Cs - Qr \times Cs$	+	$Qr \times Cv$
$Qr \times Cs - Qr \times Cv$	=	$Qbi \times Cs - Qbi \times Ci$		
$Qr(Cs - Cv)$	=	$Qbi\ (Cs - Cv)$		
Qr/Qbi	=	$(Cs - Ci)/(Cs - Cv)$		

The ideal method to measure recirculation must be accurate and reproducible. The "gold standard" for this measurement has been to obtain simultaneously a separate sample from the systemic circulation, generally the arm opposite to that used for the vascular access, and samples from the arterial and venous inlets of the dialyzer at the blood flow rate customarily used. The samples are usually obtained in the first 30 minutes of the therapy to take advantage of the large gradient between the inlet and outlet samples. Recirculation is then calculated as

$$\text{Recirculation} = \frac{[BUN]s - [BUN]i}{[BUN]s - [BUN]v} \qquad (2)$$

where the brackets denote the BUN concentration.

The measurement of recirculation using a systemic sample has always met with objection from patients since it requires a third venipuncture. To obviate this extra puncture two other methods may be used. In the first of these, recirculation is measured without a systemic sample by obtaining inlet and outlet samples at a low pump speed; then further reducing the blood pump speed to provide a minimum flow; and after 1 minute, when recirculation has presumably stopped, obtaining a new sample at the inlet, which should approximate the systemic concentration. It is critical in this method that enough time be allowed between reducing pump speed and obtaining the new "systemic" sample. In the second method recirculation is measured without dialysate flow. Samples from the inlet and outlet are obtained and dialysate flow is put on bypass. Because passage of dialysate through the dialyzer is prevented, the blood passing through it will not experience changes in concentration (i.e., the blood leaving the dialyzer will have a concentration equal to that of the systemic blood entering it). In this method it is also critical to allow sufficient time (1 minute) before obtaining the "systemic" sample at the inlet.

During high-efficiency treatments the urea clearance of the extracorporeal system may exceed the blood flow to a given part of the body (e.g., the lower extremities or splanchnic region). Therefore, if during the treatment a peripheral and/or central venous blood specimen is obtained, it may show a significant difference from the sample obtained at the dialyzer inlet, even when no recirculation is present. In high-efficiency treatments, therefore, it is incorrect to use a peripheral sample to measure recirculation. The inlet sample should be used for measuring access recirculation in treatments with a urea clearance in excess of 200 ml/min.

Monitoring of venous pressure during the treatment has been suggested as a means of detecting the presence of recirculation. This approach observation is acceptable at blood flow rates below 250 ml/min, but at higher blood flow rates venous pressure is no longer a reliable indicator of recirculation. Clinical observation of a dark venous bubble trap during hemodialysis when using a peripheral arteriovenous access (fistula or graft) is a gross indicator of recirculation.

Factors Important in the Development of Recirculation

The most important factors in increasing recirculation during the treatment are needle positioning, blood flow rate, and distal venous obstruction. Needle positioning is an important factor in generating recirculation in a vascular access even when using low blood flows and is particularly important in vascular grafts when the arterial needle is placed downstream from the graft. When recirculation varies greatly from one measurement to the other, needle placement must be carefully assessed and recorded.

There is no question that at blood flows greater than 250 ml/min, recirculation increases. The clinician's awareness of the risks of recirculation must increase proportionally with the use of high blood flow rates during the treatment.

Distal venous obstruction is the most frequent cause of recirculation. The increased resistance to flow generated in the narrow venous lumina favor backflow of blood and recirculation. Proximal obstructions to the blood flow result in ischemia during the treatment and are an infrequent cause of recirculation.

Effect on Clearance

Recirculation during the treatment will not affect dialyzer clearance per se but will have an impact in the total quantity of solutes removed from the patient over a fixed time period. The dialyzer clearance is equal to the solute mass removed in a given time divided by the plasma concentration at the blood inlet [Clearance (ml/min) = mass removed (mg/min)/Ci (mg/ml)]. Assuming that in the absence of recirculation the inlet concentration of a solute is 0.80 mg/dl and that the solute is removed at a rate of 100 mg/min, the dialyzer clearance is 125 ml/min. In the presence of 25.5 percent recirculation (Cs = 0.80, Ci = 0.70, and Cv = 0.408 mg/dl respectively), the inlet concentration is now 0.70 mg/dl, the solute removal rate is 87.5 mg/min, and the dialyzer clearance is again 125 ml/min. From the patient's point of view, during each minute 12.5 mg less solute is removed (i.e., body clearance decreases from 125 109.4 ml/min). This is the effective clearance and represents the clearance of clinical importance. Recirculation will have varying effects on the clearance of different solutes depending on their permeability characteristics and plasma concentration.

Effective Clearance

Effective clearance[4] represents the impact of recirculation on the dialyzer clearance and can be calculated by equation 3:

$$\text{Effective clearance (ml/min)} = \text{dialyzer clearance } [1 - 1.05 \times R\,(1 - Cv/Ci)] \qquad (3)$$

where R is recirculation, CV is concentration in the venous line, and Ci is concentration arterial line. In general the dialyzer clearance is reduced by slightly less than the percentage of recirculation (% decreased in dialyzer clearance = 0.85 × % recirculation + 0.98). That is, in a dialyzer with a urea clearance of 250 ml/min at a blood flow of 450 ml/min and a recirculation of 15 percent at the same blood flow will have an effective clearance decrease of about 13.7 percent, or 216 ml/min.

Table 13-1. Effects of Recirculation on Clearance and Kt/V

Amount of Recirculation	Effect of Recirculation on Dialyzer Clearance: Dialyzer 1 Clearance (ml/min)	Dialyzer 2 Clearance (ml/min)
0	200	300
10%	181	272
20%	160	246

Amount of Recirculation	Effect of Recirculation on Kt/V: Prescribed Kt/V	Actual Kt/V
0	1.0	1.0
10%	1.0	0.92
20%	1.0	0.83

Clinical Consequences of Recirculation

The most important consequences of recirculation is a reduction in the total amount of solute removed during the treatment. Recirculation will reduce the prescribed Kt/V (K = dialyzer clearance, V = volume of solute distribution, t = dialysis time) owing to the discrepancy between the dialyzer clearance and the effective clearance (Table 13-1).

What level of recirculation is acceptable? In conventional hemodialysis 10 to 15 percent has been considered acceptable. In high-efficiency hemodialysis the clearance used to calculate the dialysis prescription must be corrected for any recirculation amounting to 10 percent or more. Monthly measurement of recirculation must be a routine procedure in units practicing high-efficiency hemodialysis. An advantage of this policy is that, in addition to permitting adjustment of the dialysis prescription for recirculation, it may permit detection of distal obstruction in the vascular access, indicated by a progressive increase in recirculation over time. In our experience a progressive increase in recirculation is an indication for angiography in order to determine whether an angioplasty may correct the distal obstruction.

USE OF HIGH BLOOD FLOWS

The use of high blood flows in high-efficiency dialysis generates a series of events that are not seen in conventional hemodialysis. Most of these phenomena are the results of the hydraulic pressures generated within the extracorporeal circuit. Figure 13-2 depicts a schematic pressure profile of the extracorporeal circuit in high-efficiency hemodialysis. There are two particularly salient points in this pressure profile: the negative pressure generated in the arterial line before the blood pump and the positive pressure observed after the arterial pump.

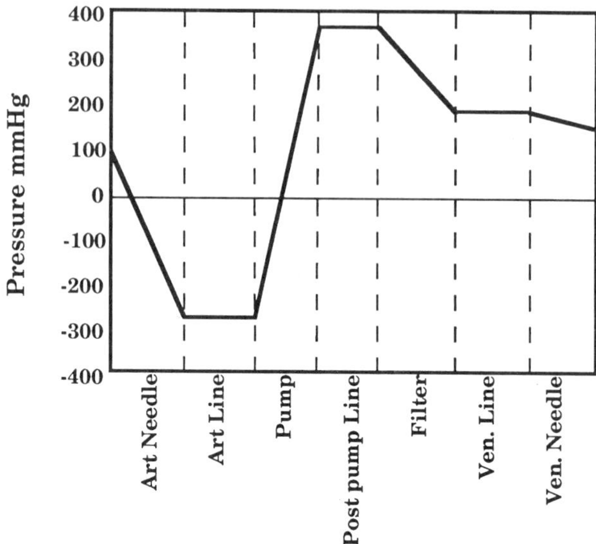

Fig. 13-2. Pressure profile in the extracorporeal circuit during high-efficiency hemodialysis.

High Negative Arterial Pressure

Figure 13-3 depicts the pressure in the arterial line before the blood pump at 300 and at 500 ml/min. It is apparent that at higher blood flows the pressure in this segment become more negative as a result of the pulling of the blood through an area of high resistance (the needle). This greater negative pressure can have two adverse consequences. First, it may lead to the generation of microbubbles due to the entry of air into the blood circuit. Blood degassing may also contribute to the generation of these microbubbles. Very small microbubbles may not be detected by the air bubble detector and thus may reach the patient. This phenomenon may be minimized by making sure that all connections in the extracorporeal circuit are airtight so that no air entry will occur even under high negative pressures. It is important that blood flow rates be compatible with needle size and that the conditions of the blood access be such that no excessive negative pressure are generated during the treatment.

The second effect of high negative arterial pressure is its interferes with the reexpansion of the blood tubing inside the blood pump segment; since the lumen is effectively decreased, the blood flow delivered is less than expected. The magnitude of this effect is shown in Figure 13-3.

High Positive Pressure after the Arterial Pump

The significant pressure gradients that are generated between the blood and dialysate paths result in a phenomenon unique to high-efficiency treatment, namely, backfiltration, which is the passage of dialysate fluid into the

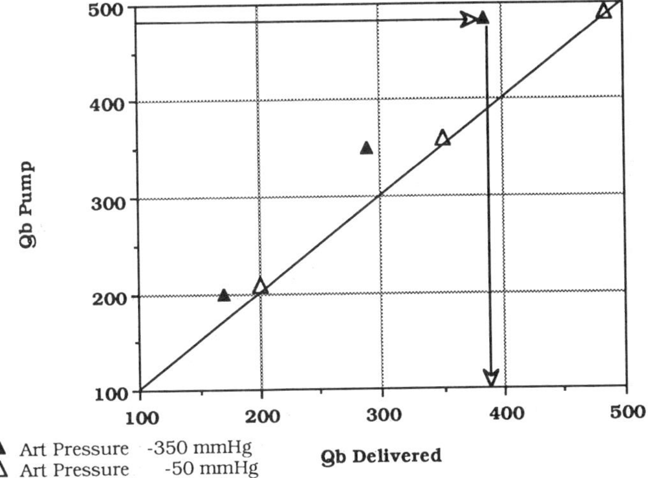

Fig. 13-3. Effect of negative pressure in the prepump segment on the delivery of blood flow during high-efficiency treatments.

blood compartment in response to a pressure gradient between the blood and dialysate paths. The practical implications of this phenomenon are that (1) the dialysate fluid gain will tend to neutralize the fluid losses from blood to dialysate (ultrafiltrate), and (2) the increased amount of ultrafiltration during the treatment will augment the total amount of solute removed during the treatment. The amount of backfiltration will depend directly on the pressure gradient between the blood and dialysate paths. The water permeability of the membrane used will also determine the volume of backfiltration during the treatment (Fig. 13-4). To avoid pyrogenic reactions, we recommend, in addition to the dialysate water standards of the Association for Advancement of Medical Instrumentation (AAMI), the filtration of the dialysate prior to enter the dialyzer. This is easily accomplished by placing two polysulfone hollow-fiber dialyzers in series in the dialysate path. These dialyzer need to be changed only after several months of use. In our unit the dialyzers are changed every 6 months.

Pump Calibration

Since in all forms of high-efficiency treatments a blood flow in excess of 350 ml/min is used, it is imperative that the blood pump of the dialysis machine is able to provide accurately the prescribed blood flow. To achieve this goal blood pumps must be calibrated on a monthly basis, and the blood tubing used must have a pump segment with a constant inside diameter. The blood pump should be calibrated at different pump speeds with fluid at body temperature and at the negative pressures measured in the prepump

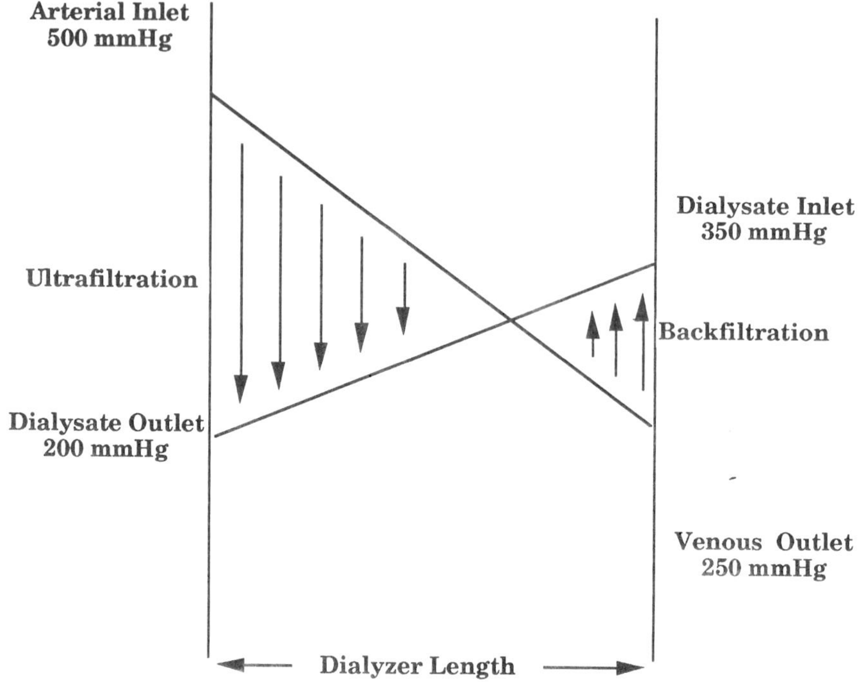

Fig. 13-4. Backfiltration in high-flux hemodialysis.

segment during the treatment. Removing the dialyzer from the circuit after clinical use and connecting the arterial line to the joined dialysate lines is a convenient method of obtaining warm fluid at a controllable negative pressure for blood pump calibration in many dialysis machines. The actual blood flow should be recorded and posted for comparison with that indicated by the digital flowmeter.

DIALYZER SELECTION: FACTORS AFFECTING DIALYZER CLEARANCE

The selection of the dialyzer for hemodialysis requires an assessment of biocompatibility, distribution and amount of solutes removed during the treatment, ultrafiltration capacity, and the cost. In high-efficiency treatments the following additional factors must be considered: (1) not all dialyzers increase their performance with augmentation of the blood or dialysate flow rate; (2) the ultrafiltration rate of some of the dialyzers commercially available may be greater than the sensitivity of the ultrafiltration control system of the dialysis equipment available; and (3) in high-efficiency dialysis the performance of the dialyzer may be enhanced by increasing the dialysate flow rate.

The clearance of a particular solute in a dialyzer is dependent on the following variables: (1) the product of the mass transfer coefficient and the area (KoA); (2) blood flow rates; (3) dialysate flow rate; and (4) the ultrafiltration coefficient of the dialyzer. In order to select the "right dialyzer" for high-efficiency treatments, it is important to understand the role of these variables.

Concept of KoA

The KoA parameter defines a property of the dialyzer determined by the surface area, membrane characteristics, and dialyzer geometry. The interrelationships between KoA, blood flow, and dialyzer clearance have been defined[5] and permit the clinician to evaluate the benefits of one dialyzer against another as well as to determine the effects of increasing blood flow and dialysate flow. The known clearance of a dialyzer at a particular blood flow rate cannot be extrapolated to determine the clearance of that device at a different blood flow and/or a different dialysate flow rate, but on the other hand, knowledge of the KoA does allow to prediction the clearance of a dialyzer at any blood or dialysate flow rate from a known clearance.

The KoA is calculated by the following steps:

1. The manufacturer has supplied the blood clearance of a given solute, generally urea, at a known blood flow rate (Qd) and dialysate flow rate (Qd) (e.g., 165 ml/min at a Qb of 200 ml/min and a Qd of 500 ml/min.
2. KoA is then calculated by the equation

$$\text{KoA} = [\text{Qb}/1 - (\text{Qb}/\text{Qd})] \ln [((\text{clearance}/\text{Qd}) - 1)/((\text{clearance}/\text{Qb}) - 1] \quad (4)$$

$$\text{If Qb} = \text{Qd}$$

$$\text{KoA} = \text{clearance}/[1 - (\text{clearance}/\text{Qb})] \quad (5)$$

3. From KoA is possible to calculate the clearance for the dialyzer at any blood or dialysate flow rate by the following equation[5]:

$$\text{D} = \text{Qb}\,[1 - \exp((\text{KoA}/\text{Qb})(1 - \text{Qb}/\text{Qd}))]/[\text{Qb}/\text{Qd} - \exp((\text{KoA}/\text{Qb})(1 - \text{Qb}/\text{Qd}))] \quad (6)$$

This calculations assume that KoA remains constant at all Qb and Qd values, which this may not be the case for high Qd.[4]

Blood Flow

Figure 13-5 shows the relationship between blood flow and clearance for different dialyzers. It is apparent that for dialyzers with a KoA below 400 (surface area below 0.8 m^2), increasing blood flow from 200 to 500 ml/min results in only a small increase in clearance (150 ml/min at Qb 200 ml/min to 200 ml/min at Qb 500 ml/min). In large dialyzers with KoA 700 or higher (surface area 1.4 m^2) increasing blood flow results in significant augmentation of the clearance of the device. This effect tends to decrease when the blood flow exceeds 500 ml/min (clearance was 172 at Qb 200 ml/min and 325 at Qb 500 ml/min) (see Fig. 13-7).

Dialysate Flow Rate

Figure 13-6 shows the effect of different dialysate flow rates on dialyzer clearance at two blood flows. It is apparent that for dialyzers with small KoA (<500) doubling the dialysate flow rate from 500 to 1,000 ml/min results in a 10 percent increase in clearance. For larger dialyzers doubling the dialysate flow rate increases clearance by 14 to 15 percent. (Tables 13-2 and 13-3).

Figure 13-7 simplifies the analysis of all these variables and may be useful in selecting a given dialyzer. From the manufacturer's clearance at a given Qb and Qd, it is easy to extrapolate the KoA. Knowing the KoA makes it possible to judge the performance at different blood flows as well as to assess the impact of increasing the dialysate flow rate.

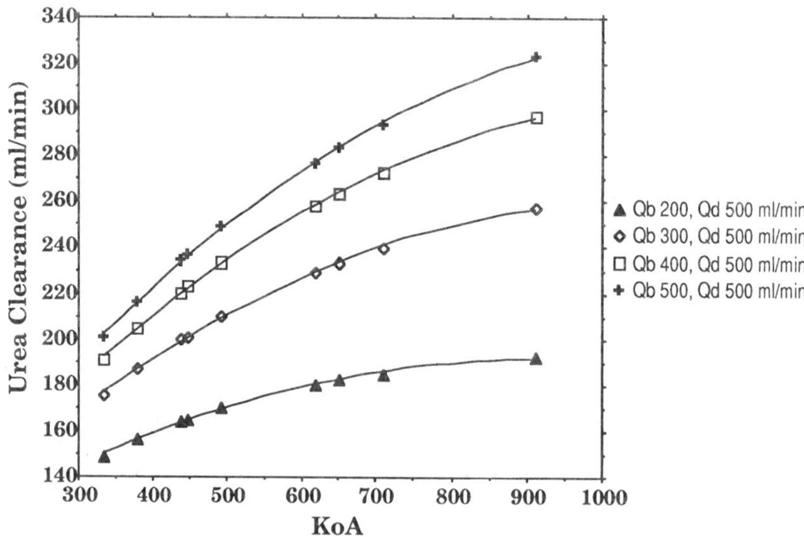

Fig. 13-5. Relationship between mass transfer coefficient–area product (KoA) and urea clearance at different blood flows.

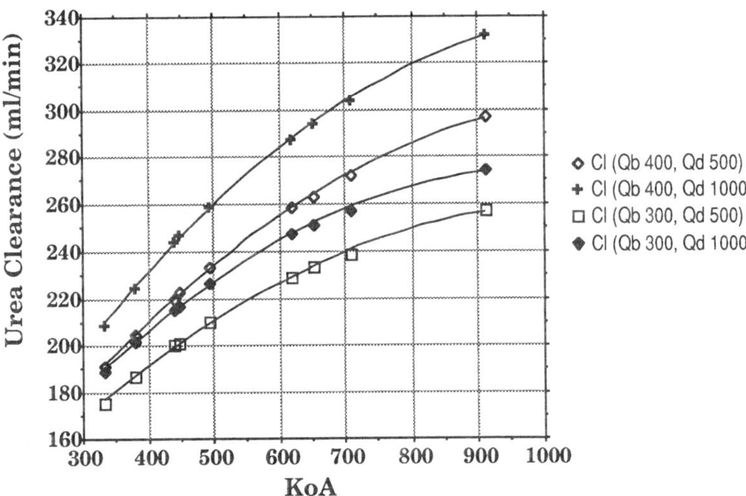

Fig. 13-6. Relationship between mass transfer coefficient–area product (KoA) and urea clearance at different blood flows and different dialysate rates (500 and 1,000 ml/min).

Ultrafiltration Rate

Ultrafiltration will increase the solute clearance to about the volume of ultrafiltration (hemofiltration) or to less than that volume (hemodiafiltration).

PATIENT COMPLIANCE

Patients and staff must be aware of the need to comply with the dialysis prescription. For the staff this entails careful monitoring of the actual treatment time (i.e., the time during which the patient is connected to the extracorporeal circulation and the blood pump has reached the prescribed blood flow). Interruptions in the treatment, due to hypotension or other causes,

Table 13-2. Hollow-Fiber Polysulfone Dialyzers, Hemoflow F-Series (High-Flux), Fresenius AG

	F40	F50	F60	F80
Surface area (m^2)	0.7	1.1	1.3	1.8
KoA	448	619	709	912
Urea clearance (Qb 400, Qd 1,000 ml/min)	246	287	304	332

Table 13-3. Parallel Plate Dialyzers, Lundia IC Series, Gambro

	2N	3N	5N	6N
Surface area (m^2)	0.8	0.8	1.1	1.6
KoA	335	380	439	652
Urea clearance (Qb 400, Qd 1,000 ml/min)	208	240	262	324

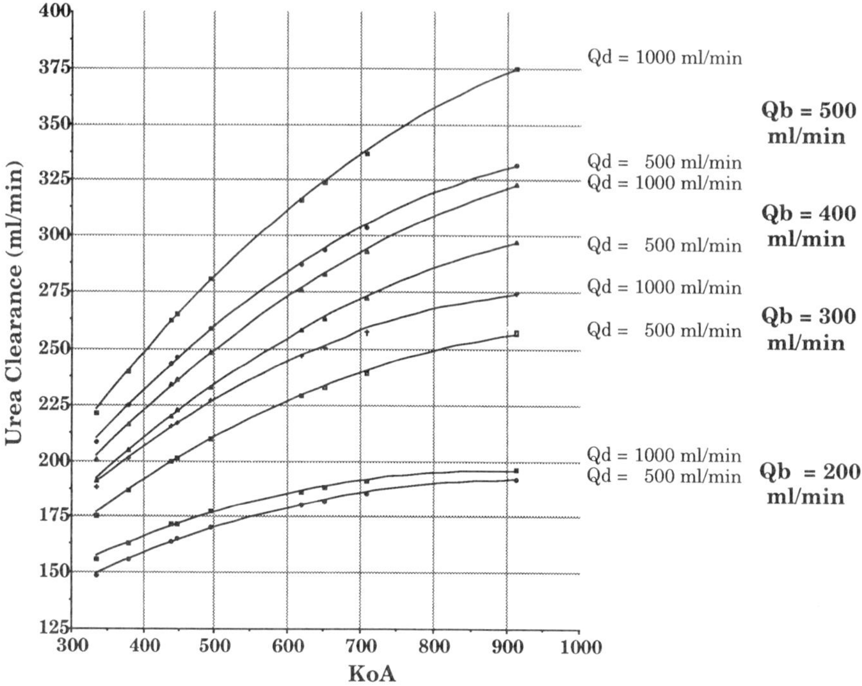

Fig. 13-7. Functional variables in the selection of a dialyzer. This chart permits prediction from a known clearance, of the performance of a dialyzer at different blood and dialysate flow rates within a KoA range of 300 to 900.

should be compensated by extending the treatment time. The time during which the patient is sitting in the dialysis chair without being connected to the extracorporeal circulation is not dialysis time. Patients must also realize the importance of complying with their prescribed treatment time. Patient must also demonstrate compliance by following dietary prescription. Fluid intake may be the most important factor limiting reduction in treatment time. A negative fluid balance greater than 25 ml/min in the majority of patients may be associated with symptomatic hypotension. In diabetic patients the rate of fluid removal may be even less. Therefore in a 3-hour treatment, the maximal amount of fluid removal without symptomatic hypotension is approximately 4.5 L. If a patient consistently gains this large amount of fluid and at the end of the session dry body weight is not reached, the patient is at risk of pulmonary edema in the interdialytic period and should not continue to receive the high-efficiency treatment.

HEPARINIZATION

In high-efficiency treatments heparin is supplied only as an initial bolus. This is important, since patients do not want to stay in the dialysis unit beyond the time required for their treatment. In our unit the policy is to give all patients a 2,000-IU bolus at the beginning of the treatment and to measure activated clotting time. In those patients who are undergoing high-efficiency hemodialysis and in whom dialyzers are not reused, 2,000 to 3,000 IU is most commonly used for a 3- to 3.5-hour treatment. Patients undergoing high-flux hemodialysis or hemodiafiltration require on the average 3,000 to 3,500 IU for a 2.5- to 3-hour treatment. In these patients dialyzers are reused.

MACHINE MAINTENANCE

In general, nephrologists have delegated the care of dialysis equipment to dialysis technicians under the supervision of the nursing staff. In many units physicians are not at all involved in equipment selection. In high-efficiency treatments, equipment performance is paramount in the delivery of the prescription. Therefore nephrologists must have knowledge of the technical factors related to the treatment, including the water treatment process; arterial and venous pressure monitors; the ultrafiltration control system; the dialysate composition, temperature and flow rate; the blood leak detector; blood pump calibration, sterilization, and rinse procedures, and electrical safety. The nephrologist does not need to be directly involved in technical maintenance but must know the issues involved and the procedures carried out to ensure adequate performance of the equipment. The monthly log of equipment testing must be reviewed by the unit director and available for the other nephrologists practicing in that unit.

DIALYZER REUSE

If dialyzer reuse is considered in high-efficiency treatments, in addition to all the established criteria for adequate and safe reprocessing of the dialyzer, special care must be taken with heparinization (see above). An adequate dose of heparin must be established for each patient so that the dialyzer can be reused adequately but no prolonged bleeding occurs at the end of the treatment. It has been accepted that if the volume of the fiber bundle of a reprocessed dialyzer is maintained within 80 percent of the reference volume, the clearance will be 90 percent or more of the reference value.[6] In prescribing the dialysis treatment, the dialyzer clearance must be assumed to be at least 5 to 10 percent less than that of a new dialyzer.

REFERENCES

1. Gotch FA: The Kidney. WB Saunders, Philadelphia, 1976, p. 1680
2. Nardi L, Bosch J: Recirculation: review, techniques for measurement and ability to predict hemoaccess stenosis before and after angioplasty. Blood Purif 6:85, 1988

3. Pederson JA, Dunlay R, Williams J, Llach F: Two-needle calculation of recirculation compared with the standard three-needle method. Clin Nephrol 33:203, 1990
4. Shinaberger JH, Miller JH, Gardner P: Short hemodialysis. p. 360. In Maher JF (ed): Replacement of Renal Function by Dialysis. 3rd Ed., Kluwer, Boston, 1989
5. Michaels AS: Operating parameters and performance criteria for hemodialyzers and other membrane separation devices. Trans Am Soc Artif Intern Organs 12:387, 1966
6. Gotch FA: Quality control tests for validation of dialyzer performance. In: Hemodilayzer Reuse: Issues and Solutions, AAMI Technology Assessment Report 10-85. Association for Advancement of Medical Instrumentation, Arlington, VA, 1985

14

Biocompatibility Issues in High-Efficiency Treatments

Lee W. Henderson

INTRODUCTION

Concern about biocompatibility of the extracorporeal circuit is as old as identification of the need for anticoagulant to prevent the clotting of blood that occurs when surface-sensitive proteins of the clotting cascade come in contact with the nonbiologic surface of the artificial organ.[1] I shall not address the issues surrounding anticoagulation in any detail, as much has been written on this subject previously and it is expected that the reader who is exploring the theory and practice of high-efficiency therapy will have a competent grasp of the subject. Rather, I will focus my comments on the implications of the spate of articles that followed the identification by Kaplow and Goffinet[2] of hemodialysis leukopenia. Colton[3] has referred to this period as the "age of discovery." The artificial kidney is identified in this age as a device that not only transports toxins out of the blood but also acts as a bioreactor, creating downstream pathophysiologic events that may have significant and at times adverse consequences for patient longevity and morbidity. In addition, these events, if thoroughly understood, might be exploited for the benefit of the patient, for example, membrane adsorption of toxins such as β_2-microglobulin.[4]

The term *biocompatibility,* as it applies to the extracorporeal circuit for blood, refers to all abnormal sequelae of the interaction between blood constituents and the nonbiologic surfaces comprised in the circuit. Blood has both cell elements and plasma proteins that may participate in this interaction. I shall address these elements according to my perception of their clinical relevance for high-efficiency treatment. This means that I will not provide a comprehensive review of the subject as it applies to conventional artificial kidney therapy. For example, I will not review all the numerous reports of blood cell perturbation occurring during extracorporeal circulation of blood but rather will describe only those that may have relevance to high-efficiency treatment.

COMPLEMENT ACTIVATION

Background

Figure 14-1 is a simplified diagram of the complement cascade. Figure 14-2 plots the release of the anaphylotoxin C3a versus duration of dialysis for several clinically relevant dialysis membranes, particularly cuprophane and polyacrylonitrile (PAN).[5] Figure 14-3 shows the correlation between plasma concentration of C3a and of C3a desArg and polymorphonuclear leukocyte concentration in the peripheral blood.[5] The alternative pathway shown in Figure 14-1 is now accepted as the predominant participant in the events that occur as a result of the triggering of C3b by a complement-activating dialysis membrane. Conventional dialysis circuit tubing, whether made of silicone rubber or polyethylene, has been shown not to trigger the complement cascade.[6] The initial view was that a covalent bonding of the complement component C3b to the hydroxyl groups on the cellulosic dialysis membrane cuprophane occurred. Subsequent studies by Cheung et al.[7,8] have shown that adsorptive binding to the membrane surface and activation of C3b occur. This adsorptive binding occurs to a greater or lesser extent with all dialysis membranes. The feature that distinguishes a "complement-kind" membrane from one that triggers the cascade is the comparative degree to which two of the complement regulatory proteins, factors B and H, are adsorbed and modulate the rate of anaphylotoxin release. Figure 14-4 is a diagram of the alternate pathway, showing the role of these regulatory proteins. Table 14-1 lists membranes in descending order (worst first) of their capacity to trigger the alternative pathway of complement activation.[9] Several general observations are worthy of note:

1. Synthetic membranes are more complement-kind than cuprophane, the most widely used cellulosic membrane.

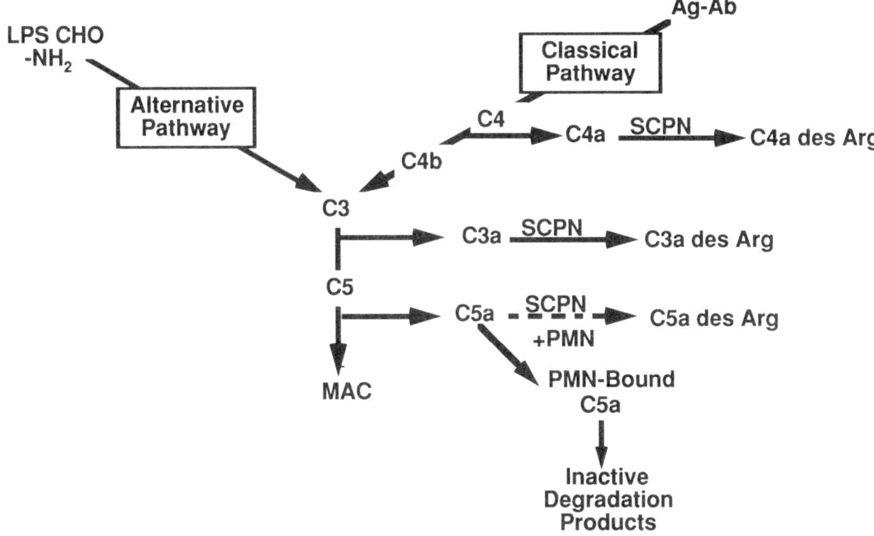

Fig. 14-1. The alternative and classical pathways of complement activation. Lipopolysaccharide (LPS) and carbohydrate moieties (CHO), such as may be found on dialysis membranes along with amino groups, have all been shown to trigger the alternative pathway. Antigen antibody complexes (Ag-Ab) trigger the classical pathway. Release of anaphylotoxins C3a and C5a occurs with the alternative pathway, whereas classical pathway activity results in the release of C4a as well. Enzymatic degradation by serum carboxypeptidase (SCPN) to their desArg forms occurs in plasma.

2. High-flux membranes, being synthetic, are more complement-kind. By *high-flux* I mean membranes that have sufficiently high hydraulic permeability to require special fluid cycling hardware in order to prevent excessive fluid loss during treatment (e.g., PAN or polysulfone).
3. Cellulosic membranes that have their hydroxyl groups modified by acetylation are more complement-kind (e.g., Hemophan, cellulose triacetate).

A notable exception to the above statements is the cellulose triacetate membrane, which is both comparatively complement-kind and high-flux. It is interesting to note that the original view[5,10] of the mechanism by which acetylation or other chemical modification of the hydroxyl groups affects the membrane's action (i.e., that acetylation simply masks all the reactive groups resulting in major reductions in complement activation) was wrong. Two observations contribute to this change in interpretation: first, the determination that specific covalent binding was not what was happening[7,8] and second, the remarkably low substitution rate that causes major amelioration of complement activation (e.g. substitution of 5 percent of the hydroxyl groups of cuprophane yields Hemophan. This latter observation argues for heterogeneity of the adsorptive sites on the membrane, with those that can cause complement activation being selectively acetylated.

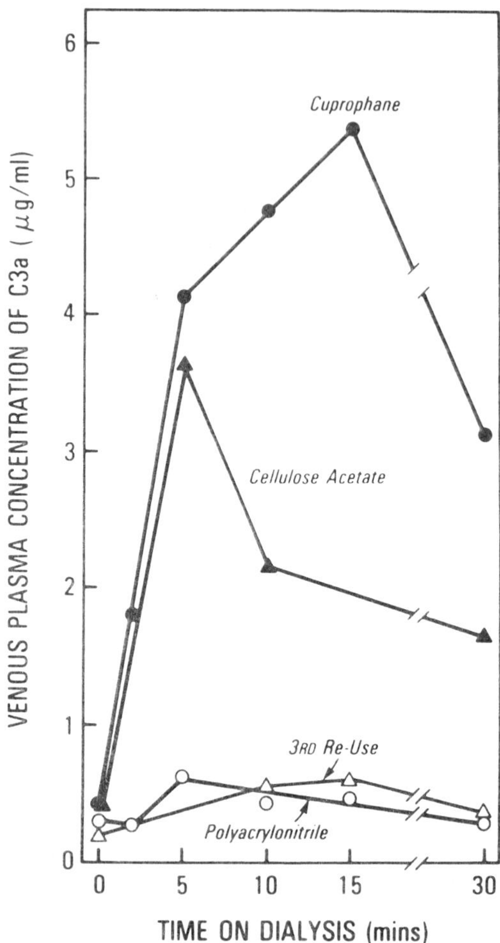

Fig. 14-2. Time-dependent generation of C3a in different dialyzers. Different dialyzers show different concentration versus time profiles in the first 30 minutes of hemodialysis. The reuse protocol carried out in this clinical study was a saline rinse with formaldehyde storage.

What about the impact of membrane area on the amount of anaphylotoxin release? One would think that these variables would be closely correlated. In the course of bench experiments under carefully controlled conditions it has become apparent that while there is a correlation, it is not a fully quantitative one (i.e., doubling the membrane area or the blood flow rate does not double the quantity or rate of release).[6,11] Membrane area and complement activation are more nearly proportional than blood flow rate, which has a much lower effect.

Finally, it should be noted that activation of complement on the membrane surface with simultaneous adsorption of the reaction products, as observed

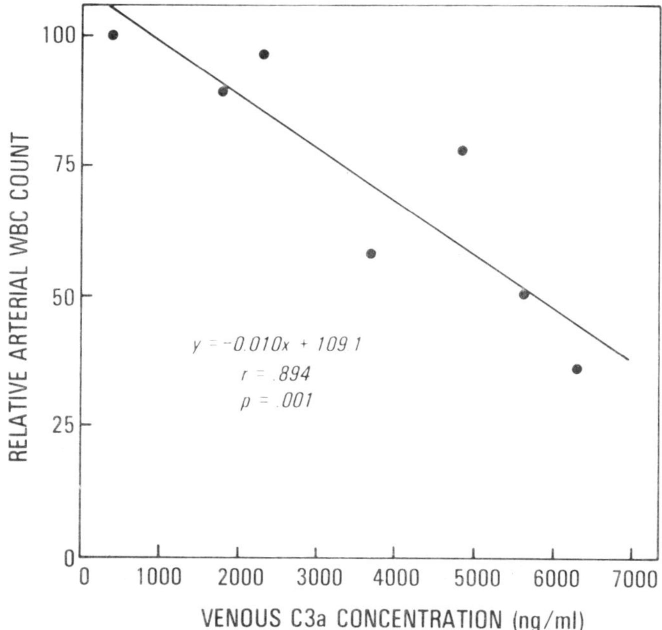

Fig. 14-3. Correlation of hemodialysis leukopenia with complement activation. The close correlation between arterial white blood cell count and venous C3a concentration is depicted. Data points are drawn from the first 20 minutes of dialysis.

with PAN membrane,[12] appears to be recorded by the body as a "nonevent," in that the biologic consequences of activation are not manifest.

Clinical Sequelae

While C3a is the preferred entity to measure as an index of the degree to which complement has been activated, it is predominantly C5a that has biologic consequences.[9] Figure 14-5 shows the biologic consequences that result from the activation of complement.[9] The release of the cytokines interleukin-1 (IL-1) and tumor necrosis factor (TNF) may result from a multiplicity of causes, which are shown diagramatically in Figure 14-6. As these mechanisms have recently been reviewed,[13,14] I shall not do so again here. Rather, I will explore some of the newer information that is important when considering high-efficiency treatment.

Recent studies by Gutierrez and associates from Bergstrom's laboratory[15,16] show that choice of the membrane used will affect the amount of metabolite that must be removed in order to achieve adequate treatment. Work in normal volunteers, in whom sham dialysis (without circulating dialysate) was carried out with (1) cuprophane, (2) PAN, and (3) cuprophane plus oral indomethacin, showed that complement activation with cuprophane correlated with increased release of amino acids from the muscles of

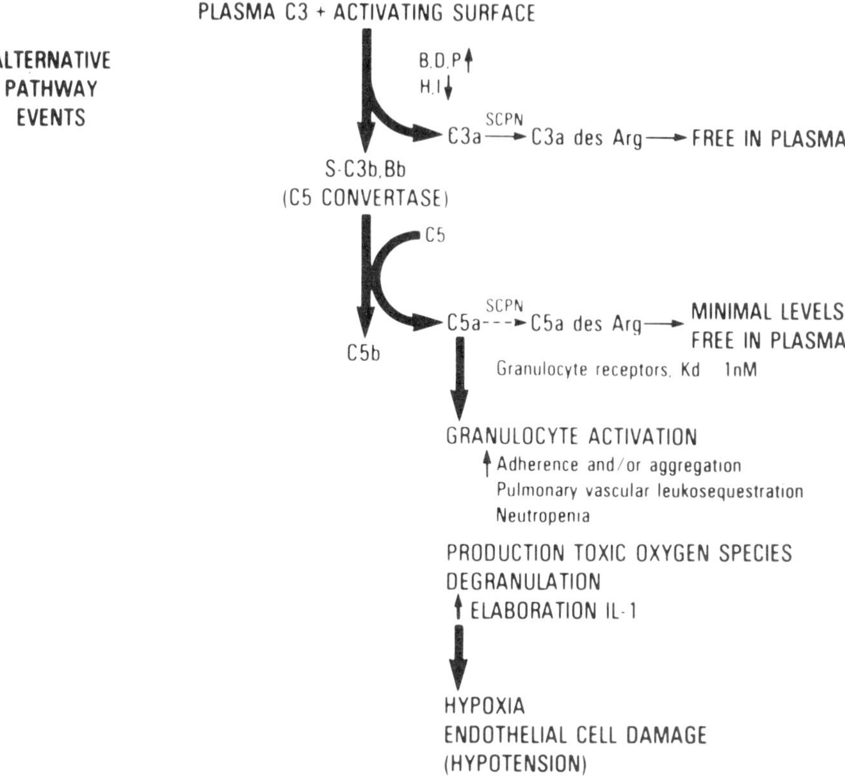

Fig. 14-4. The sequential events of complement activation and anaphylatoxin formation. Complement activation at the membrane surface is modulated by binding of the regulatory proteins for the alternative pathway (factors B, D, P, H, I). See text for further discussion of the role of complement activation in the causation of symptomatic hypotension.

Table 14-1. Activity Series—Complement Activation by Artificial Kidney Membranes[a]

1. Cellulose Hydrate (Difra Secon)
2. Cuprophane
3. Cellulose Acetate (Dow-CDAK)
4. Hemophan
5. Cellulose acetate (Baxter CA70/CA90)
6. Polycarbonate
7. Polymethylmethacrylate
8. Cellulose triacetate
9. Polysulfone
10. Reused cuprophane (saline, formalin)
11. Polyacrylonitrile

[a] Listed in descending order of their tendency to trigger anaphylotoxin release.

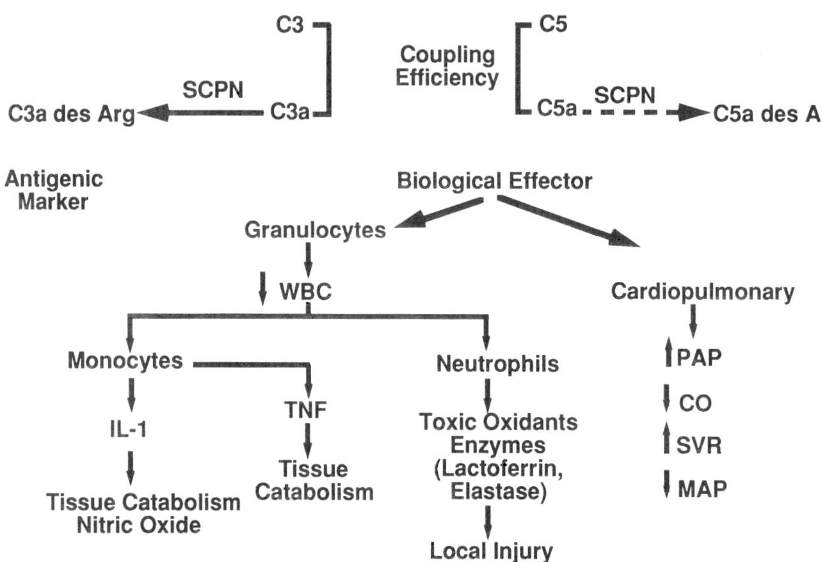

Fig. 14-5. Biologic consequences of systemic anaphylatoxin production. The anaphylatoxins C3a and C3a desArg more closely parallel the magnitude of complement activation when measured in the plasma than do the anaphylatoxins C5a and C5a desArg. The latter are swiftly bound to granulocytes and vascular endothelia and hence become poor indicators of the magnitude of complement activation. Stimulated monocytes release the two cytokines interleukin 1 (IL-1) and tumor necrosis factor (TNF).

the lower limb (femoral arterial and venous catheters were employed as vascular access). Release did not occur either when the complement-kind PAN membrane was used or when the response to IL-1 was pharmacologically blocked with indomethacin.[15] In a more recent paper,[16] this group showed that one of many amino acids released was 3-methylhistidine. This, by metabolic requirement, indicates that the increase in amino acids observed in the blood returning from the limb was the result of muscle catabolism, as opposed to the alternative explanation of reduced anabolism.[14] A possible criticism of this work may be based on the concern that normal subjects and uremic patients may not respond in the same way. In addition, the lack of "real world" analogy makes the work suspect (i.e., no dialysis was performed, as no dialysate was circulated). Why should this be comparable with clinical experience?

The validity and clinical relevance of the observations of Gutierrez and colleagues are supported by work from several laboratories using different methodology which showed that hemodialysis with a cuprophane membrane is a catabolic event.[17,18] The catabolism could not be explained by the loss of glucose into the dialysate with resulting gluconeogenesis.[17] From this work one may estimate that the additional metabolic load imposed by the need to remove urea that is the result of complement-induced catabolism is approxi-

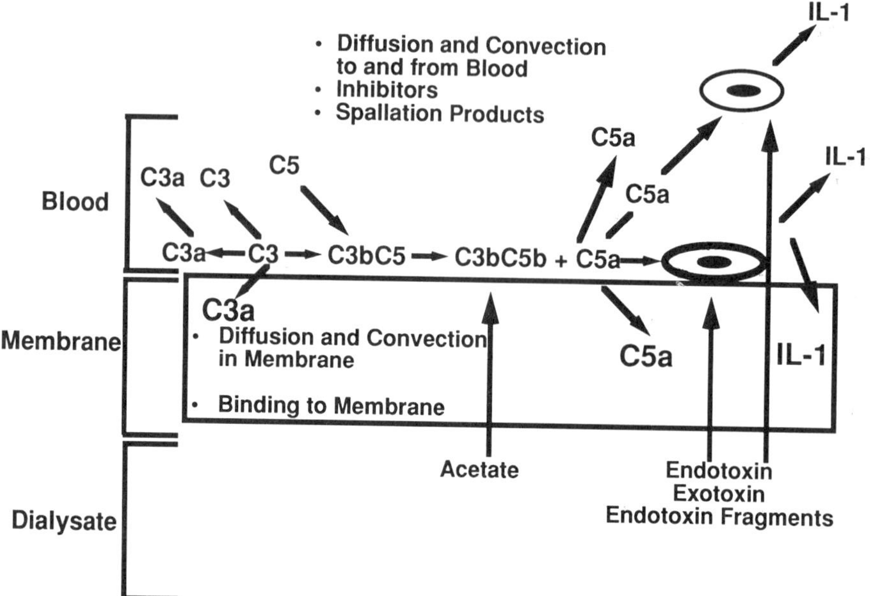

Fig. 14-6. The monokine hypothesis. The many elements that induce the monocyte to release cytokine are shown. The system is complex, involving both direct membrane stimulation and stimulation by complement activation products, acetate from the dialysis bath, and endotoxin fragments. Adsorptive properties of the membrane may modulate plasma concentrations of cytokines released at the membrane surface, as has been demonstrated for complement activation products.

mately 20 percent more than would be required without this source of urea. What is the relevance of this observation to high-efficiency therapy? Clearly, if the goal is to accomplish adequate treatment in the shortest possible time, there is a definite advantage to eliminating the "iatrogenic catabolism" that results from the prescription of a complement-activating membrane.

Chanard et al.[19] have reported that a significantly shorter treatment time (9.3 ± 0.2 hours/wk) with the PAN membrane, as contrasted with cuprophane (16.2 ± 0.3 hours/wk), can provide a lower incidence of morbid events defined as days spent in the hospital for complications [2.1 ± 0.5 versus 6 ± 1.1 days/yr ($P < .001$)]. Their study is retrospective, and the number of study subjects, while substantial (31 patients in each group, followed for nearly 2 years), raises inevitable concern about case mix differences. Further, the clarity of experimental design present in the sham dialysis conducted in the laboratory by Bergstrom's group[15,16] is lost in the clinic, where both a difference in solute clearance profile and a difference in complement activation are present. Another point of difference is that the high-flux membrane requires sophisticated machine support to manage fluid balance. As such, the incidence of symptomatic hypotension may be lower with the PAN than with the cuprophane membrane simply because fluid balance is better managed. (I will return to this topic below.) If Chanard's observation is correct—and I suspect that it is—one may pragmatically argue that this or a comparable membrane is best selected for high-efficiency treatment pending clarification of the validity of these various potential explanations. Further understanding will likely come from work in progress by Parker[20] which addresses the complex problem of distinguishing the effects of cytokine-induced catabolism, from those of solute clearance profile on clinical outcome.

SYMPTOMATIC HYPOTENSION—THE INTERLEUKIN HYPOTHESIS

Background

Why on earth should symptomatic hypotension be included in a chapter on biocompatibility? Prior to the publication of the interleukin hypothesis,[21] which speculates that cytokines bear an etiologic relationship to dialysis hypotension ("crashing"), it would not have been relevant. Crashing on dialysis remains an ugly fact of life for the dialysis patient. I do not propose to review the rather substantial literature on the multifactorial etiology of this event. I[22] and others[23] have done so in the past, and those with oversight responsibility for dialysis patients are offered a daily refresher course in this unpleasant subject.

With respect to high-efficiency treatment, the concern about achieving "dry weight" in the shorter time frame is obviously counter to achieving the necessary balance between vascular refilling rate and net ultrafiltration that sustains vascular volume and blood pressure. In fact many, I among them, believe that the limit to reducing treatment time with hemodialysis is determined not by solute transport but by fluid balance. Patients obviously vary in their tolerance of fluid removal from the vascular space. There are those with baroreflex abnormalities or other forms of autonomic neuropathy[24–26] that may or may not be explained by the presence of diabetes mellitus or other systemic diseases. These are special problems requiring special solutions. More relevant here are considerations related to the routine patient whom one wishes to place on high-efficiency treatment.

To further explore this subject, it is necessary to subdivide high-efficiency treatment into high-efficiency hemodialysis and high-flux treatments. *High-efficiency hemodialysis* is here defined as treatment with membranes of low hydraulic permeability (i.e., in the range of cuprophane). While the restoration to normal of total body water is accomplished in a shorter time frame, the predominant mechanism for solute transport remains diffusive. *High-flux treatment (hemodiafiltration)* is here defined as treatment with membranes of high hydraulic permeability, (i.e., in the range of PAN). As previously noted, this imposes the requirement of special fluid cycling equipment in order to properly manage net fluid balance. The predominant mechanism of solute transport for hemodiafiltration is that of convection.

In this scheme how does one classify therapy with a cellulose triacetate, PAN, or polysulfone membrane, all of which have high hydraulic permeability, when these membranes are used only to perform conventional "hemodialysis"? In this mode of operation there is internal filtration and also reabsorption that is due to the pressure relationships along the blood path,[27,28] and convective transport contributes to the total solute removed in proportion to the molecular weight of the solute. I consider this convective transport as hemodiafiltration, recognizing that for conventional low molecular weight uremic toxins the predominant mode of transport remains diffusive. The respective contributions of convection and diffusion in this treatment mode also depend upon the membrane chosen. The two extremes of behavior may be illustrated by contrasting the high-flux cellulose tracetate hollow fiber membrane with one composed of polysulfone. The former retains the thin fiber wall (short diffusion path) prerequisite to good diffusive transport whereas the latter has a thick spongy wall that in no way inhibits convective transport but largely prevents swift diffusive transport. Convective transport is roughly comparable in both, but the thin cellulosic wall facilitates the greater diffusive transport of small solutes.

Clinical Sequelae

The relationship of crashing and cytokine release was first explored when there was no information about cytokines in the end-stage renal disease population.[20] The subsequent flood of investigative reports on this subject will challenge the most assiduous reader. Highly relevant to the interpretation of this mass of material is the recent identification of two naturally occurring soluble inhibitors of TNF, which bind to this cytokine in the plasma, and a competitive inhibitor of IL-1.[29] This identification throws into question the meaning of simple measurements of plasma cytokine levels. It is now apparent that we have been looking at only one side of the coin. At present both sides can apparently be best examined by measuring an outcome parameter rather than a given cytokine concentration. This approach is illustrated by the work from Bergstrom's laboratory, in which the net impact of the cytokine milieu on metabolism of the muscle is assessed rather than simply the plasma cytokine levels.[15,16] To put the situation in other words, it is not possible at present to make sense out of plasma cytokine levels from the clinical perspective of "what they do to the patient."

An additional technical point may help to reconcile some of the conflicts in the literature with regard to IL-1 plasma levels. Namely, a discrepancy is introduced by the presence of a competitive inhibitor (Il-1 Ra) in the plasma, which would blunt the assay of this cytokine based on the proliferation of lymphocytes but would not affect the radioimmunoassay. One might argue that the bioassay would be properly reflective of the net impact of the cytokine and its competitive inhibitor, whereas the radioimmunoassay would not. The close similarity of both the pathophysiologic responses and the stimuli for induction and release of IL-1 and TNF[29–31] still leaves the net outcome in question. When account is taken of the concern that local tissue concentrations of these agents are probably the main determinant of their effect, the relevance of isolated measurements of plasma levels becomes far-fetched indeed.

The recent work of Beasley et al.[32] is worthy of comment. They have shown in a rat model that IL-1 is capable of releasing nitric oxide, a potent dilator of the microvascular resistance vessels. This then provides the link that was postulated but was not incorporated into the initial formulation of the interleukin hypothesis, namely, that complement activation by the dialysis membrane initiates a train of events that cause symptomatic hypotension.[21] The obvious clinical experiments are now under way by this group to measure these events in the dialysis population and to search for any correlation between measured indices of nitric oxide release and crashing.[32] The recent description by Vallance et al.[33] from the Wellcome Laboratories of a naturally occurring (endogenous) inhibitor of nitric oxide formation from L-arginine needs to be factored into this equation. Asymmetric dimethylarginine (ADMA), the inhibitor, is normally lost in the urine, and its concentration rises in parallel with that of plasma creatinine as renal failure ensues. Vallance et al. postulate that its accumulation in kidney failure may be etiologic in the hypertension so commonly seen with uremia. From our perspective, loss of ADMA from the cytokine-rich environment of dialysis by permissive enhancement of the formation of the potent vasodilator nitric oxide needs examination to determine if this mechanism does underlie crashing. ADMA has a molecular weight of approximately 230 and as such should be readily removed by diffusive transport.

An additional area of both early and recent investigation is informative about the matter of biocompatibility and crashing, namely, the difference between convective and diffusive transport as it affects vascular stability. Quellhorst et al. examined the classical hemodynamic parameters of cardiac output, peripheral vascular resistance, and blood pressure (monitored invasively) during hemodialysis and hemofiltration.[34] Their experimental design was subtle in that the same membrane was used for both techniques and patients served as their own controls. The high-flux, complement-kind PAN membrane was used, and hemofiltration was carried out in postdilution mode. An additional point of interest was that a high (150-mEq/L) and a low (130-mEq/L) sodium dialysate or reconstituting fluid were compared as well. The results of this experiment for hemodialysis were comparable with those of other studies[35–37] in that during the last hour of treatment peripheral vascular resistance failed to rise to a degree commensurate with the removal of excess body water and blood pressure fell even with a moderate rise in heart rate. This was in striking contrast to the hemofiltration mode, during which peripheral resistance rose appropriately and blood pressure was sustained. While solutions of high and low sodium content modulated these events, they did not in any way abrogate the striking difference in total peripheral resistance noted between the two modes of treatment. Clearly this cannot be due to membrane-induced cytokine release through complement activation, as the membrane was the same in both circumstances.

I wished to confirm these important experiments but at the time noninvasive hemodynamic measurements were unavailable to me. Later, with their qualification, these experiments were repeated with only minor variation.[35] Figure 14-7 is taken from that work and confirms Quellhorst et al.'s initial findings. I am obliged to conclude that differences in solute clearance profile between the two techniques underlie this difference in peripheral resistance rather than complement activation and cytokine induction and release. I do not rule out a possible additional contribution from cytokine-induced nitric oxide formation. For example, one might argue that in hemofiltration, unlike hemodialysis, there is no pyrogen-containing dialysis fluid to trigger cytokine release. I consider this an unlikely mechanism in light of the rather small amount of cytokine that has been measured in plasma experimentally in this circumstance; however, such a mechanism nonetheless must be considered.[38] Because acetate was used for both limbs of the study both by Quellhorst et al. and by Fox and myself, Bingel et al.'s potential explanation[39] based on an effect of acetate was also eliminated. The balance between cytokine-induced nitric oxide vasodilation (high-flux versus cuprophane) and the more efficient loss of ADMA with diffusion than with convection (maximal loss occurring with hemodiafiltration) does not at present allow me to form a unifying hypothesis about symptomatic hypotension. As for most investigationally resistant problems, I expect there will be many expla-

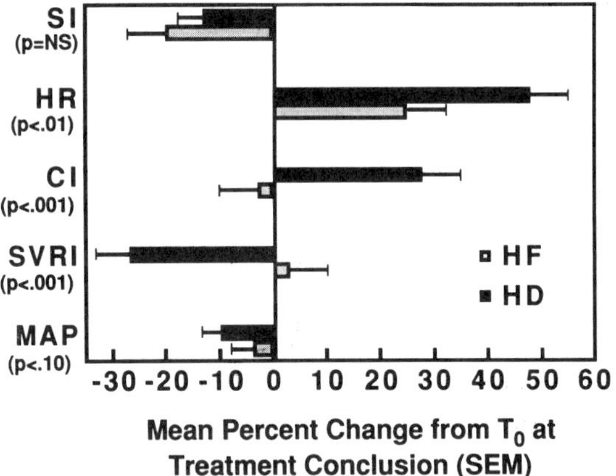

Fig. 14-7. Hemofiltration and hemodialysis are contrasted in nine patients acting as their own control when treated with polyacrylonitrile membrane (Hospal AN69). Stroke index (SI), heart rate (HR), cardiac index (CI), systemic vascular resistance index (SVRI), and mean arterial pressure (MAP) are shown. Mean values ±1 standard error of the mean are plotted as changes from predialysis values (T_0). The primary point of difference is the change from baseline in SVRI as fluid is removed during the course of treatment. The modest rise in hemofiltration is analogous to that seen in normal volunteers. (From Fox and Henderson,[35] with permission.)

nations for the phenomenon of crashing. The major one at present still escapes us and is probably not related to biocompatibility of the membrane. To reiterate, I have not included a considerable body of important and interesting work on crashing as it falls outside the scope of this chapter.

In summary and conclusion, the impact of biocompatibility in high-efficiency treatment may be seen in the areas of catabolic burden and probably symptomatic hypotension. Both areas need further investigative definition, but despite their present marginally understood status, the available information may be used in the pragmatic shaping of prescriptions for high-efficiency therapy.

REFERENCES

1. Abel JJ, Rowntree LG, Turner BB: On the removal of diffusible substances from the circulating blood of living animals by dialysis. J Pharmacol Exp Ther 5:275, 1914
2. Kaplow LS, Goffinet JA: Profound neutropenia during the early phase of hemodialysis. JAMA 203:1135, 1968
3. Colton CK: Analysis of membrane prosthesis for blood purification. J Blood Purif 5:202, 1987
4. Floege J, Granolleras C, Desholdt G et al: Hi flux synthetic versus cellulosic membranes for β-2-microglobulin removal during hemodialysis, hemodiafiltration and hemofiltration. Nephrol Dial Transplant 4:653, 1989
5. Chenoweth DE, Cheung AK, Henderson LW: Anaphylatoxin formation during hemodialysis: effects of different dialyzer membranes. Kidney Int 24:764, 1983
6. Chenoweth DE, Henderson LW: Complement activation during hemodialysis: laboratory evaluation of hemodialyzers. Artif Organs 11:155, 1987
7. Cheung AK, Parker CJ, Wilcox L, Janatova J: Activation of the alternative pathway of complement by cellulosic hemodialysis membranes. Kidney Int 36:257, 1989
8. Cheung AK, Parker CJ, Janatova J: Analysis of the complement C3 fragments associated with hemodialysis membranes. Kidney Int 35:576, 1989
9. Henderson LW, Chenoweth DE: Biocompatibility of artificial organs: an overview. J Blood Purif 5:100, 1987
10. Chenoweth DE: Complement activation during hemodialysis: clinical observations, proposed mechanisms, and theoretical implications. Artif Organs 8:281, 1984
11. Bell JL, Henderson LW: Anaphylotoxin mass generated by cuprophane membrane is not influenced by blood flow rate. Kidney Int 35:240, 1989
12. Cheung AK, Parker CJ, Wilcox LA, Janatova J: Activation of complement by hemodialysis membranes: polyacrylonitrile binds more C3a than cuprophane. Kidney Int 37:1055, 1990
13. Dinarello CA: Cytokines and biocompatibility. J Blood Purif 8:208, 1990
14. Dinarello CA: Cytokines: agents provocateurs in hemodialysis? Kidney Int 41:683, 1992
15. Gutierrez A, Alvestrand A, Wahren J, Bergstrom J: Effective in vivo contact between blood and dialysis membranes on protein catabolism in humans. Kidney Int 38:487, 1990

16. Gutierrez A, Alvestrand A, Bergstrom J: Membrane selection and muscle protein catabolism. Kidney Int 41:586, 1992
17. Borah MF, Shoenfeld P, Gotch FA et al: Nitrogen balance during intermittent dialysis therapy of uremia. Kidney Int 14:491, 1978
18. Farrell PC, Hone PW: Dialysis induced catabolism. Am J Clin Nutr 33:1417, 1980
19. Chanard J, Brunois JP, Melin JP et al: Long term results of dialysis therapy with a highly permeable membrane. Artif Organs 6:261, 1982
20. Parker TF: Interrelationships of dialysis prescription: protein catabolic rate, dialyzer compatibility and morbidity/mortality, abstracted. J Blood Purif 9:208, 1991
21. Henderson LW, Koch KM, Dinarello CA, Shaldon S: Hemodialysis hypotension: the interleukin hypothesis. J Blood Purif 1:3, 1983
22. Henderson LW: Symptomatic hypotension during hemodialysis. Kidney Int 17:571, 1980
23. Daugirdas JT: Dialysis hypotension: hemodynamic analysis. Kidney Int 39:233, 1991
24. Kersh ES, Kronfield SJ, Unger A et al: Autonomic insufficiency in uremia as a cause of hemodialysis-induced hypotension. N Engl J Med 280:650, 1974
25. Lilly J, Golden J, Stone R: Adrenergic regulation blood pressure and chronic renal failure. J Clin Invest 57:1190, 1976
26. Henderson LW: Heterogeneity of the cardiovascular response to hemofiltration. Kidney Int 28:901, 1986
27. Schmidt M, Baldamus CA, Schoeppe W: Back filtration in hemodialyzers with highly permeable membranes: an in vitro and in vivo investigation. J Blood Purif 2:108, 1984
28. Leypoldt JK, Schmidt B, Gurland HJ: Measurement of backfiltration rates during hemodialysis with highly permeable membranes. J Blood Purif 9:74, 1991
29. Dinarello CA: Production of interleukin-I and tumor necrosis factor and their naturally occurring antagonists during hemodialysis. Kidney Int 41:568, 1992
30. Schindler R, Lonnemann G, Shaldon S et al: Induction of interleukin-I and tumor necrosis factor during in vitro hemodialysis with different membranes. Contrib Nephrol 74:58, 1989
31. Schindler R, Lonnemann G, Shaldon S et al: Transcription, not synthesis, of interleukin-I and tumor necrosis factor by complement. Kidney Int 37:85, 1990
32. Beasley D, Schwartz JH, Brenner BM: Interleukin-I induces prolonged L-arginine-dependent cyclic guanosine monophosphate and nitrite production in rat vascular smooth muscle cells. J Clin Invest 87:602, 1991
33. Vallance P, Leone A, Calver A et al: Accumulation of an endogenous inhibitor of nitric oxide synthesis in chronic renal failure. Lancet 339:572, 1992
34. Quellhorst E, Schuenemann B, Hildebrand U, Falda Z: Response of vascular system to different modifications of haemofiltration and haemodialysis. Nephrol Dial Transplant 17:197, 1980
35. Fox S, Henderson LW: Disparate hemodynamic profiles during hemodialysis and hemofiltration: dissociation from thermal, catecholamine and membrane differences. Kidney Int (in press)
36. Shaldon S, Baldamus CA, Koch KM, Lysaght MJ: Of sodium symptomatology and syllogism. J Blood Purif 1:16, 1983
37. Hampl H, Paeprer H, Unger V, Kessel MW: Hemodynamics during hemodialysis: sequential ultrafiltration and hemofiltration. J Dial 3:51, 1979

38. Dinarello CA, Lonneman G, Maxwell R, Shaldon S: Ultrafiltration to reject human interleukin-I inducing substances derived from bacterial cultures. J Clin Microbiol 25:1233, 1987
39. Bingel M, Lonneman G, Koch KM et al: Enhancement of in vitro human interleukin-I production by sodium acetate. Lancet 1:14, 1987

15

Hypertension in Dialysis Patients

Manuel T. Velasquez

INTRODUCTION

Hypertension is perhaps the most common hemodynamic feature of end-stage renal disease (ESRD). It is also the most important risk factor for the development of cardiovascular complications, such as ischemic heart disease, myocardial infarction, and stroke, which are the leading causes of morbidity and mortality in dialysis patients.[1–3] Prior to initiation of dialysis therapy the prevalence of hypertension in patients with ESRD ranges from 70 to 90 percent[4–6]; however, the prevalence rate in patients undergoing maintenance dialysis is lower, averaging between 15 and 20 percent[4–8] Thus, hypertension continues to be a common serious problem among dialysis patients and requires the skills of the nephrologist not only in prescribing the proper dialysis treatment but also in controlling the blood pressure. Over the years my group's approach to the patient with ESRD and hypertension has changed as our understanding of the pathophysiology of hypertension and the uremic syndrome has improved and as more sophisticated dialysis techniques and newer antihypertensive agents have become available. This chapter discusses the current concepts of the pathogenesis of hypertension in ESRD and principles of antihypertensive therapy in dialysis patients.

PATHOPHYSIOLOGY

The regulation of arterial blood pressure is a complex process, which involves the interactions of multiple factors that influence cardiac output or total peripheral resistance (TPR). Similarly, the pathophysiology of hypertension in ESRD may be considered a multifactorial process, including volume-related factors as well as vasoconstrictor-related mechanisms (Table 15-1). Although each of these proposed factors is capable of inducing a rise in blood pressure, the relative contribution of each to the development and maintenance of hypertension in ESRD may vary, depending on the underlying disease, diet, genetic predisposition to hypertension, presence or absence of diseased kidneys, and quality of dialysis treatment.

Table 15-1. Mechanism of Hypertension in Dialysis Patients

Volume-related factors (i.e., salt and water retention)
Vasoconstrictor-related mechanisms
Activation of the renin-angiotensin system
Sympathetic nervous system overactivity
Increased vasoconstrictor hormones or peptides
Deficiency of vasodilator hormones or compounds
"Structural" factor
Divalent cation abnormalities—hypercalcemia
Pressor effects of recombinant human erythropoietin

Salt and Water Retention

Salt and water retention is considered the dominant factor contributing to the hypertension of ESRD in most patients. This is not surprising, since the kidney is the primary regulator of salt and water balance, a major determinant of arterial pressure. The inability of the diseased kidney to excrete ingested sodium and water inevitably leads to accumulation of salt and water and consequently in expansion of plasma and extracellular fluid (ECF) volumes. Expansion of plasma volume initially elevates blood pressure by increasing cardiac output. The increase in total body sodium also enhances the pressor response to vasoconstrictor hormones, which may further aggravate hypertension. Indeed, a number of studies have demonstrated an increase in plasma volume, exchangeable sodium, and ECF volume in a large group of hypertensive patients with chronic renal failure.[9–11]

In some studies exchangeable sodium or ECF volume was found to be directly correlated with the level of blood pressure.[9–12] Koomans and coworkers[13] examined the relation between increased salt intake and changes in blood pressure, blood volume, and ECF volume in patients with moderate or severe renal insufficiency. Increased dietary salt resulted in a greater expansion of blood volume and a larger increase in arterial pressure in the group with severe renal failure. Moreover, blood pressure in this group was greater for any given increase in ECF volume. Conversely, in hypertensive patients undergoing hemodialysis, restriction of dietary salt resulted in a significant decrease in blood pressure coincident with reductions in exchangeable sodium, plasma volume, and ECF volume.[14,15] Further support for the dominant role of salt and water retention in the hypertension of ESRD is provided by the observation that removal of salt and water by dialysis normalizes blood pressure in 70 to 80 percent of hypertensive uremic patients.[8,15–18]

Renin-Angiotensin System

Hypertension persists in a minority of patients with ESRD despite strict control of salt and water balance with dialysis treatment.[4,6,15–18] Plasma renin activity (PRA) is often increased in this group of patients, which suggests that such hypertension is renin-mediated.[4,6,15–17,19,20] Bilateral nephrectomy was formerly performed in some patients with resistant hypertension and increased PRA; blood pressure, TPR, PRA, and plasma angiotensin II levels all decreased after the operation,[4,15,16,19–22] and the fall in blood pressure was correlated with the reduction in PRA.[21,22] It has also been suggested that hypertension develops in patients with chronic renal failure because circulating levels of renin and angiotensin II are inappropriately high in relation to sodium status.[23,24] In a minority of patients whose hypertension cannot be controlled by dialysis, renin levels are noted to be abnormally high and may increase even further in response to sodium depletion,[23] which might explain the persistence of hypertension after dialysis in these patients. In most patients, however, blood pressure can be controlled by dialysis, and in these, renin and angiotensin II levels are lower, but their relation to exchangeable sodium is abnormal.[23] The increase in blood pressure in these patients is thought to result from a failure of normal renin suppression with sodium retention. Further evidence for the role of renin in dialysis-resistant hypertension comes from studies that have employed pharmacologic intervention of the renin-angiotensin system. Administration of the angiotensin II antagonist saralasin or inhibition of angiotensin-converting enzyme (ACE) with captopril has been found to effectively lower blood pressure in hemodialysis patients with resistant hypertension and increased PRA.[25–28]

Central Nervous System

It is well established that the central nervous system plays an essential role in the regulation of blood pressure. The sympathetic system acts to increase blood pressure by directly increasing cardiac output and peripheral vascular resistance and indirectly by stimulating the renin-angiotensin system.[29] Angiotensin II, in turn, augments central and peripheral sympathetic nervous activity.[30] Whether and to what extent neurogenic mechanisms contribute to hypertension in ESRD patients is not entirely clear. Plasma levels of norepineprine and epinephrine have been found to be normal or increased in hypertensive patients with ESRD, both in the predialysis phase and during regular hemodialysis treatment.[31–33] However, no consistent relationship between plasma norepinephrine levels and blood pressure could be demonstrated. Moreover, the value of basal plasma norepinephrine levels as an index of sympathetic nervous activity is limited in view of altered peripheral metabolism and diminished neuronal re-uptake of norepinephrine in uremia.[34,35]

Nonetheless, there are other lines of evidence that suggest the participation of neural mechanisms in at least some patients with ESRD. Marked decreases in blood pressure and peripheral vascular resistance have been demonstrated after total autonomic blockade in hypertensive patients undergoing maintenance hemodialysis.[36] Debrisoquin, a selective sympathetic neurone blocker, was shown to lower blood pressure in hypertensive but not normotensive patients maintained on long-term dialysis.[33] Substantial reductions in mean arterial pressure, heart rate, and plasma norepinephrine and epinephrine levels have been observed following the administration of clonidine in hypertensive uremic patients.[37] In all these investigations, the decrease in blood pressure occurred even though blood volume and renin levels were slightly increased. Additionally, one study has shown that administration of bromocriptine, a drug that stimulates central dopaminergic activity, reduces blood pressure and decreases plasma norepinephrine and prolactin levels in hypertensive hemodialysis patients; this suggests that dopaminergic control of sympathetic activity is impaired in hypertensive patients receiving maintenance dialysis.[38] This is in accord with the concept that a reduction in central dopaminergic activity may contribute to development of hypertension by stimulating sympathetic nervous system activity.[39]

On the other hand, there is also evidence that sympathetic nerve function is impaired in patients with ESRD. Reduced baroreflex sensitivity and signs of autonomic neuropathy have been documented in some patients with chronic renal failure.[40,41] End-organ response to catecholamines is also reduced in uremic patients.[42,43] These abnormalities have been suggested to contribute to the cardiovascular instability observed in patients during hemodialysis. In addition to the sympathetic nervous system and the renin-angiotensin system, an increasing number of vasoconstricting and vasodilating agents have been or are being investigated for their possible role in blood pressure regulation.

Vasoconstrictor Hormones or Peptides

Arginine Vasopressin

The role of arginine vasopressin (AVP) in the pathogenesis of hypertension is controversial. Plasma levels of AVP have been reported to be increased in human hypertension, especially in its severe and malignant forms.[44–46] However, a consistent feature in all these reports is the lack of correlation between blood pressure levels and circulating AVP concentrations. Recent studies using the specific vasopressin V1-vascular antagonist $d(CH_2)5$-Tyr (Me)AVP suggest that AVP may play a critical role in the maintenance of blood pressure under certain conditions. The infusion of this compound does not produce a change in blood pressure in normal well hydrated human volunteers[47] or in patients with mild essential hypertension.[48] In patients with accelerated or malignant hypertension of various causes, the V1 antagonist induced a slight fall in blood pressure when given alone; however, when the patients were pretreated with the sympatholytic agent clonidine, the AVP antagonist produced a substantial fall in blood pressure.[49] These findings are consistent with previous experimental studies in animals, which have shown AVP to assume an important pressor role when the sympathetic system is inhibited.[50] Interestingly, the same V1 antagonist was also shown to lower blood pressure significantly in ESRD patients with increased plasma AVP levels and severe hypertension.[51,52]

Parathyroid Hormone

It has been known for a long time that parathyroid hormone (PTH) possesses vasoactive properties, but its precise role in the pathogenesis of hypertensive disease has yet to be defined. If PTH does have a pressor effect, this effect may be related to its action on calcium ion metabolism.[53] There are some reports linking the action of PTH to the renin-angiotensin system[54] and to sympathetic nerve activity.[55]

Endothelin

Recent studies have shown that endothelin, a potent endothelium-derived vasoconstrictor peptide, is elevated in the plasma of undialyzed uremic patients as well as in that of patients treated with hemodialysis or continuous ambulatory peritoneal dialysis (CAPD).[56–59] Moreover, plasma endothelin levels are found to be higher in hypertensive than in normotensive patients treated by hemodialysis.[58] The physiologic significance of elevated endothelin in uremia is, however, unknown.

Vasodilator Hormones or Peptides

Renal Kallikreins, Prostaglandins, and Medullary Lipids

Since the kidney is the source of kallikrein, vasodilatory prostaglandins (PGE_2), and antihypertensive neutral renomedullary lipid (medullipin), reduced formation of these potentially antihypertensive compounds by the diseased kidney could theoretically contribute to the development of hypertension in ESRD. However, data are lacking to support this hypothesis.

Atrial Natriuretic Factor

Decreased secretion of atrial natriuretic factor (ANF), a natriuretic and vasodilator peptide, is an unlikely cause of hypertension in ESRD, since plasma levels of ANF are found to be elevated in many patients with chronic renal failure.[59–62] The increased secretion of ANF, in fact, may be a compensatory mechanism to counteract the progressive volume expansion that occurs in advanced renal failure or a secondary response to impaired cardiac function reported in some patients with ESRD.[63]

Structural Factor

Structural changes in the cardiovascular system have been regarded as one of the major factors contributing to the development and maintenance of hypertension in humans and animal models. This mechanism, advanced by Folkow,[64] applies not only to primary hypertension but also to hypertension in chronic renal failure. In fact, it was Richard Bright who in 1836 showed that chronic renal disease was characterized by wall hypertrophy in heart, arteries, and arterioles.[65] These structural abnormalities have been ascribed to adaptive responses to blood pressure elevation.[65,66] However, studies in animals and humans suggest that structural cardiovascular changes may occur in the early stages of hypertension.[67,68] These findings have both pathogenic and therapeutic significance since there is increasing evidence that cardiovascular hypertrophy can be reversed by antihypertensive drug therapy.

Calcium

The calcium ion plays a central role in blood pressure regulation by acting to modulate cardiovascular tone. An increase in free intracellular calcium ion concentration enhances vascular smooth muscle contractility, thereby increasing vascular resistance. Similarly, acute hypercalcemia evokes an increase in blood pressure due to an increase in TPR.[69–72] The pressor effect of hypercalcemia is particularly pronounced in the presence of renal failure.[72] The mechanism of hypercalcemia-induced hypertension is not entirely clear. Experimental studies have indicated that calcium ions not only are important for cardiac and arterial smooth muscle contraction but may modulate the release of neurotransmitters.[73] Increased calcium ion activity may augment the release of catecholamines from nerve terminals.[74] In a study in humans, acute hypercalcemia produced an early and progressive rise in blood pressure and a late increase in plasma norepinephrine and epinephrine.[70] These findings suggest that the initial rise in blood pressure results from a direct effect of calcium on blood vessels, whereas catecholamines released by calcium may later contribute to the sustained pressure elevation.

Increased catecholamine levels and enhanced vascular reactivity to norepinephrine have also been demonstrated in some patients with hypercalcemia and hypertension.[75] There are also studies in patients undergoing hemodialysis that suggest that raising dialysate calcium concentration diminishes the fall in blood pressure occurring during ultrafiltration and hemodialysis.[76,77] A 1989 study showed that alterations in calcium concentration within the physiologic range affect blood pressure primarily through changes in left ventricular output in stable dialysis patients.[78] Some investigators have also suggested that the incidence of hypercalcemic hypertension in dialysis patients may be increasing, perhaps as a result of therapy with calcium carbonate and/or vitamin D analogues.[72]

Recombinant Human Erythropoietin

Recombinant human erythropoietin (r-HuEpo) is used increasingly for the treatment of anemia in patients with chronic renal failure. A prominent and common side effect of r-HuEpo therapy in predialysis and dialysis patients is the development or aggravation of hypertension. The incidence of hypertension in hemodialysis patients receiving r-HuEpo therapy is reportedly as high as 30 percent.[79] A history or presence of hypertension predisposes to a further rise in blood pressure during treatment with r-HuEpo.

Several mechanisms have been proposed to explain r-HuEpo-induced hypertension, including an increase in hematocrit and blood viscosity, diminished hypoxic vasodilation, enhanced cardiac output due to better myocardial oxygenation, and insufficient adaptation of TPR due to vascular abnormalities.[80–82] Hormonal factors, such as renin, ANF, and endothelin do not appear to be involved in r-HuEpo-associated hypertension, since the plasma levels of these vasoactive hormones are not altered during r-HuEpo therapy in ESRD patients treated with CAPD.[83] In 1991 it was demonstrated that r-HuEpo induces contraction of isolated kidney and mesenteric resistance vessels in vitro.[84] This finding suggests that the hormone also has a direct on the vasculature that might contribute to its hypertensive effects.

Hemodynamic Patterns and Blood Pressure Variations

Whatever the mechanism involved in the pathophysiology of hypertension in ESRD, the hemodynamic basis for the elevation in blood pressure is an increase in cardiac output or TPR. Although cardiac output is found to be increased in many hypertensive ESRD patients, most studies indicate that the hypertension in such patients is maintained primarily by an increase in TPR.[85,86] In a 1972 study of normotensive and hypertensive patients undergoing maintenance dialysis, Kim and co-workers[85] found that cardiac indices were similar in the two groups of patients but that TPR was significantly increased in the hypertensive group. Cangiano et al.[86] also found increased blood volumes and elevated TPR in hypertensive patients with ESRD as compared with their normotensive counterparts. Moreover, bilateral nephrectomy or salt removal during dialysis resulted in significant decreases in blood pressure and TPR without a change in cardiac output. In a later (1980) study, Kim et al.[87] demonstrated four different hemodynamic patterns in ESRD patients after salt loading: (1) no change in blood pressure; (2) an increase in blood pressure and cardiac output; (3) an increase in blood pressure and TPR with no change in cardiac output; and (4) an initial increase in cardiac output and a later elevation of TPR.[87] Thus, several hemodynamic patterns may develop in hypertensive ESRD patients. In most instances, however, the hypertension is associated with an increase in TPR.

Blood pressure normally fluctuates continuously and exhibits a diurnal rhythm, with higher values during the day and lower values during the night. This diurnal pattern is also seen in patients with essential hypertension except that the entire blood pressure profile is shifted upward.[88] A 1991 study has shown that diurnal blood pressure variations are blunted in patients with advanced chronic renal failure and in patients maintained on chronic hemodialysis.[89] In some of these patients blood pressure levels during the night exceeded those during the day, resulting in severe nocturnal hypertension. Attenuation or reversal of the diurnal rhythm of blood pressure has also been observed in hypertensive conditions with plasma volume expansion, such as primary aldosteronism, Cushing's syndrome, and preeclamptic toxemia.[90–92] Thus, volume expansion may be responsible for the nocturnal rise of blood pressure in these patients. Finally, blood pressure in ESRD patients also is subject to variations during dialysis treatment. In most patients blood pressure falls during dialysis. In some hypertensive patients, however, the hypotensive response to dialysis is delayed and the maximum fall in blood pressure is usually seen 5 hours after completion of dialysis. In a few other patients blood pressure does not change or may even increase during dialysis.[93]

TREATMENT

The primary goal of antihypertensive therapy is to reduce the incidence of cardiovascular morbid events (e.g., stroke, myocardial infarction, and congestive heart failure). Many large-scale intervention studies have clearly established that antihypertensive treatment has a beneficial effect on cardiovascular morbidity and mortality in patients with essential hypertension. However, similar data are not available in hypertensive patients with ESRD. Nevertheless, reduction of blood pressure to normal or near normal levels should be one of the main objectives of therapy in such patients. Although treatment of ESRD-associated hypertension often requires individualization, certain general principles can be applied on the basis of our current knowledge of its pathophysiology.

Nondrug Therapy

Because salt and water retention is central to the pathogenesis of hypertension in patients with ESRD, control of sodium and fluid balance should be a part of their antihypertensive therapy. Therefore, initial treatment should begin with restriction of dietary sodium to 80 to 100 mEq daily. This, combined with careful removal of fluid by ultrafiltration during dialysis to achieve dry weight, is the most effective means to control blood pressure in patients receiving maintenance dialysis. Between 80 and 90 percent of long-term dialysis patients become normotensive with reduction to dry weight. Many ESRD patients are already receiving antihypertensive drug therapy when dialysis is first instituted. It may be necessary to gradually reduce and eventually withdraw these drugs in such patients while achieving reduction to dry weight.

There are reports indicating that physical exercise can have beneficial effects.[94–96] Substantial reductions in blood pressure have been observed in hypertensive hemodialysis patients who had undergone exercise training. In addition, significant improvements in hematocrit levels and coronary risk profiles have been noted in such patients. In view of these potential beneficial effects of physical exercise, an exercise training program for dialysis patients may be warranted.

Drug Therapy

In approximately 10 to 20 percent of patients, blood pressure control remains difficult despite attainment of optimum sodium balance. These patients will require addition of antihypertensive drug therapy. Presently, the range of available antihypertensive drugs has been much broadened, which makes it possible to control hypertension in virtually all patients with chronic renal disease. Different classes of drugs have been shown to be safe and effective in hypertensive hemodialysis patients. In selecting drugs, the physician should consider not only their mode of action but also several other factors particularly relevant for dialysis patients, including pharmacokinetics, dialyzability, dosing, and side effects. Table 15-2 outlines the pharmacokinetic variables of available antihypertensive drugs used in dialysis patients. Much of this information is derived from the excellent review by Bennett and co-authors[97] on drug prescribing in renal failure.

Centrally Acting Adrenergic Inhibitors

The centrally acting adrenergic inhibitors, exemplified by clonidine and methyldopa, share a common action in that they decrease sympathetic outflow to the cardiovascular system by stimulating presynaptic α_2-adrenergic receptors. These agents have been used successfully in patients with all forms of hypertension, including those with renal failure. Clonidine has been shown to effectively lower blood pressure and plasma catecholamines in patients with chronic renal failure well as in hemodialysis patients.[98] Centrally acting drugs have also been shown to cause regression of left ventricular hypertrophy, which may be especially important in severely hypertensive patients with this complication. Side effects common to all centrally acting agents are drowsiness and dry mouth. A withdrawal syndrome of sympathetic hyperactivity with rebound hypertension, sweating, tachycardia, and tremor may occur in some patients treated with clonidine if the drug is stopped suddenly.

Methyldopa may cause a positive direct Coombs test in about 20 percent of patients treated with this drug. About 60 percent of clonidine is removed by the normal kidney, and its elimination half-life is prolonged in patients with renal failure.[99] Therefore its dose should be reduced in dialysis patients. Methyldopa is also excreted by the kidney, and retention of metabolites has been noted in advanced renal failure.[100] It is readily dialyzable, and dosing following hemodialysis is recommended.

β-Adrenergic Receptor Blocking Agents

The most commonly used antihypertensive agents in dialysis patients are β-blockers, which lower blood pressure by acutely decreasing heart rate and cardiac output. However, a reduction in peripheral resistance is observed after long-term treatment with these agents. β-Blockers also inhibit sympathetically mediated renin release and mobilization of muscle glycogen. Of the many β-blockers available, all are equally effective in control of all grades of hypertension. β-Blockers are often used in combination with vasodilator agents to counter the vasodilator-induced increase in heart rate and PRA. Propranolol has proved effective in lowering blood pressure and PRA in hypertensive dialysis patients with high renin levels, who are resistant to salt depletion.[101] Some β-blockers, such as atenolol and nadolol, are primarily excreted by the kidney; hence the doses of these drugs should be reduced in dialysis patients.

Labetalol is a unique antihypertensive agent, which blocks both α- and β-adrenergic receptors. This combined action results in a reduction of peripheral resistance without reflex stimulation of cardiac output. The β effects predominate over the α effects by a 3 : 1 ratio. This drug has been shown to be useful in hypertensive patients with increased sympathetic activity, such as clonidine withdrawal and hypertension following coronary artery bypass grafting. Since labetalol is partly excreted by the kidney, the dosage should be reduced in dialysis patients to avoid severe hypotension and bradycardia.

α-Adrenergic Receptor Blocking Agents

α-Adrenergic receptor blocking agents (prazosin, terazosin, and doxazosin) exert their antihypertensive effects by vasodilatation through selective blockade of α_1-adrenoceptors at postjunctional sites in the precapillary arterioles of the peripheral circulation. This action results in a fall in peripheral vascular resistance with no change in cardiac output. Unlike direct vasodilators, these agents do not cause reflex tachycardia, in part because they do not interfere with presynaptic α_2-receptors, which modulate norepinephrine release via a direct negative feedback mechanism. Prazosin is used extensively in dialysis patients; it has proved effective in controlling hypertension in those undergoing hemodialysis.[102] Terazosin and doxazosin have lower potency on a molar basis but a longer duration of action than prazosin. α-Blockers have been reported to favorably influence plasma lipid profiles during long-term treatment of hypertension, with a tendency to improve high-density to low-very low density lipoprotein (HDL/LDL-VLDL) cholesterol ratios.[103] One major disadvantage of α-adrenergic blockers is their potential to cause orthostatic hypotension, which often occurs after the first dose of the drug. This phenomenon is probably due to dilatation of the venous vascular bed and is the basis of the so-called first-dose effect. It can be avoided by starting therapy with a very low dose (0.5 mg of prazosin) to be taken at bedtime. Prazosin and terazosin are highly bound to plasma proteins and undergo extensive metabolism in the liver so that supplemental dosing after hemodialysis is not necessary.

Table 15-2. Pharmacokinetics of Antihypertensive Drugs

Class	Major Route of Excretion	Volume of Distribution (L/kg)	Half-life Normal/ESRD (h)	Plasma Protein Binding (%)	Dosing	Removal by Dialysis	Comments
β-Adrenergic blockers							
Acebutolol	H	1.2	8–11/7–21	25	25–50% of normal	No	Active metabolite may cumulate
Atenolol	R	0.7	6–9/15–35	<5	25–50% of normal	Yes	Active metabolite may cumulate Activity unknown
Metoprolol	H	5–6	2.5–4.5/ 2.5–4.5	12	50% of normal	No (HD)	Active metabolite may cumulate Metabolite removed with HD
Nadolol	R	2.0	14–24/26–45	30–30	50% of normal	Yes	No active metabolite
Pindolol	H (R)	2.0	3–4/3–4	50–57	Normal	No	No active metabolite
Propranolol	H	3–4	3.5/2.3	90–96	Slight reduction	No (HD)	Spurious bilirubin elevation
Labetalol	H	5.6	3.5/6–8		?	?	Metabolite may cumulate
Central agonists							
Methyldopa	R (H)	0.51	1.4–5.8/3–16	<20	Dosing interval 12–24 h	Yes (HD,PD)	Active metabolite may cumulate Prolonged hypotension
Clonidine	R	3–6	6–23/39–42	20–30	25–50% of normal	No (HD)	Risk of rebound hypertension No active metabolite
Guanabenz	H	5.0	4–6/?	90		?	
Guanfacine	R	6.3	10–30	70		?	

α-Adrenergic blockers							
Prazosin	H (R)	1.2–1.7	2–3/?	97	Normal	No (HD)	Orthostatic hypotension with first dose
Doxazosin	H	?	22	90		?	
Terazosin	H (R)	?	12	98		?	
Converting enzyme inhibitors							
Captopril	R (H)	0.7	2/20	25–30	25–50% of normal	?	Active metabolite may cumulate
Enalapril	R (H)	—	11/?	60	25–50% of normal	?	Risk of hyperkalemia
Lisinopril	R		12/55	0			
Calcium channel blockers							
Verapamil	H	3–6	3–7/?	87–93	Normal	No	Metabolite may cumulate May prolong AV conduction
Diltiazem	H	3–5	2–8/–?	80–86	Normal	No	
Nifedipine	H	0.8	4–5/?	92–98	Normal	No	Effective for acute and chronic control of hypertension
Nitrendipine	H	2–6	12–24	98		No	
Vasodilators							
Diazoxide	R (H)	0.2–0.3	17–31/20–53	87–77	Normal	Yes (HD,PD)	Decreased protein binding in uremia
Hydralazine	H (NR)	0.5–0.9	2–4.5/7–16	87	Dosing interval prolonged 12–24 h	No (HD,PD)	May induce lupus-like syndrome. Very prolonged activity in slow acetylators
Minoxidil	H	2–3	2.8–4.2/3–4	0	Cautious titration	No (HD)	Prolonged hypotension Risk of pericardial effusion

Abbreviations: H, hepatic; R, renal; NR, nonrenal; HD, hemodialysis; PD, peritoneal dialysis; AV, atrioventricular. (Adapted from Bennett et al.,[97] with permission.)

Vasodilator Agents

Vasodilators act directly on vascular smooth muscle to induce relaxation. Although these agents lower blood pressure effectively, they stimulate the baroreflex, thereby producing increases in heart rate, cardiac output, and renin release. The increased heart rate with vasodilator therapy may precipitate angina or even myocardial infarction. For this reason, vasodilator drugs are usually given in conjunction with β-blockers to prevent reflex tachycardia. Other common side effects of vasodilators include headache, palpitations, and flushing. Rarely, a lupus-like syndrome has been reported in patients undergoing chronic hydralazine therapy, particularly those receiving large doses of the drug. Electrocardiographic changes, including ST segment depression and T wave flattening or inversion, have been noted in many patients treated with minoxidil. The development of pericardial effusion and in some cases cardiac tamponade has also been reported with minoxidil therapy, particularly in hemodialysis patients.[104] A common but reversible side effect of minoxidil is hypertrichosis. Hydralazine is well absorbed when given orally and undergoes extensive first-pass metabolism involving acetylation. Hydralazine accumulation may occur in patients with severely impaired renal function. This drug is not removed with hemodialysis, so supplementation postdialysis is not necessary. Minoxidil, however, is not highly protein-bound and may be removed effectively by hemodialysis; therefore, it should be given after rather than before dialysis.

Angiotensin-Converting Enzyme Inhibitors

ACE inhibitors are effective in patients with dialysis-resistant hypertension and increased PRA. These agents also can lower blood pressure in hypertensive dialysis patients with normal PRA, and the hypotensive effect is enhanced by salt depletion. Side effects of ACE inhibitors include cough, skin rash, and dysgeusia. Worsening of anemia has been observed in chronic hemodialysis patients treated with captopril or enalapril[105]; this may be related to an inhibitory effect of ACE inhibition on erythropoiesis. Enalapril has been reported to inhibit thirst, which may reduce oral fluid intake and interdialytic weight gain in hemodialysis patients.[106] All ACE inhibitors have the potential of causing hyperkalemia, particularly in those dialysis patients with residual renal function. Severe hyperkalemia has been reported in CAPD and hemodialysis patients treated with captopril.[107,108] Both captopril and enalapril are partly excreted by the kidney, and the doses of these agents should accordingly, be reduced in dialysis patients. Captopril and enalaprilat (the active metabolite of enalapril) are dialyzable.

Calcium Channel Blockers

Calcium channel blockers, by definition, act by inhibiting the influx of extracellular calcium ions into cells through the slow calcium channel in the cell membrane. This action results in a dilating effect on arterioles and a negative inotropic effect on the myocardium. Although most calcium antagonists are potent vasodilators and reduce arterial pressure by lowering TPR, their effects on the cardiovascular system differ. Thus, verapamil has the greatest negative chronotropic and inotropic effects and the dihydropyridines (nifedipine and congeners) have the least, diltiazem being intermediate. Calcium channel blockers have been used with success in both acute and chronic treatment of all grades of hypertension.[109] These agents have been shown to be most efficacious in patients with low renin levels. Nifedipine was also shown to be highly effective in hypertensive patients with chronic renal failure[110] as well as in hemodialysis patients.[111] In addition, there is increasing evidence from animal experiments and clinical studies suggesting that calcium antagonists may inhibit the development or progression of atherosclerotic lesions.[112]

SUMMARY

In conclusion, hypertension remains a common problem in patients with ESRD, contributing to the increased cardiovascular morbidity and mortality in dialysis patients. The pathogenesis of hypertension in ESRD is multifactorial and involving both volume-related factors and vasoconstrictor-related mechanisms. A rational approach to the management of hypertension in ESRD patients require careful attention to these etiologic factors.

REFERENCES

1. Friedman HS, Shah BN, Kim HG et al: Clinical study of the cardiac findings in patients on chronic maintenance hemodialysis: the relationship to coronary risk factors. Clin Nephrol 16:75, 1981
2. Degoulet P, Legrain M, Reach I et al: Mortality factors in patients treated by chronic hemodialysis. Nephron 31:103, 1982
3. Rostand SG, Kirk KA, Rutsky EA: Relationship of coronary risk factors to hemodialysis-associated ischemic heart disease. Kidney Int 22:304, 1982
4. Lazarus JM, Hampers CL, Merrill JP: Hypertension in chronic renal failure. Treatment with hemodialysis and nephrectomy. Arch Intern Med 133:1059, 1974
5. Weidmann P, Maxwell MH: The renin-angiotensin-aldosterone system in terminal renal failure. Kidney Int 8:219, 1975
6. Del Greco F, Davies WA, Simon NM et al: Hypertension of chronic renal failure: role of sodium and renal pressor system. Kidney Int, suppl. 2:S176, 1975
7. Degli Esposti E, Boero R, Chiarini C et al: Blood pressure behaviour in hemodialysis patients treated for 10 years. Int J Artif Organs 6:121, 1983
8. Sulkova S, Valek A: Role of antihypertensive drugs in the therapy of patients on regular dialysis treatment. Kidney Int, suppl. 25:S198, 1988
9. De Planque BA, Mulder E, Mees EJD: The behaviour of blood and extracellular volume in hypertensive patients with renal insufficiency. Acta Med Scand 186:75, 1969

10. Gutkin M, Levinson GF, King AS, Lasker N: Plasma renin activity in end-stage kidney disease. Circulation 40:563, 1969
11. Cannella G, Castellani A, Mioni G et al: Blood pressure control in end-stage renal disease in man: indirect evidence of a complex pathogenetic mechanism besides renin or blood volume. Clin Sci 52:19 1977
12. Dathan JRE, Johnson DB, Goodwin FJ: The relationship between body fluid compartment volumes, renin activity and blood pressure in chronic renal failure. Clin Sci 45:77, 1973
13. Koomans HA, Roos JC, Boer P et al: Salt sensitivity of blood pressure in chronic renal failure. Evidence for renal control of body fluid distribution in man. Hypertension 4:190, 1982
14. Bianchi G, Ponticelli C, Bardi U et al: Role of the kidney in "salt and water dependent hypertension" of end-stage renal disease. Clin Sci 42:47, 1972
15. Chrysanthakopolous SG, Kastagir BK, Jubiz W, Kolff W: Hypertension in patients on maintenance hemodialysis: evaluation of peripheral renin activity and bilateral nephrectomy. Am J Med Sci 264:9, 1972
16. Vertes V, Cangiano JL, Berman LB, Gould A: Hypertension in end-stage renal disease. N Engl J Med 280:978, 1969
17. Hull AR, Long DL, Prati RC et al: The control of hypertension in patients undergoing regular maintenance hemodialysis. Kidney Int, suppl. 2:S184, 1975
18. Mion C, Slingeneyer A, Canaud B: Pathophysiology and management of hypertension in continuous ambulatory peritoneal dialysis patients. Contrib Nephrol 54:202, 1987
19. Brown JJ, Curtis JR, Lever AF et al: Plasma renin concentration and the control of blood pressure in patients on maintenance hemodialysis. Nephron 6:329, 1969
20. Herrera Acosta J: Hypertension in chronic renal disease. Kidney Int 22:702, 1982
21. Medina A, Bell PRF, Briggs JD et al: Changes of blood pressure, renin and angiotensin after bilateral nephrectomy in patients with chronic renal failure. Br Med J 4:694, 1972
22. Verniory A, Potvliege P, Geertruyden JJ et al: Renin and control of arterial blood pressure during terminal renal failure treated by haemodialysis and by transplantation. Clin Sci 42:685, 1972
23. Schalekamp MA, Beevers DG, Briggs JD et al: Hypertension in chronic renal failure. Am J Med 55:379, 1973
24. Weidmann P, Beretta-Picolli C, Steffen F et al: Hypertension in terminal renal failure. Kidney Int 9:294, 1976
25. Lifschitz MD, Kirschenbaum MA, Rosenblatt SG, Gibney R: Effect of saralasin in hypertensive patients on chronic hemodialysis. Ann Intern Med 88:23, 1978
26. Mimran A, Shaldon S, Barjou P, Mion C: The effect of an angiotensin antagonist (saralasin) on arterial pressure and plasma aldosterone in hemodialysis-resistant hypertension patients. Clin Nephrol 9:63, 1978
27. Vaughn ED, Carey RM, Ayers CR, Peach MJ: Hemodialysis resistant hypertension: control with an orally active inhibitor of angiotensin-converting enzyme. J Clin Endocrinol Metab 48:869, 1971
28. Wauters MO, Waeber B, Brunner HR et al: Uncontrollable hypertension in patients on hemodialysis: long-term treatment with captopril and salt subtraction. Clin Nephrol 16:86, 1981

29. Textor SC, Gavras H, Tifft CP et al: Norepinephrine and renin activity in chronic renal failure. Evidence for interacting roles in hemodialysis hypertension. Hypertension 3:294, 1981
30. Zimmerman BG: Adrenergic facilitation by angiotensin: does it serve a physiological function? Clin Sci 60:343, 1981
31. McGrath BP, Ledingham SGG, Benedict CR: Catecholamines in peripheral venous plasma in patients on chronic hemodialysis. Clin Sci 55:89, 1978
32. Izzo JL Jr, Izzo MS, Sterns RH, Freeman RB: Sympathetic nervous system hyperactivity in maintenance hemodialysis patients. Trans Am Soc Artif Intern Organs 28:604, 1982
33. Schohn D, Weidmann P, Jahn H, Beretta-Piccoli C: Norepinephrine-related mechanism in hypertension accompanying renal failure. Kidney Int 28:814, 1985
34. Rascher W, Schomig A, Kreye VA, Ritz E: Diminished vascular response to noradrenaline in experimental chronic uremia. Kidney Int 21:20, 1982
35. Hennemann H, Hevendehl G, Herler E, Heidland A: Toxic sympathicopathy in uremia. Nephrol Dial Transplant 10:166, 1973
36. McGrath BP, Tilder DJ, Bune A et al: Autonomic blockade and the Valsalva maneuver in patients on maintenance hemodialysis: a hemodynamic study. Kidney Int 12:294, 1977
37. Izzo JL Jr, Santarosa RP, Larrabee PS et al: Increased plasma norepinephrine and sympathetic nervous activity in essential hypertensive and uremic humans: effects of clonidine. J Cardiovasc Pharmacol 10(suppl 12):S225, 1987
38. Degli Esposti E, Sturani A, Santoro A et al: Effect of bromocriptine treatment on prolactin, noradrenaline and blood pressure in hypertensive haemodialysis patients. Clin Sci 69:51, 1985
39. Van den Buuse M, Versteeg DHG, DeJong W: Role of dopamine in the development of spontaneous hypertension. Hypertension 6:899, 1984
40. Lilley JJ, Golden J, Stone RA: Adrenergic regulation of blood pressure in chronic renal failure. J Clin Invest 57:1190, 1976
41. Pickering T, Gribbin B, Oliver D: Baroreflex sensitivity in patients on long-term haemodialysis. Clin Sci 43:645, 1972
42. Canella G, Picotti GB, Movilli E et al: Plasma catecholamine response to postural stimulation in normotensive and dialysis hypotension-prone uremic patients. Nephron 27:285, 1981
43. Campese VM, Romoff MS, Levitan D et al: Mechanisms of autonomic nervous system dysfunction in uremia. Kidney Int 20:246, 1981
44. Thibonnier M, Aldigier JC, Soto ME et al: Abnormalities and drug-induced alterations of vasopressin in human hypertension. Clin Sci 61:148s, 1981
45. Cowley AW Jr, Skelton MM, Velasquez MT: Sex differences in the endocrine predictors of essential hypertension: vasopressin versus renin. Hypertension 7(suppl 1):S1151, 1985
46. Morton JJ, Padfield PI: Vasopressin and hypertension in man. J Cardiovasc Pharmacol 8(suppl 7):S101, 1986
47. Bussien JP, Waeber B, Nussberger J et al: Does vasopressin sustain blood pressure of normally hydrated healthy volunteers? Am J Physiol 246:H143, 1984
48. Waeber B, Nussberger J, Hofbauer KG et al: Studies with a vascular vasopressin antagonist. J Cardiovasc Pharmacol 8(suppl 7):S111, 1986
49. Ribeiro A, Mulinari R, Gavras H et al: Sequential elimination of pressor mechanisms in severe hypertension in humans. Hypertension 8(suppl 1):SI-169, 1986

50. Gavras H, Hatzinikolaou P, North WG et al: Interaction of the sympathetic nervous system with vasopressin and renin in the maintenance of blood pressure. Hypertension 4(suppl 3):S400, 1982
51. Gavras H, Ribeiro AB, Kohlmann O et al: Effects of a specific inhibitor of the vascular action of vasopressin in humans. Hypertension 6(suppl 1):S1156, 1984
52. Papadoliopoulou-Diamandopoulou N, Papagalanis N et al: Vasopressin in end-stage renal disease: relationship to salt, catecholamines and renin activity. Clin Exp Hypertens[A] A9:1197, 1987
53. Massry SG, Iseki K, Campese VM: Serum calcium, parathyroid hormone, and blood pressure. Am J Nephrol 6(suppl 1):S19, 1986
54. Resnick LM, Muller FB, Laragh JH: Calcium regulating hormones in essential hypertension: relation to plasma renin activity and sodium metabolism. Ann Intern Med 105:649, 1986
55. Campese VM: Calcium, parathyroid hormone and sympathoadrenal system. Am J Nephrol 6(suppl 1):S29, 1986
56. Koyama H, Tabata T, Nishzawa Y et al: Plasma endothelin levels in patients with uraemia. Lancet 1:991, 1989
57. Totsune K, Mouri T, Takahashi K et al: Detection of immunoreactive endothelin in plasma of hemodialysis patients. FEBS Lett 249:239, 1989
58. Shichiri M, Hirata Y, Ando K: Plasma endothelin levels in hypertension and chronic renal failure. Hypertension 15:493, 1990
59. Lai KN, Li PKT, Woo KS et al: Vasoactive hormones in uremic patients on continuous ambulatory peritoneal dialysis. Clin Nephrol 35:218, 1991
60. Rascher W, Tulassay T, Lang RE: Atrial natriuretic peptide in plasma of volume overloaded children with chronic renal failure. Lancet 2:303, 1985
61. Hasegawa K, Matsushita Y, Inoue T et al: Plasma levels of atrial natriuretic peptide in patients with chronic renal failure. J Clin Endocrinol Metab 63:819, 1986
62. Ando R, Matsuda O, Miyake S, Yoshiyama N: Plasma levels of human atrial natriuretic factor in patients treated by hemodialysis and continuous ambulatory peritoneal dialysis. Nephron 50:225, 1988
63. Walker RG, Swainson CP, Yandle TG et al: Exaggerated responsiveness of immunoreactive atrial natriuretic peptide to saline infusion in chronic renal failure. Clin Sci 72:19, 1987
64. Folkow B: Cardiovascular structural adaptation: its role in the initiation and maintenance of primary hypertension. The Fourth Volhard Lecture. Clin Sci 55(suppl IV):S3, 1978
65. Folkow B: Physiological aspects of primary hypertension. Physiol Rev 62:347, 1982
66. Bevan RD, van Marthens E, Bevan JA: Hyperplasia of vascular smooth muscle in experimental hypertension in the rabbit. Circ Res 38(suppl II):SII-58, 1976
67. Sivertsson R: Structural adaptation in human hypertension. Hypertension 6(suppl III):SIII-103, 1984
68. Trimarco B, Wikstrand J: Regression of cardiovascular structural changes by antihypertensive treatment: functional consequences and time course of reversal as judged from clinical studies. Hypertension 6(suppl III):SIII-150, 1984
69. Weidmann P, Massry SG, Coburn JW et al: Blood pressure effects of acute hypercalcemia: studies in patients with chronic renal failure. Ann Intern Med 76:741, 1972

70. Marone C, Beretta-Piccoli C, Weidmann P: Acute hypercalcemic hypertension in man: role of hemodynamics, catecholamines, and renin. Kidney Int 20:92, 1980
71. Bianchetti MG, Beretta-Picolli, Weidmann P et al: Calcium and blood pressure regulation in normal and hypertensive subjects. Hypertension 5(suppl II):SII-57, 1983
72. Sica DA, Harford AM, Zawada ET: Hypercalcemic hypertension in hemodialysis. Clin Nephrol 22:102, 1984
73. Rubin RP: The role of calcium in the release of neurotransmitter substances and hormones. Pharmacol Rev 22:239, 1970
74. Lane JD, Aprison MH: Calcium-dependent release of endogenous serotonin, dopamine, and norepinephrine from nerve endings. Life Sci 20:665, 1977
75. Vlachakis ND, Frederics R, Velasquez M et al: Sympathetic system function and vascular reactivity in hypercalcemic patients. Hypertension 4:452, 1982
76. Maynard JC, Cruz C, Kleerekoper M, Levin MW: Blood pressure response to changes in serum ionized calcium during hemodialysis. Ann Intern Med 104:358, 1986
77. Sherman RA, Bialy GB, Gazinski B et al: The effect of dialysate calcium levels on blood pressure during dialysis. Am J Kidney Dis 8:244, 1986
78. Fellner SK, Lang RM, Neumann A et al: Physiologic mechanisms for calcium-induced changes in systemic arterial pressure in stable dialysis patients. Hypertension 13:213, 1989
79. Ad Hoc Committee for the National Kidney Foundation: Statement on the clinical use of recombinant erythropoietin in anemia of end-stage renal disease. Am J Kidney Dis 14(3):163, 1989
80. Raine AEG: Hypertension, blood viscosity, and cardiovascular morbidity in renal failure: implications of erythropoietin therapy. Lancet 1:97, 1988
81. Nonnast-Daniel B, Creutzig A, Kuhn K et al: Effect of treatment with recombinant human erythropoietin on peripheral haemodynamics and oxygenation. Contrib Nephrol 66:185, 1988
82. Jandeleit K, Heintz B, Gross-Heitfeld E et al: Increased activity of the autonomic nervous system and increased sensitivity to angiotensin II infusion after therapy with recombinant human erythropoietin. Nephron 56:20, 1990
83. Lai KN, Lui SF, Leung JCK et al: Effect of subcutaneous and intraperitoneal administration of recombinant human erythropoietin on blood pressure and vasoactive hormones in patients on continuous ambulatory peritoneal dialysis. Nephron 57:394, 1991
84. Heidenreich S, Rahn K-H, Zidek W: Direct vasopressor effect of recombinant human erythropoietin on renal resistance vessels. Kidney Int 39:259, 1991
85. Kim KE, Onesti G, Schwartz AB et al: Hemodynamics of hypertension in chronic end-stage renal disease. Circulation 46:456, 1972
86. Cangiano JL, Ramirez-Muxo O, Ramirez-Gonzalez R et al: Normal renin uremic hypertension. Study of cardiac hemodynamics, plasma volume, extracellular fluid volume and the renin-angiotension system. Arch Intern Med 136:17, 1976
87. Kim KE, Onesti G, DelGuercio ET et al: Sequential hemodynamic changes in end-stage renal disease and the anephric state during volume expansion. Hypertension 2:102, 1980
88. Drayer JIM, Weber MA, Nakamura DK: Automated ambulatory blood pressure monitoring: a study in age-matched normotensive and hypertensive men. Am Heart J 109:1334, 1985

89. Baumgart P, Walger P, Gemen S et al: Blood pressure elevation during the night in chronic renal failure, hemodialysis and after renal transplantation. Nephron 57:293, 1991
90. Redman CWG, Beilin LJ, Bonnar J: Reversed diurnal blood pressure rhythm in hypertensive pregnancies. Clin Sci 51:S687, 1976
91. Tanaka T, Natsume, Shibata H et al: Circadian rhythm of blood pressure in primary aldosteronism and renovascular hypertension. Jpn Circ J 47:788, 1983
92. Imai Y, Abe K, Sasaki A et al: Altered circadian blood pressure rhythm in patients with Cushing's syndrome. Hypertension 12:11, 1988
93. Battle DC, von Riotte A, Lang G: Delayed hypotensive response to dialysis in hypertensive patients with end-stage renal disease. Am J Nephrol 6:14, 1986
94. Hagberg JM, Goldberg AP, Ehsani AA et al: Exercise training improves hypertension in hemodialysis patients. Am J Nephrol 3:209, 1983
95. Goldberg AO, Geltman EM, Gavin JR et al: Exercise training reduces coronary risk and effectively rehabilitates hemodialysis patients. Nephron 42:311, 1986
96. Painter PL, Nelson-Worel JN, Hill MM et al: Effects of exercise training during hemodialysis. Nephron 43:87, 1986
97. Bennett WM, Aronoff GR, Morrison G et al: Drug prescribing in renal failure: dosing guidelines for adults. Am J Kidney Dis 3:155, 1983
98. Levitan D, Massry SG, Romoff M, Campese VM: Plasma catecholamines and autonomic nervous system function in patients with early renal insufficiency and hypertension: effect of clonidine. Nephron 36:24, 1984
99. Hulter HN, Licht JH, Ilnicki LP, Singh S: Clinical efficacy and pharmacokinetics of clonidine in hemodialysis and renal insufficiency. J Lab Clin Med 94:223, 1979
100. Myhre E, Brodwall EK, Stenbeak O, et al: Plasma turnover of methyldopa in advanced renal failure. Acta Med Scand 191:343, 1972
101. Linder A, Douglas SW, Adamson JW: Propranolol effects in long-term hemodialysis patients with renin-dependent hypertension. Ann Intern Med 88:457, 1978
102. Harter HR, Delmez JA: Effects of prazosin in the control of blood pressure in hypertensive dialysis patients. J Cardiovasc Pharmacol 1:S43, 1979
103. Meltzer VN, Goldberg AP, Tindira CA et al: Effects of prazosin and propranolol on blood pressure and plasma lipids in patients undergoing chronic hemodialysis, abstracted. Am J Cardiol 53(3):40A, 1984
104. Martin WB, Spodick DH, Zins GR: Pericardial disorders occuring during open-label study of 1,869 severely hypertensive patients treated with minoxidil. J Cardiovasc Pharmacol 2(suppl 2):S217, 1980
105. Hirakata H, Onoyama K, Hori K, Fujishima M: Participation of the renin-angiotensin system in the captopril-induced worsening of anemia in chronic hemodialysis patients. Clin Nephrol 26:27, 1986
106. Oldenburg B, MacDonald GJ, Shelley S: Controlled trial of enalapril in patients with chronic fluid overload undergoing dialysis. Br Med J 296:1089, 1988
107. Atkin SL, Tomson CR, Venning MC: Life-threatening captopril-induced hyperkalemia in a patient on continuous ambulatory peritoneal dialysis (letter). Nephrol Dial Transplant 4:1084, 1989
108. Papadimiriou M, Zamboulis C, Alexopoulos E et al: Alarming hyperkalaemia during captopril administration in patients on regular hemodialysis. Nephrol Dial Transplant 14:473, 1985

109. Heidland A, Riegel W, Horl W et al: Calcium antagonists: hypotensive and humoral actions in different forms of hypertension. Contrib Nephrol 49:201, 1985
110. Ambroso GC, Como G, Scalamogna A et al: Treatment of arterial hypertension with nifedipine in patients with chronic renal insufficiency. Clin Nephrol 23:41, 1985
111. Kubo K, Shiraishi K, Muto H et al: Treatment of hypertension in hemodialysis patients with nifedipine. Hypertension 5(suppl II):S109, 1983
112. Keogh AM, Schroeder JS: The antiatherogenic effects of calcium antagonists. Am J Hypertens 4:512S, 1991

16

Metabolic Alkalosis in Patients with End-Stage Renal Disease

Susie Q. Lew

INTRODUCTION

Metabolic alkalosis results from accumulation of base or loss of acid. If unaccompanied by another acid-base disturbance, metabolic alkalosis manifests as an elevation in arterial blood pH (alkalemia) and in plasma bicarbonate concentration and a reciprocal reduction in plasma chloride.

Acid-base disturbances are common in patients with end-stage renal disease (ESRD) as a result of the kidney's impaired capacity to respond to either an acid or a base load. Metabolic acidosis is frequently observed and is the result of the kidney's inability to generate bicarbonate and/or to excrete hydrogen ions. Once metabolic alkalosis is generated, patients with impaired renal function are unable to excrete the excess base, and thus alkalosis is maintained.

The blood pH is maintained within the physiologic range by compensatory mechanisms involving the kidney and the lung. The arterial carbon dioxide pressure ($PaCO_2$) and plasma bicarbonate move in the same direction to minimize pH shifts, as predicted by the Henderson-Hasselbalch equation. In the presence of nonfunctioning kidneys the Henderson-Hasselbalch equation would predict wide shifts in pH since the kidney cannot buffer either changes due to alterations in $PaCO_2$ or variations in plasma bicarbonate concentration resulting from addition of either acid or base.

This chapter focuses on the causes, clinical manifestations, and management of metabolic alkalosis in patients with ESRD.

CAUSES

Metabolic alkalosis has been reported to be the most common acid-base disturbance in hospitalized patients.[1] The etiologies of this condition[2,3] are listed in Table 16-1. As in patients without renal disease, metabolic alkalosis in patients with ESRD can be divided into two phases. The first phase is the generation of alkalosis by addition of base or loss of acid; however, the mechanism of urinary acid loss does not apply to patients with nonfunctioning kidneys. The second phase is maintenance of alkalosis by the kidney.

Generation of Metabolic Alkalosis

Exogenous Administration of Base

Alkali administration. Exogenous base may be administered in the form of bicarbonate or as base equivalents such as acetate, carbonate, or citrate. Sodium bicarbonate is administered as an antacid or in the treatment of metabolic acidosis. Patients ingest varying quantities of base before and after the development of ESRD in the form of calcium acetate, calcium carbonate, or calcium citrate as antacids, phosphate binders, or calcium supplements to prevent renal osteodystrophy. Potassium bicarbonate may be given as a potassium supplement.

In subjects with functioning kidneys, an elevation in plasma bicarbonate may be observed only after administration of large quantities of these substances, since the kidneys should be able to excrete the excess base. However, in patients with nonfunctioning kidneys, any base administered that is not

Table 16-1. Causes of Metabolic Alkalosis

Generation of Metabolic Alkalosis

- Exogenous base administration
  - Bicarbonate
    - Sodium bicarbonate
    - Dialysate
  - Carbonate
    - Antacids
    - Milk-alkali syndrome
    - Calcium supplements
  - Acetate
    - Hyperalimentation
    - Dialysate
  - Citrate
    - Anticoagulation (blood transfusion)
- Gastrointestinal acid loss
  - Gastric
    - Vomiting
    - Nasogastric suction
  - Stool
    - Chloridorrhea
- Urinary acid loss
  - Increased tubular flow rate or sodium delivery
  - Increased mineralocorticoid activity
    - Hyper-reninemic states
      - Extracellular volume contraction
      - Magnesium deficiency
      - Bartter syndrome
    - Hyporeninemic states
      - Primary hyperaldosteronism (adenoma, hyperplasia, carcinoma)
      - Cushing syndrome or disease
        - Ectopic adrenocorticutropic hormone
        - Adrenal carcinoma
        - Adrenal adenoma
        - Primary pituitary
    - Adrenal enzymatic defects
      - 11β-Hydroxylase deficiency
      - 17α-Hydroxylase deficiency
  - Increased tubule lumen negativity
    - Non-reabsorbable anions
  - Increased PCO_2
    - Posthypercapnia
  - Decreased parathyroid hormone or hypercalcemia
  - Other
    - Licorice
    - Carbenoxolone
    - Chewing tobacco
    - Nasal spray
    - Liddle syndrome

Maintenance of Metabolic Alkalosis

- Decreased glomerular filtration rate
- Volume contraction
- Hypokalemia
- Hypochloremia
- Steroid excess

consumed in neutralizing acid results in addition to the base pool, since the kidneys cannot excrete the excess.

Dialysis-related exogenous base. Another source of exogenous bicarbonate or base equivalent in patients with ESRD is acetate or bicarbonate dialysis. Mass transfer of base depends on concentration gradient between plasma and dialysate, membrane surface area, temperature, and a constant, defined as diffusivity, which depends on the membrane material and its interface with the solute and solvent under consideration. The latter factors are relatively stable in clinical dialysis. Thus, the concentration gradient and surface area of the membrane are the major determinants of mass transport.

In standard acetate hemodialysis, the acetate concentration in the dialysate is approximately 37 mEq/L. The plasma concentration of acetate is low to nonexistent. During acetate hemodialysis the acetate moves from the dialysate to the plasma and is subsequently metabolized to bicarbonate in the Krebs cycle. The rate of conversion of acetate to bicarbonate has been demonstrated to vary from 2.5 to 5.5 mmol/min, with a mean value of 5 mmol/min in nonuremic subjects and 3 mmol/min in uremic subjects.[4–6] Approximately 20 percent of this bicarbonate replenishes body stores.[7] In acetate dialysis there is simultaneous movement of bicarbonate from the plasma to a dialysate that contains no bicarbonate. Since the acetate concentration gradient between the dialysate and the plasma is greater than the bicarbonate concentration gradient, there is a net gain of acetate or base equivalent during an acetate hemodialysis treatment.

In bicarbonate hemodialysis, movement of bicarbonate depends on the concentration gradient between dialysate and plasma. Generally, plasma bicarbonate losses do not occur when bicarbonate dialysate is used since the dialysate/plasma bicarbonate concentration ratio is greater than unity. Metabolic alkalosis has been reported in patients who underwent dialysis against a dialysate that had a very high bicarbonate concentration as a result of intent, human error, or mechanical malfunction.[8,9] If the dialysate/plasma bicarbonate concentration ratio is less than unity, there may be bicarbonate loss to the dialysate.

Bicarbonate dialysate contains carbon dioxide, which may be the result of carbon dioxide insufflation into a closed system or of its production from the chemical reaction of bicarbonate with small quantities of acetic acid. These processes are used to maintain a chemically stable dialysate. The dialysate/plasma carbon dioxide concentration gradient generally favors carbon dioxide movement from dialysate to plasma during hemodialysis. The dissolved carbon dioxide entering the plasma is neutral and thus does not interfere with acid-base balance. The excess plasma carbon dioxide is finally excreted by the lungs.[10]

In addition to the base (acetate and bicarbonate) transport mentioned above, there is transport of other base equivalents, namely organic acid anions such as lactate, β-hydroxybutyrate, and acetoacetate. These anions are normally neutralized by oxidation to carbon dioxide and water. If the anions are removed by dialysis, the fact that the oxidation now does not take place results in a net accumulation of hydrogen ion.[11]

In mass balance studies, total infusion of acetate per dialysis treatment have varied from 780 ± 61 to 1,165 ± 49 mmol of acetate, depending on dialyzer surface area, dialysate and blood flow rates, and acetate concentration of the dialysate.[12–15] Bicarbonate losses have varied from 550 to 900 mmol per dialysis treatment. Additional loss of alkaline equivalents such as lactate and β-hydroxybutyrate has ranged from 50 to 100 mmol per treatment,[15] the calculated weekly net base balances being slightly positive or at least near zero. In the study by Gotch et al.[15] on bicarbonate dialysis, the weekly hydrogen ion generation was 352 mmol and weekly β-hydroxybutyrate and lactate losses were 37 and 55 mmol/week, respectively. Bicarbonate mass transfer was 618 mmol/wk (206 mmol per dialysis treatment), and the net base gain was 175 mmol/wk.

The final acid-base balance at the end of a dialysis treatment depends on (1) the predialysis acid-base status; (2) movements of dialysate acetate or bicarbonate, plasma organic acid anions and bicarbonate, and dialysate and plasma PCO_2; and (3) endogenous acid production and consumption of buffers to neutralize the acid during the treatment.

To illustrate the changes in pH, $PaCO_2$, and bicarbonate during acetate and bicarbonate hemodialysis, pre- and post-treatment arterial blood gases (ABGs) were obtained from patients with ESRD who underwent dialysis against dialysate containing acetate or bicarbonate.

The mean values for bicarbonate, $PaCO_2$, and pH before and after acetate hemodialysis and bicarbonate hemodialysis are shown in Table 16-2. A higher pretreatment bicarbonate level and greater gain in bicarbonate is noted in bicarbonate hemodialysis than in acetate hemodialysis.

Figure 16-1 depicts individual studies performed during bicarbonate hemodialysis, with the prebicarbonate level plotted on the abscissa and the difference between the post- and pre-bicarbonate level on the ordinate. Figure 16-2 is a similar graph of data obtained during acetate hemodialysis.

Table 16-2. Comparison of Pre- and Postdialysis Valves in Bicarbonate and Acetate Hemodialysis

	Bicarbonate (n = 51)	Acetate (n = 52)
Predialysis bicarbonate	21.63 ± 3.22	17.75 ± 4.02
Postdialysis bicarbonate	27.11 ± 3.36[a]	19.34 ± 3.75[b]
Predialysis $PaCO_2$	37.34 ± 4.97	31.94 ± 6.72
Postdialysis $PaCO_2$	39.42 ± 6.27	29.92 ± 4.93[c]
Predialysis pH	7.38 ± 0.05	7.36 ± 0.05
Postdialysis pH	7.45 ± 0.06[a]	7.42 ± 0.05[a]

[a] $P < .0001$.
[b] $P < .001$.
[c] $P < .007$.

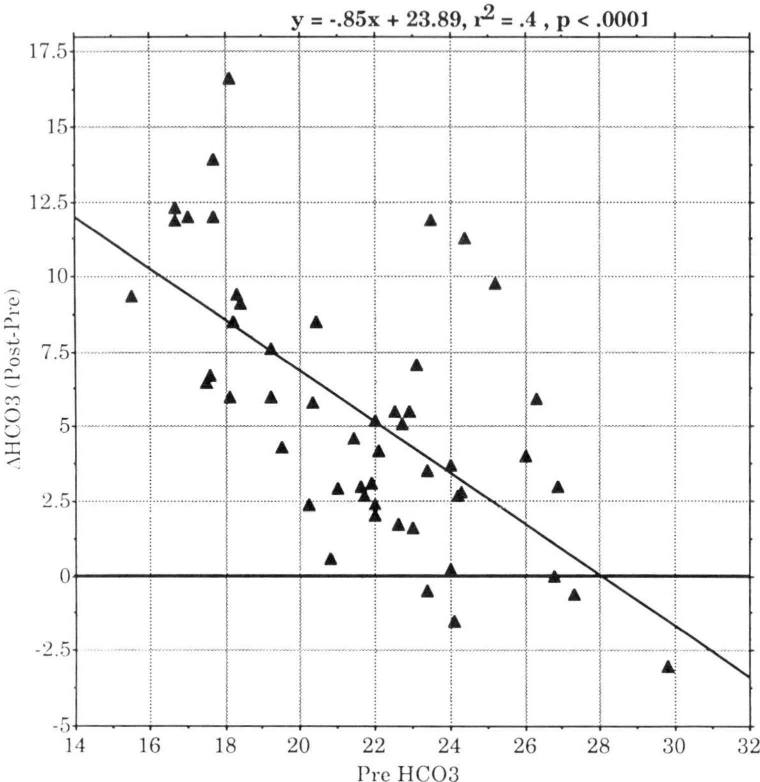

Fig. 16-1. Changes in plasma bicarbonate concentration after bicarbonate hemodialysis. The pretreatment bicarbonate level is plotted on the abscissa, and the change produced (difference between post- and pretreatment level) is plotted on the ordinate. ($r = .7$, $P < .002$.)

Both graphs represented the best fitted curve. Changes in bicarbonate concentration tend to be mostly positive with bicarbonate hemodialysis but tend to be variable with acetate hemodialysis. If acetate conversion to bicarbonate is problematic, the bicarbonate level may fall, remain unchanged, or increase slightly. These graphs may be used to predict the change in bicarbonate level as a result of either a bicarbonate or an acetate hemodialysis treatment. For example, if the pretreatment bicarbonate level is 18 mEq/L, the expected increment in bicarbonate level would be 8 mEq/L at the end of a bicarbonate hemodialysis treatment but only 1.5 mEq/L from an acetate hemodialysis treatment. The pretreatment bicarbonate level at which no change in bicarbonate level would be expected is 28 mEq/L for bicarbonate hemodialysis and 21.5 mEq/L for acetate hemodialysis. This is consistent with the observed higher pretreatment bicarbonate level in patients receiving bicarbonate hemodialysis, which may be associated with better correction of acid-base disorders in ESRD patients.

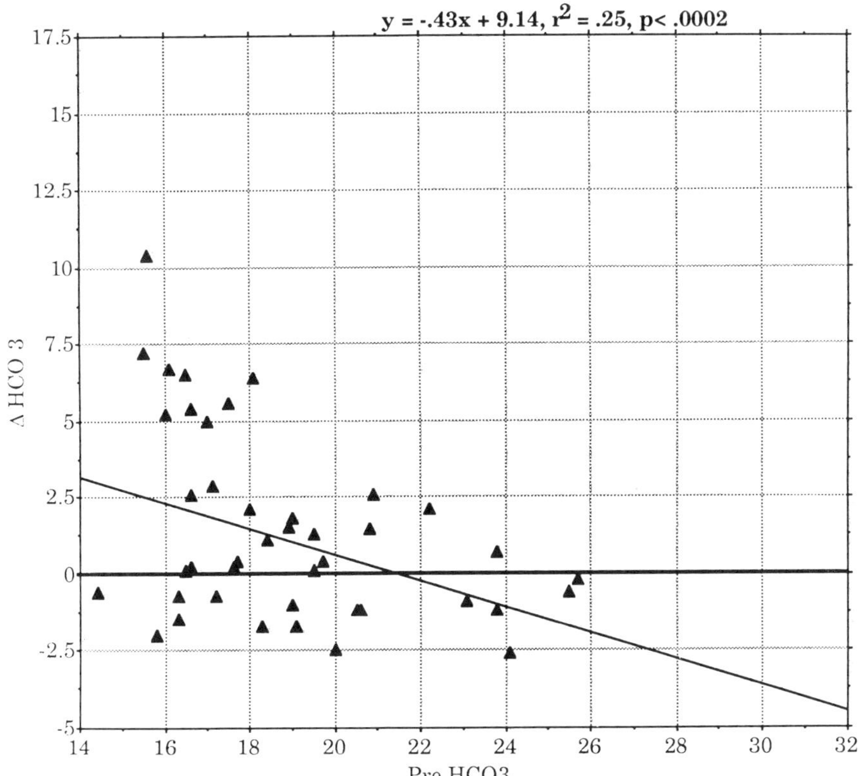

Fig. 16-2. Changes in plasma bicarbonate concentration after acetate hemodialysis. The pretreatment bicarbonate level is plotted on the abscissa, and the postdialysis change is plotted on the ordinate. ($r = .55$, $P < .002$.)

The changes in $PaCO_2$ during bicarbonate hemodialysis (Fig. 16-3) and acetate hemodialysis (Fig. 16-4) are presented similarly to the changes in bicarbonate level, with pretreatment $PaCO_2$ values on the abscissa and changes in $PaCO_2$ after treatment on the ordinate. For a pretreatment $PaCO_2$ of 40 mmHg, the expected fall in $PaCO_2$ is negligible during bicarbonate hemodialysis and amounts to 6 mmHg during acetate hemodialysis. The pretreatment $PaCO_2$ at which the expected change in $PaCO_2$ is minimal is 40 mmHg for bicarbonate hemodialysis compared with 28 mmHg for patients receiving acetate hemodialysis.

Once the variables of pretreatment plasma bicarbonate and $PaCO_2$ are known, the expected changes can be predicted from Figures 16-1 through 16-4. The direction in which the pH will be altered can be predicted from Figure 16-5, which represents the relationship involving plasma bicarbonate (abscissa), PCO_2 (ordinate), and pH (diagonal). The intersection of two points, namely, plasma bicarbonate and PCO_2, predicts the pH. The pre- and post-treatment coordinates determine the final pH. For example, for a patient

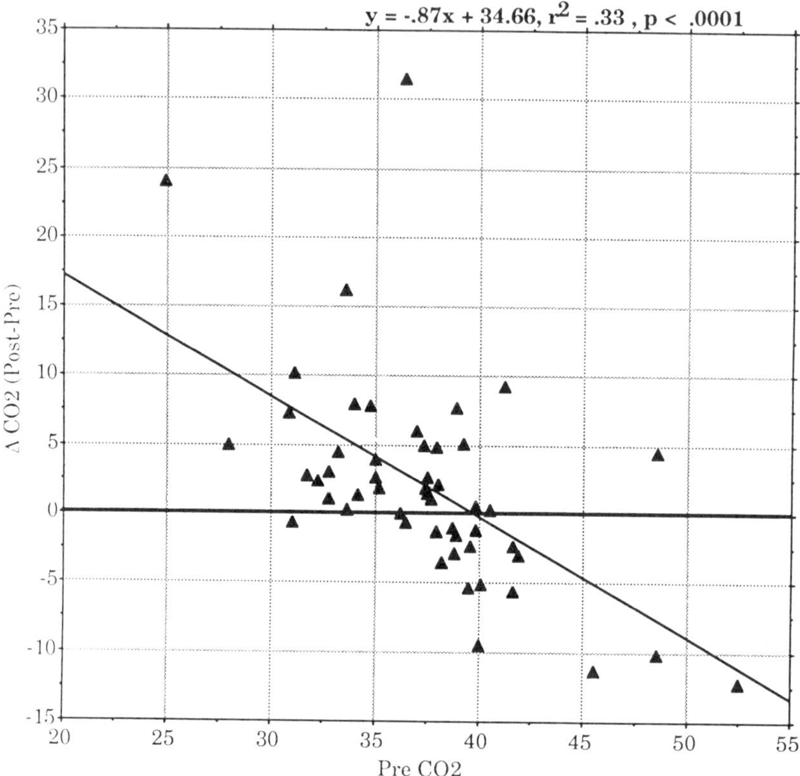

Fig. 16-3. Changes in $PaCO_2$ after bicarbonate hemodialysis. The pretreatment $PaCO_2$ is plotted on the abscissa, and the change after hemodialysis is plotted on the ordinate. ($r = .55$, $P < .015$.)

presenting to hemodialysis with ABG values of pH 7.5, $PaCO_2$ 35 mmHg, and bicarbonate 26 mEq/L who receives acetate hemodialysis (A), the predicted final ABG values would be pH 7.53, $PaCO_2$ 31 mmHg, and bicarbonate 24 mEq/L (dashed line). If this patient receives bicarbonate hemodialysis (B), the predicted final ABG values would be pH 7.50, $PaCO_2$ 39 mmHg, and bicarbonate 28 mEq/L (solid line). The increase in pH at the end of the treatment may be harmful to the patient. Thus, one can choose the type of dialysate appropriate for a patient's dialysis treatment on the basis of the pretreatment ABG values in such manner that post-treatment pH extremes can be avoided.

Hemofiltration. The acid-base balance in postdilutional hemofiltration is the difference between the base lost in the ultrafiltration (i.e., bicarbonate, organic anions, and part of the buffer infused intravenously) and the amount of base administered to the patient in the substitution fluid. Base removal in the ultrafiltrate, as well as carbon dioxide removal, occurs by convection only. The substitution fluid usually contains acetate or lactate as a base

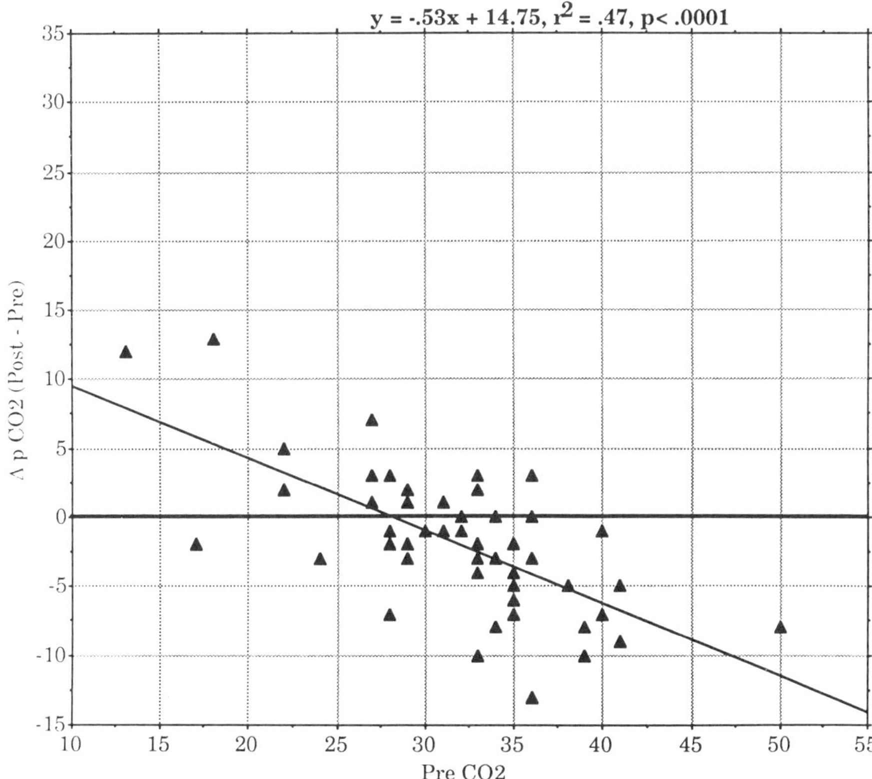

Fig. 16-4. Changes in $PaCO_2$ after acetate hemodialysis. The pretreatment $PaCO_2$ is plotted on the abscissa, and the change after hemodialysis is plotted on the ordinate. ($r = .7$, $P < .001$.)

equivalent at an average concentration of 40 mmol/L. Substitution fluids containing bicarbonate have been used experimentally.[16] The plasma pH, bicarbonate concentration, arterial oxygen pressure (PaO_2), and $PaCO_2$ behave in a fashion similar to that seen in acetate dialysis[17]—that is, PO_2 decreases moderately, $PaCO_2$ remains stable, and pH and bicarbonate increases progressively during the hemofiltration treatment. It appears that the $PaCO_2$ and plasma bicarbonate concentration are significantly higher in hemofiltration than in acetate hemodialysis. Similar results have been demonstrated when lactate-containing substitution fluid was used.[18] No cases of metabolic alkalosis have been reported to date; however, it is conceivable that if the base concentration in the substitution fluid is high and exceeds that in the ultrafiltrate, eventually the plasma bicarbonate concentration will approach the base concentration in the substitution fluid, resulting in metabolic alkalosis.

Hemodiafiltration and rapid dialysis. Highly efficient dialyzers permit large quantities of base equivalents to be transported across the membrane

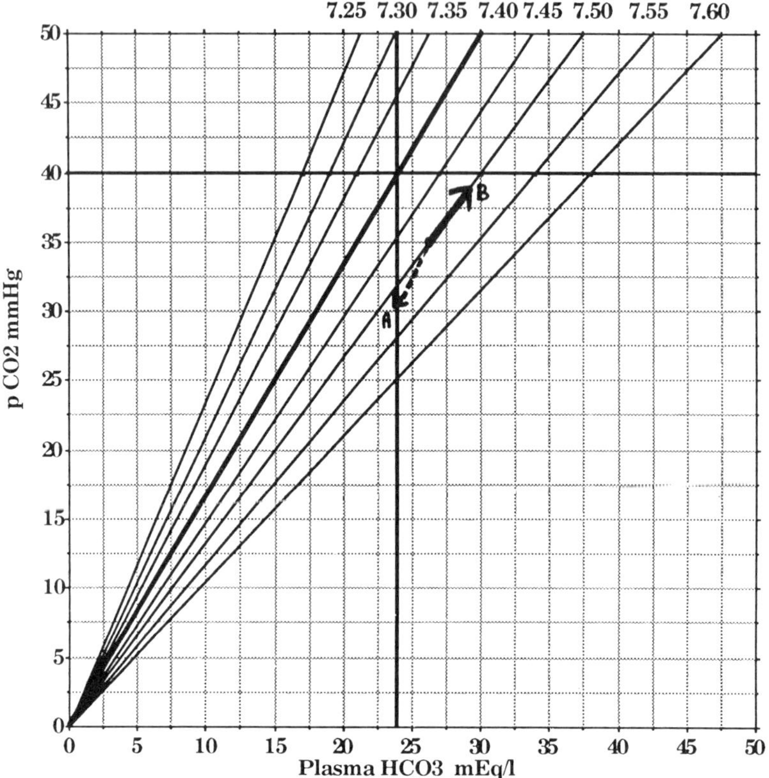

Fig. 16-5. The relationship among plasma bicarbonate, PCO_2, and pH. This graph may be used to predict the expected change in pH. A = acetate dialysate, B = bicarbonate dialysate.

by both diffusive and convective processes. The quantity of acetate delivered to plasma from dialysate exceeds the maximal metabolic capacity of the body to convert it to bicarbonate, which may result in acidosis. As a result, bicarbonate dialysate is preferred. It has been shown that in hemodiafiltration using acetate dialysate and lactate substitution fluid, patients do not reach the positive net overall buffer flux necessary to achieve optimal interdialytic acid-base balance[20]; however, such optimal interdialytic balance can be achieved at clinically used ultrafiltration rates when bicarbonate substitution fluid and dialysate are used. Additionally, bicarbonate dialysate provides cardiovascular stability, which acetate and lactate cannot do.[19,21]

Peritoneal dialysis. Metabolic alkalosis is not limited to hemodialysis. Peritoneal dialysis-associated metabolic alkalosis has been reported as a result of water being removed in excess of bicarbonate when a 7 percent dextrose peritoneal dialysis solution was used.[22] Movement of acetate from the dialysate to the plasma and of bicarbonate from the plasma to the dialysate is similar to that occurring in hemodialysis. The amount transported depends on the acetate and bicarbonate concentration gradients between plasma and dialysate and the duration of peritoneal dialysate dwell.

Other forms of alkalemia associated with dialysis. It is important to differentiate dialysis-associated alkalemia from true metabolic alkalosis as described in the previous paragraphs. Alkalemia is defined as blood pH higher than 7.45. Metabolic and respiratory causes may operate separately or in concert to produce alkalemia. Patients with ESRD may exhibit hypocapnia as part of a compensatory respiratory mechanism in response to the fall in plasma bicarbonate associated with metabolic acidosis. Alternatively, hypocapnia may be a primary respiratory event in which the respiratory rate is fixed and/or rapid. Patients receiving mechanical ventilation and those who hyperventilate because of a central nervous system disorder, pulmonary abnormality, or anxiety are representative examples of patients who have respiratory alkalosis. Normally, respiratory alkalosis would trigger renal compensatory mechanisms that lower the plasma bicarbonate level to protect the body from severe alkalemia. In patients with nonfunctioning kidneys, the kidneys are unable to increase urinary bicarbonate excretion or further decrease acid excretion. When patients presenting to hemodialysis with hypocapnia are unable to decrease ventilation as plasma bicarbonate increases during the hemodialysis treatment, a mixed acid-base disturbance develops with at least a component of respiratory alkalosis. Severe alkalemia has been reported in patients receiving either hemodialysis or peritoneal dialysis.[23]

The hemodialysis treatment itself can result in an increase in pH due to alteration in carbon dioxide tension (PCO_2). Carbon dioxide mass balance determinations in acetate hemodialysis show that carbon dioxide is lost from the plasma to the dialysate.[24] This loss of carbon dioxide occurs not only by diffusion but to a lesser extent also by convection due to ultrafiltration. Since the dialysance of carbon dioxide is identical to that of blood urea nitrogen (BUN), carbon dioxide removal will be as efficient as BUN removal. Rapid urea removal in high-efficiency hemodialysis has not been shown to be deleterious. However, if carbon dioxide removal and hydrogen ion generation exceed acetate conversion to bicarbonate, plasma bicarbonate concentration may fall and acetate concentration increase. The final pH would reflect a fall in PCO_2 and bicarbonate. When bicarbonate dialysate is used, plasma bicarbonate concentration is dependent on bicarbonate transport across the dialyzer membrane and not on a metabolic step in which a base equivalent is converted to bicarbonate. In addition, carbon dioxide movement from blood to dialysate would be less, since the carbon dioxide gradient is attenuated. It has been shown that $PaCO_2$ levels remain stable[25,26] or increase moderately.[27]

Gastrointestinal Acid Loss

Vomiting results in the loss of acid from the gastrointestinal tract. Patients with ESRD frequently vomit, since this is a complication of uremia. The chemoreceptor trigger center in the floor of the fourth ventricle and the vomiting center in the medulla are integrated to produce vomiting. One or more of the uremic toxins can stimulate the trigger zone to activate the vomiting center.[28] Patients vomit during hemodialysis in response to shifts in electrolytes or to hypotension, and in those with diabetes mellitus, diabetic gastroparesis is a common cause of vomiting.

Vomiting in patients with renal disease rarely leads to severe metabolic alkalosis. The serum bicarbonate concentration rarely exceeds the normal range since the increase in serum bicarbonate must offset the low serum bicarbonate associated with renal metabolic acidosis. In patients with normal renal function, the volume depletion associated with vomiting enhances the metabolic alkalosis. This additional factor is generally not seen in patients with ESRD, but if oral intake does not exceed urinary and gastrointestinal losses, volume depletion may enhance the metabolic alkalosis.

However, when metabolic alkalosis does occur from gastric acid losses, it is severe, with bicarbonate values exceeding 50 mEq/L. Bicarbonate ions generated by the gastric mucosa during hydrogen ion secretion are unopposed by hydrogen ion absorption when gastric acid losses occur. Additionally, pancreatic bicarbonate secretion is reduced in the absence of the acid stimulus of duodenal contents. Both these factors contribute to the increase in plasma bicarbonate concentration.[29]

Urinary Acid Loss

Urinary acid loss is not discussed here since this event is not applicable to patients with ESRD.

Maintenance of Metabolic Alkalosis

The addition of base or loss of acid by itself usually will not lead to significant metabolic alkalosis. The normal kidney rapidly excretes the excess bicarbonate within 1 hour of oral or parenteral bicarbonate administration. Urinary bicarbonate excretion is maximal at 24 to 48 hours.[30] Therefore, to maintain metabolic alkalosis, impaired renal bicarbonate excretion must be present. Factors that affect renal bicarbonate excretion are (1) decreased glomerular filtration rate, (2) volume contraction, (3) hypokalemia, (4) hypochloremia, and (5) steroid excess.[31] Of these factors only the first is applicable to patients with ESRD. Metabolic alkalosis is maintained by the kidney's inability to filter and excrete bicarbonate. Any bicarbonate administered or generated that is not used to buffer acid is retained by the kidney to maintain the metabolic alkalosis.

CLINICAL MANIFESTATIONS

Several physiologic compensatory mechanisms are activated to decrease the plasma bicarbonate in persons with acute and chronic metabolic alkalosis and thereby to maintain the pH within an acceptable range.

Physiologic Pulmonary Response

The lung compensates immediately with a response that takes minutes. This response consists of hypoventilation with subsequent retention of carbon dioxide and occasional hypoxemia.

Several calculations are available to predict the $PaCO_2$ in response to metabolic alkalosis:

$PaCO_2 = 0.73\ [HCO_3^-] + 20 \pm 5\ (r = 0.9)$ (ref. 32)

$PaCO_2$ increases by 0.7 mmHg (range 0.2 to 0.9 mmHg) for each mEq/L increment in the plasma bicarbonate concentration. (ref. 3)

$PaCO_2 = 0.9\ [HCO_3^-] + 9$ (ref. 33)

$PaCO_2$ rises linearly with elevation of serum bicarbonate up to 75. (ref. 34)

Respiratory compensation in response to the metabolic disorder prevents severe changes in blood pH.[35–43]

Respiratory failure with hypercapnia and hypoxemia has been observed in patients with metabolic alkalosis.[32,35,36,41] Compensatory hypoventilation in severe metabolic alkalosis was commonly thought to be limited by hypoxemia. However, alkalosis has been shown to reduce the sensitivity of peripheral chemoreceptors to hypoxia,[44] and compensatory decreased alveolar ventilation can produce $PaCO_2$ values as high as 60 to 75 mmHg.[36–39] Alkalosis causes a shift in the oxygen-hemoglobin dissociation curve to the left. The diminished oxygen release from hemoglobin to the tissue together with hypoxemia makes severe alkalosis a serious medical problem.

Blood pH increases minimally in patients with metabolic alkalosis and renal failure owing to a greater effectiveness of respiratory compensation. In individuals with normal renal function, the respiratory compensation for alkalemia is partially offset by PCO_2-induced renal bicarbonate synthesis.[45] However, in uremic patients, the failure of PCO_2 to enhance the renal synthesis of bicarbonate leaves the pH lowering effect of hypercapnia unopposed.

Physiologic Renal Response

The kidney plays a major role in the compensation of metabolic alkalosis by excreting an alkaline urine. The renal response to extrarenal causes of acute metabolic alkalosis is characterized by an increase in urine pH and bicarbonate excretion and a decrease of net acid excretion. An acute rise in plasma bicarbonate increases the filtered bicarbonate level above the reabsorptive capacity of the proximal tubule. The subsequent increased bicarbonate delivery to the distal nephron increases sodium and potassium excretion. In chronic metabolic alkalosis the urine pH is low (paradoxical aciduria), potassium excretion will remain elevated, and urinary sodium and chloride excretion is low. Patients with renal disease have impaired urinary bicarbonate excretion. Since these patients have alterations in glomerular filtration rate and tubular secretory and reabsorptive abilities, metabolic alkalosis takes longer to correct because bicarbonate can not be excreted. Thus, medical interventions are usually required to lower the plasma bicarbonate.

Morbidity and Mortality

Severe metabolic alkalosis is associated with high morbidity and mortality.[46,47] Wilson et al.[46] showed that the mortality rate paralleled pH when pH was greater than 7.55 in critically ill surgical patients.

Associated Clinical Symptoms

Many of the symptoms associated with metabolic alkalosis are related to concurrent hypocalcemia or hypokalemia.[48,49] (Table 16-3). Alkalosis decreases the plasma potassium and calcium ion concentrations. Neuromuscu-

Table 16-3. Clinical Manifestations of Metabolic Alkalosis

Changes in central nervous system function
Mental confusion
Obtundation
Seizures
Changes in peripheral nervous system function
Paresthesias
Muscle cramps
Tetany
Cardiovascular
Cardiac arrhythmias
Increased sensitivity to digitalis
Hypotension
Myocardial necrosis
Pulmonary
Alveolar hypoventilation
Hypercarbia
Hypoxia
Respiratory depression
Increased difficulty in weaning patients from assisted ventilation
Neuromuscular
Increased release of acetylcholine
Metabolic
Shift of oxyhemoglobin dissociation curve to the left (limiting oxygen release at the tissue level)
Decrease in the plasma level of ionized calcium
Facilitation of glycolysis with increased lactate production
Hypokalemia
Hypophosphatemia
Symptoms related to hypokalemia
Muscle weakness
Polyuria
Polydipsia
Increased neuromuscular excitability
Paresthesias
Carpopedal spasm
Lightheadedness

lar symptoms, including paresthesias, tetany, muscle twitching, and myoclonus, are commonly reported in severe metabolic alkalosis.[50–53] Alterations in mental status may be severe. Generalized or focal seizures are not easily suppressed with anticonvulsants.[51,54] Coma may not be resolved for several days after alkalemia is corrected.[36,54] Cerebrospinal fluid alkalosis and decreased cerebral blood flow have been demonstrated in patients with metabolic alkalosis.[55]

Clinical Effect during Hemodialysis

When ESRD patients present for hemodialysis with metabolic alkalosis and respiratory compensation, it is important to consider the effects of the dialysis treatment on plasma bicarbonate, $PaCO_2$, and pH.

The postdialysis plasma bicarbonate concentration may be unchanged, increased, or decreased, depending on the type and concentration of base in the dialysate and the rate of transport of base as determined by the concentration gradients between the dialysate and the plasma. In general, the hemodialysis treatment is an alkalinizing therapy and thus results in an increase in plasma bicarbonate concentration. However, if a patient presents to hemodialysis with a plasma bicarbonate concentration higher than the dialysate bicarbonate concentration, there will be net removal of bicarbonate and a fall in plasma bicarbonate concentration.

The plasma $PaCO_2$ reflects carbon dioxide production and net gain or loss to the dialysate during dialysis and plays a significant role in the final acid-base status of the patient. Carbon dioxide moves between plasma and dialysate depending on the concentration gradient. The $PaCO_2$ will fall as a result of carbon dioxide losses through the dialyzer. Acetate dialysis will result in a greater carbon dioxide loss than bicarbonate dialysis since carbon dioxide is present in the bicarbonate dialysate but not the acetate dialysate. Thus, alkalemia due to metabolic and respiratory causes is made worse by dialysis because of the loss of carbon dioxide.

CORRECTION AND MANAGEMENT

Correction of Underlying Cause

The first step in the correction of metabolic alkalosis is to determine the etiology of the metabolic disorder. Correction of the underlying disorder usually will correct the acid-base disturbance. Cessation of exogenous base administration or gastrointestinal acid loss in general is adequate to correct the metabolic alkalosis. States of urinary acid loss, such as increased tubular flow rate and sodium delivery, increased mineralocorticoid activity, increased tubule lumen negativity, and increased peritubular PCO_2 are not applicable to patients with ESRD.

Chloride Replacement

In chloride-sensitive patients with normal renal function, replacement with chloride provides another anion besides bicarbonate for the kidney to reabsorb. These patients present with urine chloride concentrations less than 10 mEq/L. Chloride repletion is the single most important step for the correction of metabolic alkalosis[56] and can be accomplished independently of the volume or potassium status of the subject or of diminished glomerular filtration rate. Chloride is usually administered as a sodium chloride infusion, although potassium chloride and hydrochloric acid may be used. Normal saline infusion results in volume expansion with subsequent bicarbonaturia. These routine treatments cannot be used in patients with ESRD.

The nonfunctioning kidney cannot excrete bicarbonate, and the addition of sodium chloride will result in volume overload. Similarly, potassium chloride administration cannot enhance bicarbonate excretion in a nonfunctioning kidney. Moreover, administration of potassium to a patient with renal failure can result in life-threatening hyperkalemia.

Acid Administration

Previously, management of severe metabolic alkalosis involved administration of acidifying agents such as ammonium chloride, arginine hydrochloride, or even hydrochloric acid intravenously.[57–59] Arginine hydrochloride, lysine hydrochloride, and ammonium chloride are no longer commercially available because of their multiple side effects. Arginine hydrochloride administration is associated with hyperglycemia and hyperkalemia, and ammonium chloride infusion carries the risk of ammonia toxicity. Both these compounds deliver an additional nitrogenous load, resulting in an elevation of the patient's BUN level. Hydrochloric acid is still available but infrequently used. It is usually infused as a 0.1 N solution into a central vein at a rate not exceeding 25 mEq/h. Frequently, the hospital pharmacy may not have the desired acidifying agent available. In anuric patients treatments such as spironolactone, acetazolamide, ammonium chloride, or arginine monohydrochloride are risky or useless.[60,61]

H_2-Receptor Antagonists

In patients who develop metabolic alkalosis from upper gastrointestinal acid loss, the use of histamine H_2-receptor antagonists can suppress acid secretion and thus decrease acid loss.[59,62]

Renal Bicarbonate Removal

Although this approach is not applicable to patients with renal failure, metabolic alkalosis can be corrected by inducing renal bicarbonate excretion with acetazolamide. Carbonic anhydrase inhibitors decrease bicarbonate reabsorption in the proximal tubule, causing increased bicarbonate excretion. The use of this diuretic will deplete extracellular volume and potassium. Both extracellular volume and potassium depletion further exacerbate metabolic alkalosis.

Dialysis

An additional treatment modality to correct metabolic alkalosis in patients with ESRD is hemodialysis.[35,63,64] In a patient whose plasma bicarbonate concentration (35 mEq/L) was markedly elevated, a gradient between the plasma and dialysate bicarbonate concentrations was effective in lowering the plasma concentration.[35] In less severe cases or when a lower plasma bicarbonate concentration is desired, glacial acetic acid may be added to the dialysate fluid or the dialysis machine can be adjusted to a lower bicarbonate setting. Acetate dialysis is not advisable. The $PaCO_2$ is lowered to a greater extent than the plasma bicarbonate during an acetate dialysis, which results in a worsening of the alkalemia. The PCO_2 in bicarbonate- and acetate-containing dialysates was found to be 46.7 and 2.4 mmHg, respectively.[35]

Ponce et al.[63] used hemodialysis to simultaneously remove plasma bicarbonate and deliver chloride isovolumetrically. The dialysate had a chloride concentration of 143 mEq/L. After 90 minutes of acid dialysis, the changes in acid-base balance and electrolyte were as follows: pH, from 7.65 to 7.37; PCO_2, from 36 to 30.4 mmHg; bicarbonate, from 40.9 to 18.1 mmol/L; sodium, from 141 to 133 mmol/L; potassium, from 3.1 to 3.6 mmol/L; and chloride, from 61 to 88 mmol/L. The patient was hemodynamically and neurologically stable throughout treatment. These authors pointed out that if intravenous hydrochloric acid as a sterile solution of 100 to 150 mEq/L at a maximum infusion rate of 0.2 mEq/kg/h had been used to bring the pH from 7.65 to 7.37, it would have taken at least 40 hours and 2,000 ml to achieve a similar correction of metabolic alkalosis. They further pointed out that use of high-chloride, low-acetate dialysis therapy obviates the need for extra volume infusion, avoids the administration of a sclerosing solution such as hydrochloric acid, and eliminates the additional nitrogen load of ammonium chloride or arginine hydrochloride in patients with renal failure.

REFERENCES

1. Hodgkin JE, Soeprone FF, Chen DM: Incidence of metabolic alkalemia in hospitalized patients. Crit Care Med 8:725, 1980
2. Cogan MG, Liu FY, Berger BE et al: Metabolic alkalosis. Med Clin North Am 67:903, 1983
3. Cogan MG, Rector FC Jr: Acid-base disorders. p. 737. In Brenner BM, Rector FC Jr (eds): The Kidney. 4th Ed. WB Saunders, Philadelphia, 1991
4. Richards RH, Vreman HJ, Zager PH et al: Acetate metabolism in normal human subjects. Am J Kidney Dis 2:47, 1982

5. Lewis EJ, Tolchin N, Roberts JL: Estimation of the metabolic conversion of acetate to bicarbonate during hemodialysis. Kidney Int 18 (suppl 10):S51, 1980
6. Kveim M, Nesbakken R: Utilisation of exogenous acetate during hemodialysis. Trans Am Soc Artif Intern Organs 21:138, 1975
7. Mioni G, Gropuzzo M, Farazza A et al: La reazione di attivazione dell'acetato nel trattamento emodialitico [The reaction of acetate activation during hemodialysis treatment.] Minerva Nefrol 29:137, 1979
8. Graziani G, Casati S, Passerini P et al: Pathophysiology and clinical consequences of metabolic alkalosis in hemodialyzed patients. Arch Ital Urol Nefrol Androl 59:105, 1987
9. Sethi D, Curtis JR, Topham DL et al: Acute metabolic alkalosis during haemodialysis. Nephron 51:119, 1989
10. La Greca G, Fabris A, Feriani M et al: Acid-base homeostasis in clinical dialysis. p. 808. In Maher JF (ed): Replacement of Renal Function by Dialysis. 3rd Ed. Kluwer, Boston, 1989
11. Christensen HN: General concepts of neutrality regulation. Am J Surg 103:286, 1962
12. Vreman HJ, Assomull VM, Kaiser BA et al: Acetate metabolism and acid-base homeostasis during hemodialysis: influence of dialyzer efficiency and rate of acetate metabolism. Kidney Int 18 (suppl 10):S62, 1980
13. Tolchin N, Roberts JL, Hayashi J et al: Metabolic consequences of high mass-transfer hemodialysis. Kidney Int 11:366, 1977
14. Kishimoto T, Yamamoto T, Yamamoto K et al: Acetate kinetics during hemodialysis and hemofiltration. Blood Purif 2:81, 1984
15. Gotch FA, Sargent JA, Keen ML: Hydrogen ion balance in dialysis therapy. Artif Organs 6:388, 1982
16. Feriani M, Biasioli S, Fabris A et al: Calcium and bicarbonate containing solutions for peritoneal dialysis and hemofiltration. p. 277. In Nose Y, Kjellstrand C, Ivanovich P (eds): Progress in Artificial Organs. International Society for Artificial Organs Press, Cleveland, 1986
17. Bosch JP, Lauer A: Acid-base balance in hemofiltration. p. 147. In Henderson LW, Quellhorst EA, Baldamus CA, Lysaght MJ, (eds): Hemofiltration. Springer-Verlag, Berlin, 1986
18. Schaefer K, Ryzlewicz T, Sandri M et al: Effect of hemofiltration on acid-base status and ventilation. Contrib Nephrol 32:69, 1982
19. Scheider H, Liorinin E, Streicher E: Hemodynamic studies of diffusive and convective procedures using a polysulphone membrane. Contrib Nephrol 46:134, 1985
20. Feriani M, Biasioli S, Bragantini L et al: Buffer balance in bicarbonate hemodiafiltration. Trans Am Soc Artif Intern Organs 32:422, 1986
21. Feriani M, Ronco C, Biasioli S et al: Effect of dialysate and substitution fluid buffer on buffer flux in hemodiafiltration. Kidney Int 39:711, 1990
22. Gault MH, Ferguson EL, Sidhu JS: Fluid and electrolyte complications of peritoneal dialysis. Ann Intern Med 75:253, 1971
23. Kenamond TG, Graves JW, Lempert KD et al: Severe recurrent alkalemia in a patient undergoing continuous cyclic peritoneal dialysis. Am J Med 81:548, 1986
24. Bosch JP, Glabman S, Moutoussis G et al: Carbon dioxide removal in acetate hemodialysis: effects on acid base balance. Kidney Int 25:830, 1984
25. Man NK, Fournier G, Thireau P et al: Effect of bicarbonate-containing dialysate on chronic hemodialysis patients: a comparative study. Artif Organs 6:421, 1982

26. Nissenson AR: Prevention of dialysis-induced hypoxemia by bicarbonate dialysis. Trans Am Soc Artif Intern Organs 26:339, 1980
27. Graefe U, Milutinovich J, Follette WC et al: Less dialysis-induced morbidity and vascular instability with bicarbonate in dialysate. Ann Intern Med 88:332, 1978
28. Quintanilla A, Singer I: Metabolic alkalosis in the patient with uremia. Am J Kidney Dis 17:591, 1991
29. Harrington J, Kassirer J: Metabolic alkalosis. p. 227. In Cohen JJ, Kassirer JP (eds): Acid-Base. Little, Brown, Boston, 1982
30. Toto RD: Metabolic acid-base disorders. p. 229. In Kokko JP (ed): Fluids and Electrolytes. WB Saunders, Philadelphia, 1986
31. Sabastini S, Kurtzman NA: The maintenance of metabolic alkalosis: factors which decrease bicarbonate excretion. Kidney Int 25:357, 1984
32. Javaheri S, Kazemi H: Metabolic alkalosis and hypoventilation in humans. Am Rev Respir Dis 136:1011, 1987
33. Narins RG, Emmett M: Simple and mixed acid-base disorders: a practical approach. Medicine (Baltimore) 59:161, 1980
34. Harrington JT: Metabolic alkalosis. Kidney Int 26:88, 1984
35. Blank M, Lew SQ: Hypoventilation in a dialysis patient with severe metabolic alkalosis: treatment by hemodialysis. Blood Purif 9:109, 1991
36. Lavie CJ, Crocker EF, Key KJ et al: Marked hypochloremic metabolic alkalosis with severe compensatory hypoventilation. South Med J 79:1296, 1986
37. Tuller MA Mehdi F: Compensatory hypoventilation and hypercapnia in primary metabolic alkalosis. Am J Med 70:281, 1971
38. Lifshitz MD, Brasch R, Cuome AJ et al: Marked hypercapnia secondary to severe metabolic alkalosis. Ann Intern Med 77:405, 1972
39. Fulop M: Hypercapnia in metabolic alkalosis. N Y State J Med 76:19, 1976
40. Olivia PB: Severe alveolar hypoventilation in a patient with metabolic alkalosis. Am J Med 52:817, 1972
41. Jarboe TM, Penman RW, Luke RG: Ventilatory failure due to metabolic alkalosis. Chest 61:61S, 1972
42. Stone DJ: Respiration in man during metabolic alkalosis. J Appl Physiol 17:33, 1962
43. Goldring RM, Cannon PJ, Heinemann HO et al: Respiratory adjustment to chronic metabolic alkalosis in man. J Clin Invest 47:188, 1968
44. Hornbein TF, Roos A: Specificity of H concentration as a carotid receptor stimulus. J Appl Physiol 13:580, 1983
45. Rector FC Jr, Seldin DW, Roberts AD Jr et al: The role of plasma CO_2 tension and carbonic anhydrase activity in the renal reabsorption of bicarbonate. J Clin Invest 39:1706, 1960
46. Wilson RF, Gibson D, Percievel AK et al: Severe alkalosis in critically ill surgical patients. Arch Surg 105:197, 1972
47. Mennen M, Slovis CM: Severe metabolic alkalosis in the emergency department. Ann Emerg Med 17:354, 1988
48. Oster JR, Vaamonde CA: Metabolic alkalosis. p. 3,130. In Massry SG, Glassock RJ (eds): Textbook in Nephrology. Williams & Wilkins, Baltimore, 1983
49. Sabatini S, Kurtzman NA: Metabolic alkalosis. p. 691. In Maxwell MH, Kleeman CR, Narins RG (eds): Clinical Disorders of Fluid and Electrolyte Metabolism. McGraw-Hill, New York, 1987
50. Lubash GD, Cohen BD, Young CW et al: Severe metabolic alkalosis with neurologic abnormalities. N Engl J Med 258:1050, 1958

51. Rotheram ED, Safar P, Robin ED: CNS disorders during mechanical ventilation in chronic pulmonary disease. JAMA 189:993, 1964
52. Edmondson JW, Brashear RE, Ting-Kai L: Tetany: quantitative interrelationships between calcium and alkalosis. Am J Physiol 228:1082, 1975
53. Grace WJ, Barr DP: Complications of alkalosis. Am J Med 4:331, 1948
54. Goldman MA, Lisak R, Matz R et al: Hypochloremic alkalosis with symptoms of seizure disorder. N Y State J Med 70:306, 1970
55. Posner JB, Swanson AJ, Plum F: Acid-base balance in cerebrospinal fluid. Arch Neurol 12:479, 1965
56. Rosen R, Julian B, Dubovsky E et al: On the mechanism by which chloride corrects metabolic alkalosis in man. Am J Med 84:449, 1988
57. Shavelle HS, Parke R: Postoperative metabolic alkalosis and acute renal failure: rationale for the use of hydrochloric acid. Surgery 78:439, 1975
58. Williams DB, Lyons JH Jr: Treatment of severe metabolic alkalosis with intravenous infusion of hydrochloric acid. Surg Gynecol Obstet 150:315, 1980
59. Rowlands BJ, Tindall SF, Elliott DJ: The use of dilute hydrochloric acid and cimetidine to reverse severe metabolic alkalosis. Postgrad Med J 54:118, 1978
60. Swartz RD, Rubin JE, Brown RS et al: Correction of postoperative metabolic alkalosis and renal failure by hemodialysis. Ann Intern Med 86:52, 1977
61. Harrington J: Metabolic alkalosis. Kidney Int 26:88, 1984
62. Barton CH, Vaziri ND, Ness RL et al: Cimetidine in the management of metabolic alkalosis induced by nasogastric drainage. Arch Surg 114:70, 1979
63. Ponce P, Santana A, Vinhas J: Treatment of severe metabolic alkalosis by "acid dialysis." Crit Care Med 19:583, 1991
64. Ayus JC: Alkalemia associated with renal failure: correction by hemodialysis with low-bicarbonate dialysate. Arch Intern Med 140:513, 1980

17

Amyloid and β_2-Microglobulin: Metabolism and Kinetics

Babatunde Fariyike
Nathan W. Levin

INTRODUCTION

β_2-Microglobulin has assumed a prominent place in nephrology as the precursor to a common disease affecting chronic dialysis patients, namely, dialysis amyloidosis (a condition in which amyloid is deposited in synovia, bones, and rarely, visceral organs). The kinetics of β_2-microglobulin are affected by the nature and degree of renal dysfunction, the modalities of treatment, and the type of dialysis membrane used. Knowledge of these kinetics in health and in renal failure and of the effects of various dialysis treatment modalities is relevant to understanding the pathogenesis and the progression of dialysis amyloidosis.

β_2-Microglobulin, a normal constituent of plasma, was characterized initially in the urine of patients with Wilson's disease and workers with chronic cadmium poisoning.[1] This substance, originating from the surface of nearly all cells as the constant portion of the light chain of the major histocompatibility complex class I antigens of humans, has since been found in many biologic fluids. β_2-Microglobulin is not present on mature erythrocytes and trophoblastic cells of the placenta, but lymphoid cells, macrophages, and endothelial cells, rich in human leukocyte antigens (HLA), contain it in substantial quantities.

β_2-Microglobulin, with a molecular weight of about 11,800 consists of a polypeptide chain of 99 residues with a disulfide bridge. It is devoid of glycosylation sites and since it does not contain or form hydrophobic residues, it cannot be associated with the lipid bilayer of cell membranes.[2] In healthy subjects nearly 98 percent of immunoreactive β_2-microglobulin circulates as an intact monomer without evidence of formation of aggregates or fragments.[3] The remaining β_2-microglobulin is associated with HLA heavy chains or is complexed with autoantibodies present in normal serum and in greater amounts in sera from patients with autoimmune disease.[4] However, dimers and polymers of β_2-microglobulin have been described in the synovial fluid of patients receiving long-term hemodialysis.[5] Table 17-1 summarizes levels and kinetics of β_2-microglobulin in health, renal disease, and the effects of dialysis.

HEALTHY SUBJECTS

In healthy subjects the turnover of β_2-microglobulin is apparently consistent, and diurnal and day-to-day variation is small. The normal range of plasma concentration in adults is 1.1 to 2.7 mg/L.[6] Turnover studies with iodine 125-labeled β_2-microglobulin in normal adults indicate a production rate of the order of 0.11 to 0.18 mg/kg/h or 150 to 200 mg/d.[4] The substance distributes as the unbound monomer in at least two extracellular compartments, namely, plasma and interstitial fluid.[7,8] β_2-Microglobulin has been used as an indicator of renal tubular maturation in infants born from the thirty-second to the forty-first gestational week.[9] Proximal tubular maturation lags behind glomerular function, so that glomerulotubular balance for β_2-microglobulin is reached at about 35 weeks[9]. This explains why the serum level is high at birth, falling thereafter to lower values until puberty, when it rises transiently. Thereafter, the level increases gradually with age to that seen in normal adults. The higher concentrations may be related to gradual reduction in glomerular filtration rate with advancing age.

Table 17–1. Summary of Kinetics of β_2-Microglobulin in Health and Renal Disease and Effect of Dialysis Types[a]

Measurement	Normal	Renal Disease	Conventional HD (cellulosic)	High-Flux HD	Hemofiltration	CAPD
Generation rate (mg/d)	150–200[12]	150–200[12]	May be increased	150–200[12]	150–200[12]	140–210[26]
Volume of distribution (% of body weight)	17[12, 25]	20[8]	17[25]	24[20]	20[8]	20[13]
Serum levels (mg/L)	1.1–2.7[10]	6–9.7[4]	12.5–92[25] 20–60[26]	5.4–11.8[22]	15–25[32]	35–57[45] 20–35.2[19]
Catabolism (mg/d)	Renal 148.5–198 Extrarenal 15–20	Reduced, therefore serum levels rise	Virtually none because of loss of renal function	Virtually none because of loss of renal function	Virtually none because of loss of renal function	Virtually none because of loss of renal function
Excretion (mg/d)	Urinary 0.12–0.37	Urinary loss >1 in tubular disorders[46]	No loss via dialysis membrane	57–71[39]	100–128[20]	33–34[26] 16–36[19]

Abbreviations: HD, hemodialysis; CAPD, continuous ambulatory peritoneal dialysis.
[a] Superscripts are reference numbers.

β_2-Microglobulin can be measured with commercially available radioimmunoassay (RIA) kits or enzyme-linked immunosorbent assay (ELISA) kits. These methods are most reliable. Other methods of β_2-microglobulin measurement include immunoelectrophoresis, radio immunodiffusion, and nephelometric assays.

The serum concentration of the protein is determined by the *rates* of synthesis and disappearance, which in turn depend upon degradation and excretion. If the synthesis rate is constant, changes in the serum level reflect alterations in the elimination rate. Although iodinated β_2-microglobulin studies have shown extrarenal excretion, most β_2-microglobulin is metabolized and excreted by the kidneys[10]. The protein is readily filtered by the glomerulus and is subsequently almost completely reabsorbed in the proximal tubules. Tubular cellular uptake occurs by a pinocytotic mechanism common to low molecular weight proteins.[11] After internalization, the protein is transferred to lysosomal structures and degraded to amino acids.[10] The normal kidney reabsorbs about 99.9 percent of the filtered β_2-microglobulin, which means that very little (120 to 370 μg per 24 hour,) is excreted in the urine.[12]

PATIENTS WITH NONRENAL DISEASES

β_2-Microglobulin concentrations may be significantly elevated in patients with inflammatory disorders, liver diseases, acquired immunodeficiency syndrome (AIDS), or malignant diseases, especially lymphoproliferative disorders such as multiple myeloma, B-cell lymphomas and chronic lymphocytic leukemia, in which cell turnover may be increased.[12] In these cases the plasma levels of β_2-microglobulin are disproportionately elevated regardless of the glomerular filtration rate. Levels up to 20 mg/L are observed.[13] The increase in β_2-microglobulin is caused by activation of inflammatory and lymphoid cells; in the neoplastic diseases tumor cells turn over more rapidly, resulting in greater amount of β_2-microglobulin entering the extracellular fluid space. Monitoring the serum level of β_2-microglobulin may be useful in the clinical management of multiple myeloma and lymphoma. Severe reduction in proliferative activity can be gauged by changes in β_2-microglobulin concentrations.[14]

RENAL DISEASE PATIENTS

In intrinsic glomerular disease the rate of β_2-microglobulin synthesis is unchanged, but the serum level is elevated because of reduced glomerular filtration. In the absence of specific tubular functional abnormalities, an inverse correlation exists between plasma β_2-microglobulin concentration and glomerular filtration rate (GFR). However, progression of renal failure does not result in continuously increasing blood levels, which is compatible with tissue deposition or, less probably, with extrarenal excretion.

β_2-Microglobulin urinary concentrations may rise when there is damage to the proximal tubule secondary to diminished reabsorption. In particular, elevated urinary excretion of β_2-microglobulin is typical of early Balkan nephropathy and following exposure to cadmium, cyclosporine, gold, or mercury. Urinary β_2-microglobulin excretion of more than 5 mg/d may occur in the presence of tubular abnormalities. A constant elevation of urinary β_2-microglobulin is characteristic of toxins (e.g., cadmium). Other causes include aminoglycoside antibiotics, amphotericin B, chronic renal transplant rejection, vancomycin, and cyclosporine in low doses. In these settings urinary β_2-microglobulin excretion begins to rise after 5 to 10 days of exposure to the substance and may not reach peak levels for several days. Concomitant changes in GFR complicate interpretation.

In acute tubular necrosis urinary excretion of β_2-microglobulin rises until the GFR declines, then falls as serum creatinine levels rise. Presumably, since β_2-microglobulin in urine depends in part on the filtered load, the cessation of glomerular filtration reduces the amount reaching the urine even with renal tubules capable of reabsorbing it.[15]

Serum β_2-microglobulin is reduced significantly after successful renal transplantation so that frequent determination of levels has been suggested as a means of assessing glomerular and tubular function in the transplanted kidney.[16,17] However, as in other settings, coexistent changes in GFR make interpretation difficult.

DISTRIBUTION AND KINETICS OF β_2-MICROGLOBULIN

Double-pool kinetics of β_2-microglobulin have been verified by use of radioisotopic iodine-labeled β_2-microglobulin both in normal subjects and in patients with renal failure.[4,18] (see Table 17-1). In normal subjects the volume of distribution of β_2-microglobulin is about 17 percent of body weight, which is similar to the 18 percent estimated from β_2-microglobulin kinetics during hemofiltration and the estimated 20 percent of body weight in renal failure.[8] All these values correspond approximately to the extracellular fluid volume.

In addition to renal metabolism, a small extrarenal metabolic clearance of β_2-microglobulin has been identified, which approximates 2 ml/min (3 to 10 mg/d). A second extrarenal removal pathway in the patient with renal failure is the generation of β_2-microglobulin amyloid, the quantitative kinetics of which are largely obscure. Up to a 10-fold increase in serum β_2-microglobulin concentration is seen in renal patients not treated by dialysis, obviously as a result of loss of glomerular filtration rate and renal catabolic activity.

Residual renal function strongly influences serum β_2-microglobulin concentrations in dialysis patients. Although urinary volume provides only a rough indication of residual renal catabolic activity, patients with urine volumes of over 400 ml/d have been observed to have significantly lower levels of β_2-microglobulin than anuric patients treated by continuous ambulatory peritoneal dialysis (CAPD) or hemodialysis.[19]

EFFECTS OF DIALYSIS

Hemodialysis, Hemofiltration, and Hemodiafiltration

Conventional cellulosic membranes are completely impermeable and cellulose acetate membranes used for rapid high-efficiency dialysis variably impermeable to β_2-microglobulin, so that there is little of it is removed during dialysis with these dialyzers.[20] Thus, if renal clearance is zero and since production of β_2-microglobulin continues, removal of extracellular β_2-microglobulin is accomplished by extrarenal deposition, so that very high levels of serum β_2-microglobulin exist and presumably generation of β_2-microglobulin amyloid occurs. Even though little is known about the critical parameters determining the rate of amyloid β_2-microglobulin generation, it has been shown that almost half of the amino acid units in the β_2-microglobulin molecule participate in large B-pleated structures, making the molecule ideally suited to polymerization into amyloid fibrils.[21]

Serum amyloid P, a normal plasma glycoprotein that generally constitutes 10 to 15 percent of the structure of β_2-microglobulin, may play an important role in determining the nidus of polymerization. Elevated aluminum levels may also facilitate polymerization when serum levels of β_2-microglobulin are high.[21–23]

Up to a 50-fold increase above normal in the level of serum β_2-microglobulin in dialysis patients is common, possibly mainly as a result of nearly complete loss of renal function, and is therefore a precondition to dialysis amyloidosis.[12,24] Stable elevated serum levels over many years (usually over 8 years) are almost always an indication of substantial depositions.[25]

With conventional dialyzers, several investigators have reported increases in β_2-microglobulin concentrations varying from 10 to 40 percent after correcting for ultrafiltration losses during dialysis, as measured by increases in hematocrit, serum albumin, or total protein.[17,18,26] Others have argued that correction of postdialysis levels should be based instead on the contraction of the extracellular volume, in which case no anomalous increase in β_2-microglobulin levels is seen.[27] However, rises in serum β_2-microglobulin levels to an extent greater than can be explained by hemoconcentration have been reported.[28]

β_2-Microglobulin generation may be increased by hemodialysis as a result of mechanical damage following the fall in plasma osmolality during dialysis, the use of nonsterile dialysate during dialysis,[4] and the effect of cellulosic membranes.[29] Evidence for the induction of β_2-microglobulin synthesis by cellulosic membranes has been provided by studies that showed an increase in β_2-microglobulin-specific mRNA when these membranes were incubated with lymphocytes.[30] This did not occur with synthetic membranes.

An increase of β_2-microglobulin during dialysis with cuprophane membranes has led to the speculation that membranes with poor biocompatibility, as defined by complement activation and cellular activation, may cause shedding of β_2-microglobulin from involved cells. Others have theorized that there may be an increased de novo synthesis of β_2-microglobulin and/or shedding or cellular release of β_2-microglobulin. However, an increase of cellular β_2-microglobulin seems unlikely to occur within 1 hour of exposure on the basis of in vitro data.[31] β_2-Microglobulin has been demonstrated in granules of human neutrophils, which suggests the existence of an intracellular pool, and 14 to 16 β_2-microglobulin molecules per cell have been estimated to be present on the cell membranes of various cultured human cells. Thus, the possibility for rapid intracellular to extracellular movement or cell membrane shedding of proportionate amount exists. Similar rises in serum β_2-microglobulin during isovolemic cellulosic dialysis occur with either sterile acetate or bicarbonate dialysate.[29] Serum β_2-microglobulin concentration rose with both sterile dialysate and nonsterile dialysate, which suggests that the common inducing factor was the cuprophane membrane. However, the question of sterility may be important when synthetic membranes were used.[32] Higher β_2-microglobulin levels were observed with cuprophane than with polysulfone when nonsterile dialysate was used. However, with polysulfone dialyzers, β_2-microglobulin production was significantly lower when sterile dialysate was used.[32]

The development of open, synthetic membranes such as polyacrylonitrile (PAN) (e.g., AN69), polymethylmethacrylate (PMMA), and polysulfone has made it possible to provide substantial dialyzer clearances of β_2-microglobulin and to gain further insight into its kinetics.[33]

Jorstad et al.[20] reported that polysulfone and polyacrylonitrile membranes were the most effective in removing β_2-microglobulin from patients' plasma during hemofiltration, the former because of high sieving into the dialysate and the latter largely because of high adsorbence on the membrane.

Floege et al.[34] compared the removal of β_2-microglobulin by three different membranes during hemofiltration namely, AN69 (polyacrylonitrile), F60 (polysulfone), and Duoflux (cellulose acetate). Removal amounted to 393 $\pm$ 135 mg, 316 $\pm$ 35 mg, and 242 $\pm$ 79 mg per treatment, respectively. The differences between the dialyzers were significant. Several characteristics explain these differences, including the sieving properties of the membranes, their capacity to adsorb β_2-microglobulin, the water shifts, and the possible generation of β_2-microglobulin that they induce.

Adsorption of proteins on polysulfone and particularly on PMMA and AN69 membranes, has been previously reported. This action contributes to the formation of the "second" membrane, which modifies the sieving coefficient for large proteins in the course of dialysis.[35] Since low-flux polysulfone does not reduce β_2-microglobulin concentration significantly, adsorption on high-flux polysulfone probably occurs in the deeper layers of the membrane. Although AN69 is more efficient than high-flux polysulfone in adsorbing β_2-microglobulin, postdialysis β_2-microglobulin serum levels are significantly lower with high-flux polysulfone owing to higher filtration rates. During hemodialysis with PMMA membrane, plasma β_2-microglobulin clearance in the earlier part is largely dependent on adsorption on the membrane.[36] As dialysis progresses, the amount of β_2-microglobulin adsorbed is reduced, while transmembrane removal increases. Substantial removal by high-flux dialyzers has been demonstrated by von Albertini et al.[37] Even though dialytic therapy was performed with two high-flux dialyzers in series, the three membranes (i.e., PAN, PMMA, and polysulfone) performed similarly, removal of β_2-microglobulin occurring mostly in the first of the serial dialyzers.

The evidence for the transmembranous transfer of β_2-microglobulin lies in its recovery in significant amounts in the dialysate after hemodialysis with highly permeable membranes such as polysulfone or PAN.[34,38] The absolute amount removed depends on factors such as plasma concentration, blood flow, and filtration rate. Larger amounts are transferred with hemofiltration than with hemodiafiltration or hemodialysis.[31–33,39,40] For example, Quellhorst and Schunemann[32] recorded a mean removal of 167 ± 51 mg per treatment by hemofiltration with polysulfone membranes compared with 71 ± 26 mg by hemodialysis.

In principle, reprocessing of high-flux dialyzers might reduce the β_2-microglobulin removal rates. However, Diaz et al.[41] reported that the clearance of β_2-microglobulin improved when reprocessed polysulfone dialyzers were used. The mechanism behind this phenomenon is unknown, but increased openness of the membranes as a result of the process seems possible.

When serum β_2-microglobulin was serially measured in patients before, during, and after high-flux dialysis with polysulfone dialyzers, rebound was demonstrated after the intradialytic decline in serum levels of β_2-microglobulin.[7] Gotch et al.[7] postulated possible mechanisms for this observation as follows:

1. An immunologic response to dialysis with increased shedding of β_2-microglobulin from immunocompetent cells
2. Cellular catabolism known to occur postdialysis
3. Mobilization of β_2-microglobulin from the regions of active β_2-microglobulin polymerization due to the abrupt drop in serum β_2-microglobulin (possibly analogous to the effect of allopurinol in tophaceous gout)

A further possibility is the effect of nonsterile dialysate, as noted earlier.[32]

In regard to increased generation of β_2-microglobulin, Floege et al. showed no change in generation rate in patients undergoing high-flux dialysis.[42] A transient increase during or after dialysis is possible. Rebound due to slow equilibration with the plasma volume cannot be excluded.

Continuous Ambulatory Peritoneal Dialysis

CAPD has not proved to be an effective means of clearing β_2-microglobulin, its efficiency being less than that of high-flux hemodialysis, but not surprisingly, it is more effective than conventional cellulosic hemodialysis.

Residual renal function is of substantial importance—even when the GFR is about 3 ml/min daily urinary excretion of β_2-microglobulin is almost double the daily peritoneal excretion.[19] CAPD removal rates have been recorded as 239 mg/wk.[43]

Previous reports of lower serum β_2-microglobulin concentrations in CAPD patients may largely be due to preservation of residual function in the latter. However, given the possible deleterious effect of dialysis membranes and of nonsterile dialysate, relatively reduced production may be a possibility with CAPD therapy.

In CAPD patients there is no detectable change in serum concentration of β_2-microglobulin after enhanced transperitoneal removal with glucose polymer as compared with glucose.[13] Since serum concentration of β_2-microglobulin at a given time represents the balance between the rates of generation, elimination, and deposition, enhancing the clearance of β_2-microglobulin may have no discernible effect if the amount removed is trivial as compared with the body pool. This situation may occur if net elimination is independent of dialysis-related clearance or if generation from cells or from already polymerized β_2-microglobulin occurs simultaneously.

RELATIONSHIP OF DIALYSIS KINETICS TO DIALYSIS AMYLOIDOSIS

Long-standing dialysis patients (i.e., generally those treated for over 8 years) are at risk of developing dialysis amyloidosis secondary to accumulation of β_2-microglobulin. High-flux dialysis may reduce the rate of β_2-microglobulin accumulation and therefore amyloid but cannot keep up with the production rate. The body burden therefore grows with all methods of dialysis, including high-flux. Although high-flux dialysis may alleviate pain associated with dialysis amyloidosis, it cannot reverse the bony lesions[32]

A retrospective multicenter study reported in 1991 assessed the influence of dialysis membranes on the prevalence of the radiologic signs of dialysis amyloidosis and carpal tunnel syndrome. Patients undergoing dialysis with PAN (AN69) membranes had a lower incidence of amyloid bone disease than those treated with cellulosic membranes.[44] This is compatible with the concept of delay in the establishment of amyloid disease. However, hemodiafiltration and hemofiltration are more effective in reducing the body load and delaying the clinical syndrome of dialysis amyloidosis.

The role of increased β_2-microglobulin generation associated with cellulosic dialyzers is uncertain. Prospective long-term evaluation comparing conventional with biocompatible, equally low-flux dialyzers will be needed to answer this question.

CONCLUSION

In summary, once renal function is lost, β_2-microglobulin accumulates in the body over time, causing a variety of serious problems as the result of amyloid formation. In dialysis patients it appears that factors such as the sterility of the dialysate and the composition of the membrane may affect the rate of synthesis by their effects on mononuclear cells. However removal of β_2-microglobulin, albeit partial, may be important in delaying symptomatic disease and depends on the ability of the more open membranes to adsorb, filter, and permit diffusion of this molecule.

REFERENCES

1. Berggard I, Bearn AG: Isolation and properties of a low molecular weight β_2-microglobulin occurring in human biological fluids. J Biol Chem 243:4095, 1968
2. Revillard JP, Vincent C: Structure and metabolism of beta$_2$-microglobulin. Contrib Nephrol 62:44, 1988
3. Gagnon RF, Sommerville P, Thomson DM: Circulating form of beta$_2$-microglobulin in dialysis patients. Am J Nephrol 8:379, 1988
4. Karlsson FA, Groth T, Sege K et al: Turnover in humans of beta$_2$-microglobulin; the constant chain of HLA antigens. Eur J Clin Invest 10:293, 1980
5. Linke RP, Hampl H, Bartel-Schwarze S, Enlitz M: Beta$_2$-microglobulin, different fragments and polymers thereof in synovial amyloid in long term hemodialysis. Biol Chem Hoppe Seyler 368:137, 1987
6. Evrin PE, Wibell L: The serum levels and urinary excretion of β_2-microglobulin in apparently healthy subjects. Scand J Clin Lab Invest 29:69, 1972
7. Gotch F, Levin NW, Zasuwa G, Tayeb J: Kinetics of beta$_2$-microglobulin in hemodialysis. Contrib Nephrol 74:132, 1989
8. Odell RA, Slowiaczek P, Moran JE, Schindhelm K: Beta$_2$-microglobulin kinetics in end stage renal failure. Kidney Int 39:909, 1991
9. Aperia A, Broberger U: Beta$_2$-microglobulin, an indicator of renal tubular maturation and dysfunction in the newborn. Acta Pediatr Scand 68:669, 1979
10. Schardijin GHC, Statius Van Eps LW: Beta$_2$-microglobulin; its significance in the evaluation of renal function. Kidney Int 32:635, 1987
11. Bernier GM, Conrad ME: Catabolism of human β_2-microglobulin by the rat kidney. Am J Physiol 217:1359, 1969
12. Karlsson FA, Wibell L, Evrin PE: Beta$_2$-microglobulin in clinical medicine. Scand J Clin Lab Invest 40(suppl 154):S27 1980
13. Mistry CD, O'Donoghue DJ, Nelson S et al: Kinetic and clinical studies of beta$_2$-microglobulin in CAPD; influence of renal and enhanced peritoneal clearances using glucose polymer. Nephrol Dial Transplant 5:513, 1990

14. Hagberg H, Killander A, Simonsson B: Serum beta$_2$-microglobulin in malignant lymphoma. Cancer 51:2220, 1983
15. Schentag J, Plant M: Patterns of urinary beta$_2$-microglobulin excretion by patients treated with aminoglycosides. Kidney Int 17:654, 1980
16. Firlit CF, Gleenslade T, Bashoor R: The prognostic value of β_2-microglobulin in pediatric renal transplantation. Proc Dial Transplant Forum 8:219, 1978
17. Robert JL, Lewis EJ: Serum and urine beta$_2$-microglobulin and lysozyme concentrations in transplant rejections. Proc Dial Transplant Forum 9:145, 1979
18. Vincent C, Pozet N, Revillard JP: Plasma beta$_2$-microglobulin turnover in renal insufficiency. Acta Clin Belg 35(suppl 10):S1, 1980
19. Scalamogna A, Imbasciati E, De vecchi A et al: Beta$_2$-microglobulin in patients on peritoneal dialysis and hemodialysis. Perit Dial Int 9:37, 1989
20. Jorstad S, Smeby LC, Balstad T, Wideroe ET: Removal, generation, absorption of beta$_2$-microglobulin during hemofiltration with five different membranes. Blood Purif 6:96, 1988
21. Gorevic PD, Munoz PC, Casey TT et al: Polymerisation of intact β_2-microglobulin in tissue causes amyloidosis in patients on chronic hemodialysis. Proc Natl Acad Sci USA 83:7908, 1986
22. DiRaimondo CR, Stone WA: β_2-Microglobulin amyloidosis. Int J Artif Organs 10:281, 1987
23. Hawkins PN, Lavender JP, Pepys MB: Evaluation of systemic amyloidosis by scintigraphy with 123 iodine-labelled serum amyloid P component. N Engl J Med 323:508, 1990
24. Ballardie FW, Kerr DNS, Tennent G, Pepys MB: Hemodialysis vs CAPD: equal predisposition to amyloidosis? Lancet 1:795 1986
25. Vincent C, Revillard JP, Galland M, Traeger J: Serum beta$_2$-microglobulin in hemodialysed patients. Nephron 21:260, 1978
26. Blumberg A, Burgi W: Behavior of β_2-microglobulin in patients with chronic renal failure undergoing hemodialysis, hemofiltration, hemodiafiltration and CAPD. Clin Nephrol 27:245, 1987
27. Bergstrom J, Wehle B: No change in corrected β_2-microglobulin concentration after cuprophane hemodialysis, letter. Lancet 1:628, 1987
28. Shaldon S, Koch KM, Dinarello CA et al: Beta$_2$-microglobulin and hemodialysis. Lancet 1:925, 1987
29. Granolleras C, Deschodt G, Shaldon S et al: The rise of plasma beta$_2$-microglobulin during cuprophane hemodialysis is real but is not due to cuprophane per se. Blood Purif 5:285, 1987
30. Jahn B, Betz M, Deppisch R et al: Stimulation of beta$_2$-microglobulin synthesis in lymphocytes after exposure to cuprophane dialyser membranes. Kidney Int 40:285, 1991
31. Floege J, Granolleras C, Bingel M et al: Beta$_2$-microglobulin kinetics during hemodialysis and hemofiltration. Nephrol Dial Transplant 1:223, 1987
32. Quellhorst E, Schunemann B: Dialysis Amyloidosis. Wichtig Editore, Milan, 1989
33. Floege J, Granolleras C, Deschodt G et al: High flux synthetic versus cellulosic membranes for β_2-microglobulin removal during hemodialysis, hemodiafiltration and hemofiltration. Nephrol Dial Transplant 4:653, 1989
34. Floege J, Wilks M, Shaldon S, et al. β_2-microglobulin kinetics during hemofiltration. Nephrol Dial Transplant 3:784, 1988
35. Rockel A, Hertel J, Fiegel P et al: Permeability and secondary membrane formation of a high flux polysulfone hemofilter. Kidney Int 30:429, 1986

36. Ohmi T, Muto C, Nishibori F et al: Investigation of plasma clearance of beta$_2$-microglobulin in hemodialysis with PMMA membrane. Jpn J Artif Organs 20:116, 1991
37. Von Albertini B, Barlee V, Bosch JP, Phillips TM: Beta$_2$-microglobulin removal in high flux hemodiafiltration. Am Soc Artif Intern Organs—Abstracts: 87, 1991
38. Zingraff J, Beyne P, Urena P et al: Influence of hemodialysis membrane on beta$_2$-microglobulin kinetics; in vivo and in vitro studies. Nephrol Dial Transplant 3:284, 1988
39. Chanard J, Lavaud S, Toupance O et al: β_2-microglobulin associated amyloidosis in chronic hemodialysis patients. Lancet 1:1212, 1986
40. Klinke B, Röckel A, Perschel W et al: Transmembranous transport and adsorptive capacity of beta$_2$-microglobulin in different hemofilters, abstracted. Blood Purif 6:379, 1988
41. Diaz RJ, Washburn S, Cauble LA et al: The effect of reprocessing polysulfone dialyzers on the removal of β_2-microglobulin and urea clearance, abstracted J Am Soc Nephrol 2:321, 1991
42. Floege J, Bartsch A, Schulze M et al: Clearance and synthesis rates of β_2-microglobulin in patients undergoing hemodialysis and in normal subjects. J Lab Clin Med 118:153, 1991
43. Lysaght MJ, Pollock CA, Moran JE et al: Beta$_2$-microglobulin removal during CAPD. Perit Dial Int 9:29, 1989
44. Van Ypersele de Strihou C, Jadoul M, Malghem J et al: Effect of dialysis membrane and patient's age on signs of dialysis-related amyloidosis. Kidney Int 39:1012, 1991
45. Gagnon RF, Sommerville P, Kaye M: β_2-microglobulin serum levels in patients on long term dialysis. Perit Dial Bull 7:29, 1987
46. Wibell L, Evrin PE, Berggard I: Serum beta$_2$-microglobulin in renal disease. Nephron 10:320, 1973

SUGGESTED READINGS

Klinke B, Röckel A, Perschel W et al: Beta$_2$-microglobulin handling in dialysis. Contrib Nephrol 74:139, 1989

Zingraff J, Beyne P, Uzan M et al: Beta$_2$-microglobulin and hemodialysis membranes; in vivo and in vitro studies. Kidney Int 31:248, 1987

18

Sleep Disorders in Hemodialysis Patients

Paul L. Kimmel

INTRODUCTION

Studies regarding the prevalence and diagnosis of sleep disorders in patients with renal disease are limited, but interest in such abnormalities has increased over the last several years as dialytic techniques have improved and nephrologists have become more interested in enhancing the quality of life of stable long-term hemodialysis patients. Uremia has long been associated with "day-night reversal," a late symptom of advanced renal disease in the predialysis era. Patients with renal disease classically exhibited daytime somnolence and nighttime wakefulness. Disturbed sleep has also been recognized as a common complaint among patients with renal failure undergoing hemodialysis since the institution of viable chronic renal replacement therapies for patients with endstage renal disease (ESRD).[1–3]

Satisfaction with sleep is an important determinant of assessment of quality of life for hemodialysis patients.[4] Poor sleep may be a factor in the well documented poor rehabilitation and quality of life of patients chronically treated with hemodialysis for ESRD.[1,2,5] If sleep disorders in ESRD patients cannot be treated effectively, the rehabilitative potential of any dialytic therapy is necessarily limited.

One study demonstrated that 63 percent of patients treated with hemodialysis complained of disturbed sleep.[3] Symptomatic and asymptomatic patients were similar in age, personality, and medication regimen. More recently, over 40 percent of stable chronic patients treated with hemodialysis in one center complained of disturbed sleep.[4]

Disordered sleep in patients with renal disease may be secondary to psychological factors.[4,6–8] Psychological distress has been documented in such patients and may in fact be associated with some cases of poor sleep.[9] Stress, anxiety, and the effects and interactions of numerous medications, such as tranquilizers and β-blockers, and the use of alcohol[10] can result in poor sleep. Alternatively, depression in the ESRD population[9] may be in some part secondary to sleep disorders.

Several early studies, however, demonstrated abnormalities in electroencephalographic (EEG) patterns of patients with chronic renal failure and ESRD who were treated with hemodialysis, suggesting a neurologic basis for symptoms of insomnia or excessive somnolence.[11,12] Recent polysomnographic studies have demonstrated that by far the largest group of ESRD patients with such symptoms have a specific disorder, the sleep apnea syndrome (SAS).[13,14] SAS is characterized by periodic episodes of cessation of airflow during sleep, accompanied by symptoms of excessive daytime sleepiness, fatigue, headaches, depression, irritability, and cognitive dysfunction. The similarity of such nonspecific symptoms to those of uremia is striking and may contribute to the confounding of the diagnosis of the sleep disturbance. The diagnosis of this disorder can be established by polysomnography.

DIAGNOSIS

Sleep is divided into active or rapid eye movement (REM) and quiet or non-rapid eye movement (non-REM) periods. Non-REM sleep is divided into four stages based on EEG findings.[15] Stage I (a transitional phase between wakefulness and sleep) and stage II (which accounts for the greatest portion of total sleep time in the adult) comprise light sleep. Stages III and IV constitute slow or delta wave sleep. Sleep progresses in sequential fashion through these stages into REM sleep, which usually ends with a brief awakening. REM sleep occupies approximately 20 percent of total sleep time in the adult. The cycle normally repeats, starting from stage I, five or six times a night. As the night progresses, cycle length tends to decrease and the proportion of REM sleep increases.[16]

REM sleep is characterized by marked, generalized decreased muscle tone. The musculature of the neck is most profoundly affected. This diminution in upper airway muscle tone predisposes to inspiratory narrowing in the supraglottic region,[17] resulting in increased dependence on diaphragmatic motion for inspiration in REM sleep. Arousal increases the tone of the upper airway muscles and allows unobstructed breathing. The threshold for arousal is increased in REM as compared with non-REM sleep. During non-REM sleep, breathing is stimulated by hypoxia and hypercarbia, the latter being more effective in causing arousal. In REM sleep, however, ventilation is less responsive to metabolic and autonomic stimuli; hypoxia is its major determinant.[18] Respiration in non-REM sleep is slow and regular, in contrast to the variable, rapid, and irregular breathing of REM sleep.[17]

Abnormalities of the regulation of sleep or physiologic abnormalities peculiar to sleep are termed *sleep disorders,*[16] which are usually divided into four major categories.[16,19]: disorders of initiating and maintaining sleep (DIMS), or insomnias; disorders of excessive somnolence (DOES), or excessive daytime sleepiness; disorders of sleep-wake schedule; and parasomnias. Psychological and psychiatric disturbances and drug and alcohol dependence are causes of both insomnia and excessive daytime somnolence. Sleep apnea figures prominently in both these groupings and may be the most common disorder associated with chronic excessive daytime somnolence. For precise diagnosis of a sleep disorder, however, evaluation of a patient by polysomnography in a sleep laboratory is necessary. Polysomnography identifies and quantifies the time elapsed in each particular stage and phase of the patient's sleep by simultaneously recording the EEG, electro-oculogram, submental electromyogram, nasal and oral airflow, respiratory effort, and gas exchange.[20]

Monitoring respiratory effort and airflow at the nose and mouth permits the differentiation of obstructive, central, and mixed apneas. *Obstructive* apnea is defined as the cessation of airflow at the nose and mouth in the presence of respiratory effort[20] (Fig. 18-1). As airway muscle tone diminishes,

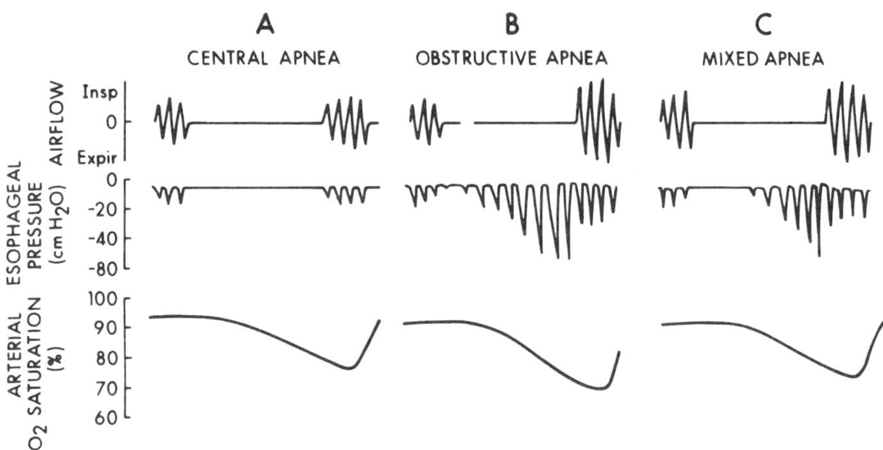

Fig. 18-1. Polysomnograph demonstrating types of apnea. Esophageal pressure measures chest respiratory efforts. (**A**) Central apnea: Note cessation of both airflow and chest respiratory efforts. (**B**) Obstructive apnea: Note cessation of airflow but continuing chest respiratory efforts. (**C**) Mixed apnea: Note initial central apnea followed by obstructive apnea. (From Orr,[20] with permission.)

particularly during REM sleep, the airway becomes occluded, with resulting increased resistance to airflow. Arterial hemoglobin desaturation often results. Anatomic abnormalities of the jaw and airway can often be demonstrated in such patients. The pharynx is the primary site of obstruction in most patients, but the airway at any level may be involved.[21] *Central* apnea is characterized both by the cessation of airflow and the absence of respiratory effort, with abrupt simultaneous resumption of the two (Fig. 18-1). A *mixed* apnea is a combination of central and obstructive apneas occurring during a single cessation of airflow. These different types of apneic events may coexist in an individual patient.[20]

An *apnea* has been defined as complete cessation of nasal and oral airflow for at least 10 seconds, accompanied by a drop in arterial oxygen saturation of at least 4 percent. Hypopnea may be defined as diminution in airflow to less than one-third of control values for at least 10 seconds, accompanied by similar oxygen desaturation. Apneas and hypopneas are disordered breathing events (DBEs). Sleep apnea has been variously defined as at least 5 DBEs per hour or at least 30 DBEs per night.

SAS is commonly complicated by systemic hypertension. Other, less common complications include pulmonary hypertension, cor pulmonale, arrythmias, and polycythemia. Perhaps the most debilitating consequences of the syndrome are the symptoms of sleepiness, fatigue, headache, and personality or intellectual changes, which may interfere seriously with a patient's sense of well-being and the ability to carry on the activities of daily life. When sleep apnea is severe, it may manifest with sleepiness while the patient is occupied at a task such as driving, eating, or talking. Patients may be aware or unaware of snoring, but bed partners will be aware of snoring, gasping, restless movements, and arousals through the night. A patient may awaken many times during the night with a sense of gasping, anxiety, or a choking sensation and may be unable to fall asleep again easily. Alternatively, the majority of such episodes may occur without the patient's conscious awareness. The great majority of patients are male.[21]

The diagnosis of sleep apnea can be suggested by nonspecific symptoms such as daytime hypersomnolence, restless sleep, snoring, or abnormalities of the pharynx on physical examination. However, clinical features do not accurately discriminate between symptomatic patients with and without SAS.[22]

Another sleep disorder, nocturnal myoclonus, is characterized by the intermittent occurrence of stereotyped, abrupt contractions of leg muscles exclusively in sleep. These jerking leg movements, usually bilateral, appear as repetitive contractions with a relatively constant relaxed interval. Such episodes may last up to 1 hour and may occur three or more times during a night's sleep.[16] Patients are typically unaware of these leg movements, although they may be aware of associated frequent awakenings.[16]

Nocturnal myoclonus is similar to the restless legs syndrome, a neurologic complication of uremia, often attributed to inadequate dialysis.[23] The restless legs syndrome may have a prevalence of up to 40 percent in patients with chronic renal disease.[24] Patients complain of uncomfortable dysesthesias, which may interfere with sleep, and an often irresistible urge to move their legs to relieve the sensation. Such leg movements often occur during wakefulness as well. This condition may coexist with nocturnal myoclonus.

PREVALENCE OF SLEEP APNEA IN HEMODIALYSIS PATIENTS

A study of 29 male hemodialysis patients[25] showed that 12 (41 percent) had complaints associated with SAS: headaches, depression, nocturnal awakenings, and restless sleep. In the subpopulation of eight symptomatic subjects who underwent polysomnography, 75 percent had evidence of obstructive sleep apnea. Testosterone administration was not related to the pathogenesis or severity of SAS in these patients, although such therapy has been implicated in causing sleep apnea in a patient without renal disease.[26]

In another study polysomnography was performed on 20 subjects with ESRD treated with standard maintenance hemodialysis.[27] Of these patients 17 were symptomatic, with complaints of daytime sleepiness, disturbed nocturnal sleep, restlessness during sleep, and morning headaches; the remaining three were asymptomatic controls. Polysomnography was performed on the night immediately following a midweek hemodialysis session, at the patients' dry weight, to ensure comparability. Twelve (71 percent) of the symptomatic patients but none of the controls had sleep apnea. The percentage of hemodialysis patients with sleep apnea was significantly higher in the symptomatic than in the asymptomatic group, in spite of the small number of subjects and control patients evaluated. Nine of the twelve symptomatic males and three of the five symptomatic female hemodialysis patients but none of the three asymptomatic hemodialysis patients had sleep apnea.

The majority of patients studied had obstructive sleep apnea. In non-REM sleep, obstructive events comprised approximately two-thirds of the DBEs. In REM sleep, however, the proportion of obstructive disordered breathing approached 80 percent, with obstructive apnea alone accounting for half of the DBEs (Fig. 18-2). There was no correlation of carbon dioxide pressure (PCO_2), blood hydrogen ion concentration, or age with total DBEs in the studied population. Patients had a substantial number of periodic leg movements during sleep. The asymptomatic control subjects, however, also had a high frequency of periodic leg movements.

In a 1990 study of 11 chronic hemodialysis patients,[28] 7 (64 percent) had symptoms suggestive of a sleep disorder, 8 (73 percent) had DBEs, and 6 (55 percent) had SAS diagnosed by polysomnography. There was little improvement in subjective quality of sleep or in parameters of disordered sleep in patients on the night following treatment with standard chronic bicarbonate hemodialysis as compared with a nondialysis night, in spite of increased

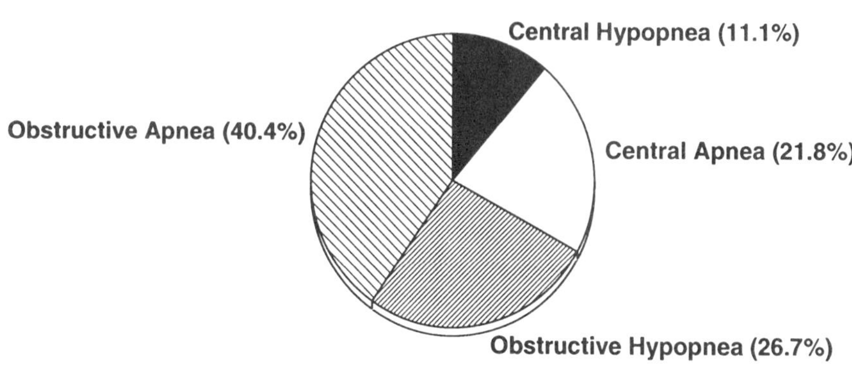

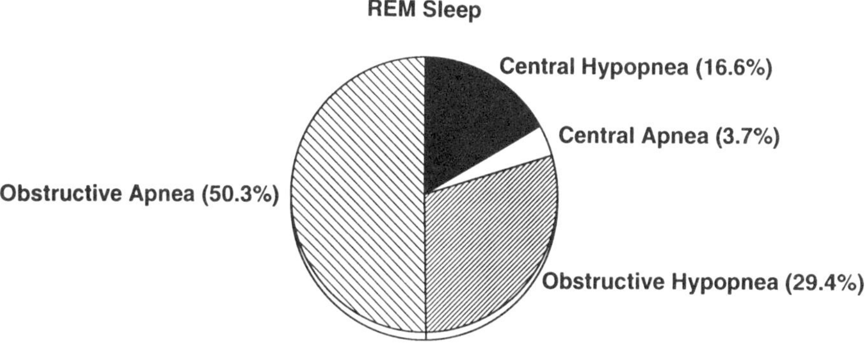

Fig. 18-2. Distribution of disordered breathing events (DBEs) in 12 ESRD patients, treated with hemodialysis, who were symptomatic for sleep apnea. (**A**) Non-REM sleep; (**B**) REM sleep. (Data from Kimmel et al.[27])

systemic pH,[22] although there was an increase in the percentage of DBEs comprising obstructive apneas after dialysis.

The results of these studies suggest that sleep apnea is a common problem in both men and women with ESRD treated by hemodialysis. The prevalence of complaints suggestive of sleep apnea in a chronic hemodialysis setting appears to be in the range of 40 to 50 percent. Consistently, 60 to 80 percent of a tested, symptomatic ESRD population treated with hemodialysis has shown polysomnographic evidence of SAS. Therefore on the basis of symptomatology and incidence rates in hemodialysis populations, the prevalence of SAS in ESRD patients treated with hemodialysis may be as high as 30 percent. A more conservative minimum estimate of 7 to 9 percent has been suggested,[27] but this figure is probably low, since it is based on studies in which not all symptomatic patients were evaluated by polysomnography. Disappointingly, chronic standard maintenance hemodialysis has not been shown to improve sleep architecture or symptoms on a short- or long-term basis.

ETIOLOGY

The reasons for the high prevalence of SAS in patients with ESRD treated with hemodialysis are obscure. One possible explanation is the chronic metabolic acidosis of renal disease, associated with lowered blood pCO_2. Hypocarbia may be insufficient to stimulate respiration and thus may be associated with the occurrence of central apnea. This situation may be exacerbated in patients who have near normal blood pH (typical of chronic renal failure) and a propensity to autonomic neuropathy. However, the results of two studies[27,28] suggest that acid-base balance cannot be an overriding determinant of the severity of SAS in ESRD patients.

Another possibility is that uremia itself predisposes to sleep disorders. This is consistent with the neurologic abnormalities that have been documented in patients with uremia, and in patients under treatment with various dialytic modalities.[23] Several studies have demonstrated correlation of the complaint of sleep disturbance with urea levels in hemodialysis patients.[4,25]

Sleep disorders associated with renal failure may be mediated by the effect of uremic toxins on the central nervous system, which results in the development of SAS by several mechanisms. Excessive reduction of airway muscle tone during sleep may result from uremic myopathy. Alternatively, instability of respiratory control secondary to central effects of uremia, which is a form of uremic neuropathy, may be present. A study in one patient[29] suggested that sleep apnea might be a reversible consequence of acute renal failure, improved by intensive hemodialysis. One polysomnographic study showed correlation of patients' predialysis blood urea nitrogen (BUN) and creatinine levels with DBEs, thus providing indirect evidence that the severity of uremia may modulate the severity of sleep apnea.[25] This finding is controversial.[28] Negative findings in the latter study may be related to the use of a small study group, which included asymptomatic as well as symptomatic subjects.

A 1991 study showed that symptomatic hemodialysis patients, without sleep apnea, had less REM sleep and poorer sleep quality (assessed as prolongation in time to fall asleep and reduced time spent in sleep) than normal controls.[30] Interestingly, an infusion of branched-chain amino acids (BCAA) increased the percent of REM sleep toward normal and stimulated nocturnal respiration (assessed by a reduction in end-tidal CO_2) in these patients.[30] In one patient with SAS who was assessed in this study, BCAA infusion resulted in a marked decrease in the total number of obstructive apneic episodes. Since patients with chronic renal disease may have decreased circulating levels of BCAA,[31,32] this study also suggests a metabolic basis for sleep disturbances in hemodialysis patients. Such findings may be affected by factors such as dietary protein intake, length of ESRD therapy, and the presence of malnutrition, which may have multifactorial effects that influence the quality of sleep. The effect of high-flux therapies on amino acid metabolism, are however, largely unknown.

Recent studies, both in vitro and in patients, have suggested that hemodialysis may increase production of interleukins 1 and 2 (IL-1 and -2), substances that could theoretically play a role in the sleep disturbances of renal failure.[33–35] Abnormal cellular IL-1 and -2 production has been demonstrated in patients with chronic renal insufficiency and in ESRD patients treated with both peritoneal dialysis and hemodialysis.[36] Since IL-1 promotes slow wave sleep[37,38] and therapy with pharmacologic doses of IL-2 has resulted in clinical somnolence,[39] perhaps renal replacement therapies or the uremic state itself may predispose to excessive sleepiness through immunologic pathways.

If sleep apnea is related to uremic toxins, treatment of ESRD should improve symptoms and laboratory parameters of sleep disorders. This has not been consistently demonstrated to be the case. It is well appreciated, however, that these markers may be poor substitutes for the adequacy, quantity, or quality of dialytic treatment administered. Alternatively, perhaps more intensive treatment of uremia than that provided by standard outpatient hemodialysis may be necessary to improve the disordered sleep in patients with ESRD. There has been no study assessing the effects of newer high-flux and high-efficiency dialysis treatments on the prevalence and severity of SAS in patients with ESRD. Conceivably, greater clearance by these techniques of uremic toxins of large molecular size could result in improvement in the quality of sleep. It is also possible, as with some types of uremic neuropathy, that the disorder may be irreversible or relatively refractory to treatment once it is established.[23]

Clearly, further studies are necessary to identify sleep-inducing or promoting substances in patients with ESRD treated with various hemodialysis techniques. Characterizing possible differences in subjective and objective parameters of disturbed sleep would be of value, as would pursuing investigations regarding the clearance of sleep-promoting substances in patients treated with different renal replacement therapies and with different Kt/V levels (K is urea clearance, t is dialysis time, and V is volume of distribution of urea).

TREATMENT

If the diagnosis of obstructive sleep apnea is made, a thorough search for surgically correctable conditions such as tonsillar hypertrophy, micrognathia, macroglossia, and deviation of the nasal septum should be undertaken. Evaluation for concurrent metabolic disorders such as hypothyroidism should also be made. The simplest treatment modality for obstructive sleep apnea in the obese patient is weight loss, which may improve hypersomnolence, apnea time, and oxygen desaturation.[40–42] However, this approach may not lead to correction of the problem in all patients.[43]

Other possible therapeutic interventions include discontinuation of sedative drugs and alcohol[10] and avoidance of supine posture during sleep. Oxygen therapy can prolong apnea duration[44] but has also resulted in a decreased proportion of total sleep time spent in apnea. Because of the possibility of blunting hypoxemia and arousal responses, the use of oxygen therapy in patients with sleep apnea and renal disease is currently controversial.

Pharmacologic therapy may increase ventilatory drive. Protryptiline, a nonsedating tricyclic antidepressant, reduces the proportion of time spent in REM sleep. This medication has improved symptoms and parameters of disordered sleep in both uncontrolled and controlled trials.[45–47] Its mechanism of action is incompletely understood, and its clinical effect in patients is variable. Anticholinergic side effects and arrythmias may limit the usefulness of this drug.

Progesterone is a respiratory stimulant, and medroxyprogesterone acetate increases minute ventilation and chemoreceptor sensitivity in normal subjects.[48,49] Its use in those with obstructive sleep apnea has been less well defined, but it may be worth a clinical trial in selected patients. Nasal vasoconstrictors or decongestants may prove useful in some patients.[50]

Tongue-retaining devices and nasopharyngeal tubes have been employed with variable success in patients with obstructive sleep apnea, but their use is limited by discomfort.[51] The use of such mechanical devices has not been systematically studied in patients with ESRD.

Continuous positive airway pressure (CPAP) breathing[52] has proved to be an effective therapy for patients with SAS. A tightly fitting mask, with a large-bore, low-resistance tube attached to an air compressor fitted through an inspiratory port, is placed over the patient's nose. Tubing emerging from an expiratory port in the mask narrows to a fixed or variable resistance, resulting in the delivery of a regulated airway pressure.[51] Several investigations have shown CPAP to have dramatic short-term therapeutic effects and have demonstrated long-term benefit in patients with obstructive sleep apnea, which may persist after CPAP is discontinued.[50] Current commercially available devices are more sophisticated and less cumbersome than earlier devices. The newer CPAP systems are compact, lightweight, and easy for patients to use (Fig. 18-3). Nasal CPAP has become the treatment of choice for the majority of patients with obstructive sleep apnea. Continuous airflow (7 to 15 L/min) through nasal prongs may also be of value, but while less cumbersome, it may also be less effective.[17]

Ear, nose, and throat disorders, pneumothorax, and pneumomediastinum are potential complications of positive airway pressure therapy. Patients must be cooperative and well motivated to employ these therapies effectively. The use of such devices has resulted in improvement of symptoms and parameters of sleep-disordered breathing in patients with obstructive sleep apnea. The mechanism of action of positive airway pressure modalities is incompletely understood.

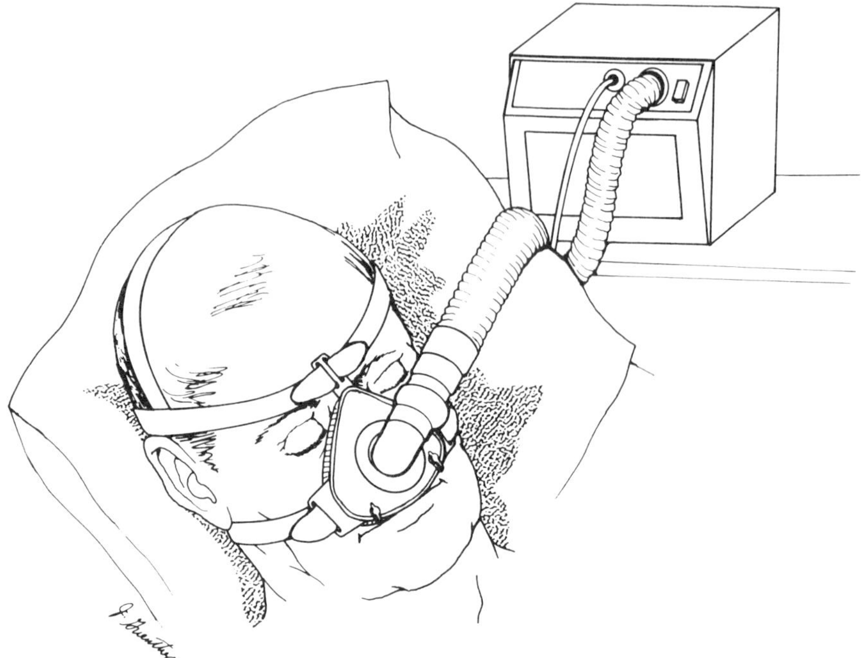

Fig. 18-3. Continuous positive airway pressure system. (From Kimmel,[14] with permission.)

There are few studies on the effect of treatment of sleep disorders in patients with SAS and ESRD. A recent report, however, suggests a beneficial effect of therapy with CPAP in ESRD patients treated with hemodialysis.[53] Further studies, specifically in patients with ESRD, are needed to evaluate the effects of such therapy.

Surgical therapy of obstructive sleep apnea may be indicated for patients who do not respond to nonpharmacologic or medical maneuvers. Surgery is directed at bypassing the site of obstruction or preventing the collapse of soft tissue structures. Uvulopalatopharyngoplasty and tonsillectomy have been employed to remove excessive soft tissue in the oropharynx. Good results have been reported,[54,55] although the response is variable. Overweight patients and subjects with severely narrowed airways tend to exhibit the best response.

Other procedures directed at reducing soft tissue obstruction have also been employed.[56–58] Tracheotomy is an effective treatment for obstructive SAS but should be reserved for patients who have failed to respond to conservative nonpharmacologic, medical, and surgical therapy and who have debilitating hypersomnolence or other serious complications of the sleep disorder. The procedure bypasses the area of obstruction and is often followed by dramatic improvement in symptoms and parameters of disordered sleep.[58] Complications related to surgery, speech impairment, and difficulties in postoperative psychological adjustment and rehabilitation may occur. Potential complications must be carefully weighted against the proposed benefits before proceeding with this operation.[13,14,50]

Treatment of the restless legs syndrome may involve increasing dialysis time or clearance, although the efficacy of this approach has never been clearly studied. Clonazepam (0.5 mg at bedtime) has been employed with variable success in treating nocturnal myoclonus and the restless legs syndrome.[59,60] Other studies have suggested opiates such as codeine and propoxyphene, and carbidopa/levodopa may diminish the magnitude of periodic leg movements.[61,62] Such evaluations have not been performed in patients with ESRD.

SUMMARY

Sleep apnea is prevalent in ESRD patients but is probably widely unrecognized. Symptoms seem to be highly predictive of the disorder in ESRD patients, perhaps in contrast to patients without renal disease.[22,25,27] A good clinical history of symptoms such as restless sleep, snoring, headaches, depression, irritability, or cognitive or personality changes and an interview with the bed partner will serve to identify ESRD patients who have a high probability of having sleep apnea. In symptomatic patients a search for anatomically correctable, drug-induced, psychological, psychiatric, or metabolic causes should be initiated. The nephrologist should ascertain that the patient is indeed well dialyzed. The use of polysomnography in a sleep laboratory should provide the clinician with an accurate diagnosis of the sleep disorder, if present.

Therapy must be individualized for each patient.[13,14,51] It is important for the nephrologist to take precautions such as avoiding the use of drugs that may suppress ventilation (such as tranquilizers, alcohol, and narcotics) in hemodialysis patients who have symptoms suggestive of a sleep disorder. CPAP breathing is an effective treatment for patients with obstructive sleep apnea. Effective diagnosis and treatment of sleep disorders is imperative if we wish to improve the quality of life of ESRD patients.

REFERENCES

1. De-Nour AK, Shanan J: Quality of life of dialysis and transplanted patients. Nephron 25:117, 1980
2. Evans RW, Manninen DL, Garrison LP et al: The quality of life of patients with end-stage renal disease. N Engl J Med 312:553, 1985
3. Strub B, Schneider-Helment D, Gnirss F, Blumberg A: Sleep disorders in patients with chronic renal insufficiency in long-term hemodialysis treatment. Schweiz Med Wochenschr 112:824, 1982

4. Barret BJ, Vavasour HM, Major A, Parfrey PS: Clinical and psychological correlates of somatic symptoms in patients on dialysis. Nephron 55:10, 1990
5. Gutman RA, Stead WW, Robinson RR: Physical activity and employment status of patients on maintenance hemodialysis. N Engl J Med 304:309, 1981
6. Richmond JM, Lindsay RM, Burton HJ et al: Psychological and physiological factors predicting the outcome on home hemodialysis. Clin Nephrol 17:109, 1982
7. Brown DJ, Craick CC, Davies SE et al: Physical, emotional and social adjustment to home dialysis. Med J Aust 11:245, 1978
8. Livesley WJ: Factors associated with psychiatric symptoms in patients undergoing chronic hemodialysis. Can J Psychiatry 8:562, 1981
9. Sacks CR, Peterson RA, Kimmel PL: Perception of illness and depression in chronic renal disease. Am J Kidney Dis 15:31, 1990
10. Roth T, Roehrs T, Zorick F, Conway W: Pharmacological effects of sedative-hypnotics, narcotic analgesics, and alcohol during sleep. Med Clin North Am 69:1281, 1985
11. Passouant P, Cadilhac J, Baldy-Moulinier M, Mion C: Nocturnal sleep in chronic uremic patients undergoing extrarenal detoxification, abstracted. Electroencephalogr Clin Neurophysiol 25:91, 1968
12. Reichenmiller HE, Reinhard U, Durr F: Sleep EEG and uraemia, abstracted. Electroencephalogr Clin Neurophysiol 30:263, 1971
13. Kimmel PL: Sleep disorders in chronic renal disease. J Nephrol 1:59, 1989
14. Kimmel PL: Sleep disorders in end-stage renal disease. Semin Dial 4:52, 1991
15. Rechtschaffen A, Kales A: A manual of standardized terminology, techniques, and scoring system for sleep stages of human subjects. Brain Information Service, Brain Research Institute, Los Angeles, 1968
16. Baker TL: Introduction to sleep and sleep disorders. Med Clin North Am 69:1123, 1985
17. Ingbar DH, Gee BL: Pathophysiology and treatment of sleep apnea. Annu Rev Med 36:365, 1985
18. Irsigler GB, Severinghaus JW: Clinical problems of ventilatory control. Annu Rev Med 31:109, 1980
19. Roffwarg HP, Chairman: Sleep Disorders Classification Committee, Association of Sleep Disorders centers. Sleep 2:1, 1980
20. Orr WC: Utilization of polysomnography in the assessment of sleep disorders. Med Clin North Am 69:1153, 1985
21. Guilleminault C: Obstructive sleep apnea. Med Clin North Am 69:1187, 1985
22. Viner S, Szalai JP, Hoffstein V: Are history and physical examination a good screening test for sleep apnea? Ann Intern Med 115:356, 1991
23. Fraser C, Arieff AI: Nervous system complications in uremia. Ann Intern Med 109:143, 1988
24. Raskin NH, Fishman RA: Neurologic disorders in renal failure. N Engl J Med 294:204, 1976
25. Millman RP, Kimmel PL, Shore ET, Wasserstein A: Sleep apnea in hemodialysis patients: the lack of testosterone effect on its pathogenesis. Nephron 40:407, 1985
26. Sandblom RE, Matsumoto AM, Schoene RB et al: Obstructive sleep apnea syndrome induced by testosterone administration. N Eng J Med 308:508, 1983
27. Kimmel PL, Miller G, Mendelson WB: Sleep apnea syndrome in chronic renal disease. Am J Med 86:308, 1989

28. Mendelson WB, Wadhwa NK, Greenberg HE et al: Effects of hemodialysis on sleep apnea syndrome in end-stage renal disease. Clin Nephrol 33:247, 1990
29. Fein AM, Niederman MS, Imbriano L, Rosen H: Reversal of sleep apnea in uremia by dialysis. Arch Intern Med 147:1355, 1987
30. Soreide E, Skeie B, Kirvela O et al: Branched-chain amino acid in chronic renal failure patients: respiratory and sleep effects. Kidney Int 40:539, 1991
31. Gulyassy PF, Aviram A, Peters JH: Evaluation of amino acid and protein requirements in chronic uremia. Arch Intern Med 126:885, 1970
32. Counahan R, El-Bishti M, Cox BD et al: Plasma amino acids in children and adolescents on hemodialysis. Kidney Int 10:471, 1976
33. Bingel M, Lonnemann G, Shaldon S et al: Human interleukin-1 production during hemodialysis. Nephron 43:161, 1986
34. Port FK, VanDeKerkhove KM, Kunkel SL, Kluger MJ: The role of dialysate in the stimulation of interleukin-1 production during clinical hemodialysis. Am J Kidney Dis 10:118, 1987
35. Luger A, Kovarik J, Stummvoll H-K et al: Blood-membrane interaction in hemodialysis leads to increased cytokine production. Kidney Int 32:84, 1987
36. Kimmel PL, Phillips TM, Phillips E, Bosch JP: Effect of renal replacement therapy on cellular cytokine production in patients with renal disease. Kidney Int 38:129, 1990
37. Dinarello CA, Mier JW: Lymphokines. N Engl J Med 317:940, 1987
38. Obal F Jr, Opp M, Cady AB et al: Interleukin 1 alpha and an interleukin 1 beta fragment are somnogenic. Am J Physiol 259:R439, 1990
39. Rosenberg SA, Lotze MT, Muul LM et al: A progress report on the treatment of 157 patients with advanced cancer using lymphokine-activated killer cells and interleukin-2 or high dose interleukin-2 alone. N Engl J Med 316:889, 1987
40. Harman EM, Wynne JW, Block AJ: The effect of weight loss on sleep disordered breathing and oxygen desaturation in normal men. Chest 82:291, 1982
41. Walsh RE, Michaelson ED, Harkleroad LE et al: Upper airway obstruction in obese patients with sleep disturbance and somnolence. Ann Intern Med 76:185, 1972
42. Browman CP, Sampson MG, Yolles SF et al: Obstructive sleep apnea and body weight. Chest 85:435, 1984
43. Guilleminault C, Eldridge FL, Tilkian A et al: Sleep apnea syndrome due to upper airway obstruction: a review of 25 cases. Arch Intern Med 137:296, 1977
44. Martin RJ, Sanders MH, Gray BA: Acute and long term ventilatory effects of hyperoxia in the adult sleep apnea syndrome. Am Rev Respir Dis 125:175, 1983
45. Conway WA, Zorick F, Piccioni P, Roth T: Protriptyline in the treatment of sleep apnea. Thorax 37:49, 1982
46. Brownell LG, West P, Sweatmen P et al: Protriptyline in obstructive sleep apnea: a double blind trial. N Engl J Med 307:1037, 1982
47. Stepanski EJ, Conway WA, Young DK et al: A double-blind trial of protryptyline in the treatment of sleep apnea syndrome. Henry Ford Hosp Med J 36:5, 1988
48. Zwillich CW, Natalino MR, Sutton FD, Weil JV: Effects of progesterone on chemosensitivity in normal men. J Lab Clin Med 69:262, 1978
49. Skatrud JB, Dempsey JA, Kaiser DG: Ventilatory response to medroxyprogesterone acetate in normal subjects: time course and mechanism. J Appl Physiol 44:939, 1978
50. Strohl KP, Cherniack NS, Gothe B: Physiologic basis of therapy for sleep apnea. Am Rev Respir Dis 134:791, 1986

51. Lombard RM, Zwillich CW: Medical therapy of obstructive sleep apnea. Med Clin North Am 69:1317, 1985
52. Sullivan CE, Berthon-Jones M, Issa FG: Reversal of obstructive sleep apnea by continuous positive airway pressure applied through the nares. Lancet 1:862, 1981
53. Benz RL, Pressman MR, Schliefer CR, Peterson DD: Sleep disorder profiles in chronic renal failure patients: successful intervention with nasal continuous positive airway pressure, abstracted. Am J Kidney Dis 20:A1, 1992
54. Fujita S, Conway WA, Sicklesteel JM et al: Evaluation of the effectiveness of uvulopalatopharyngoplasty. Laryngoscope 95:70, 1985
55. Simmons FB, Guilleminault C, Miles LE: The palatopharyngoplasty operation for snoring and sleep apnea: an interim report. Otolaryngol Head Neck Surg 92:375, 1984
56. Motta J, Guilleminault C, Schroeder JS, Dement WC: Tracheostomy and hemodynamic changes in sleep-induced apnea. Ann Intern Med 89:454, 1978
57. Guilleminault C: Obstructive sleep apnea: a review. Psychiatr Clin North Am 10:607, 1987
58. Thawley SE: Surgical treatment of obstructive sleep apnea. Med Clin North Am 69:1337, 1985
59. Jennekens FGI, Jennekens-Schinkel A: Neurological aspects of dialysis patients. p. 730. In Drukker W, Parsons FM, Maher J (eds): Replacement of Renal Function by Dialysis. 2nd Ed. Martinus Nijhoff, Boston, 1983
60. Mitler MM, Browman CP, Menn SJ et al: Nocturnal myoclonus: treatment efficacy of clonazepam and ternazepam. Sleep 9:385, 1986
61. Trzepacz PT, Violette EJ, Sateia MJ: Response to aploids in three patients with restless legs syndrome. Am J Psychiatry 141:993, 1984
62. Sandyk R, Bernick C, Lee SM et al: L-dopa in uremic patients with the restless legs syndrome. Int J Neurosci 35:233, 1987

19

Cytokines: Relevance in the Treatment of Dialysis Patients

Terry M. Phillips

INTRODUCTION

The term *cytokine* is used to characterize a collection of low molecular weight glycosylated peptides that can either activate or regulate a number of different cell types and a diversity of different biologic functions and pathways. Cytokines are part of the body's intercellular chemical communication system and may interact with cells possessing specific membranes receptors. In this manner cytokines can become both cell growth regulators and chemoattractive agents for other cells. Their regulatory functions appear to be threefold: (1) autocrine, in their regulation of their own production; (2) paracrine, in their influences over adjacent cells; and (3) endocrine, in their effects on other tissues and organs.[1] Although these entities are involved in many normal mechanistic pathways, one of their most important activities is their role in several important pathologic reactions associated with host defense mechanisms, such as inflammation and hypersensitivity.[2]

CLASSIFICATION OF CYTOKINES

Cytokines are usually classified by families, which include the interleukins (of which IL-1 to IL-8 are well defined), the colony-stimulating factors (CSF), interferons (IFN), and tumor necrosis factor (TNF). In addition, there are a number of growth factors that act as cell growth and activation regulators, such as platelet-derived growth factor (PDGF), epidermal growth factor (EGF), fibroblast growth factor (FGF), insulin-like growth factor 1 (ILGF-1 or somatomedin), transforming growth factor (TGF), and endothelin. An overview of these cytokine families and the cells responsible for their production is given in Table 19-1. However, when studying specific cytokine-associated processes such as inflammation or cell-mediated immunity, it is often more practical to classify cytokines by their cellular origin, as outlined below.

Macrophage-Derived Cytokines

Phagocytic monocytes or macrophages are a large family of circulating and tissue-resident cells (i.e., Kupffer, Langerhans [skin] and mesangial cells), which are involved in host defense mechanisms. Macrophages are capable of producing a large series of cytokines, which can act both as intercellular signals, used for cell recruitment, and as regulators of several physiologic processes.[3] Activated macrophages can secrete a wide variety of cytokines belonging to the interleukin (IL-1, IL-6, IL-8), interferon (IFN-α), colony-stimulating factor (G-CSF, M-CSF), growth factor (TGF-β, PDGF, EGF, FGF, ILGF-1), and tumor necrosis factor (TNF-α) families. The secretion of the cytokines augments both specific and nonspecific host responses to a variety of different stimuli.

Lymphocyte-Derived Cytokines

During specific immune responses, antigens are presented to thymus-derived or T lymphocytes by macrophages. Following recognition of the human leukocyte antigen (HLA) class II complex, the T lymphocytes respond

Table 19–1. Cytokine Families and their Major Cell Sources

Cytokine Family	Cellular Origin
Interleukins	
IL-1α/β	Many different cells, including macrophages, fibroblasts, and mesangial cells
IL-2	T lymphocytes
IL-3	T lymphocytes
IL-4	T lymphocytes and mast cells
IL-5	T lymphocytes
IL-6	Many different cells, including macrophages, T lymphocytes, fibroblasts, endothelial cells, and mesangial cells
IL-7	Bone marrow stomal cells and T lymphocytes
IL-8	Macrophages and endothelial and mesangial cells
Tumor Necrosis Factors	
TNF-α	Macrophages, T lymphocytes, fibroblasts, and mesangial cells
TNF-β	T and B lymphocytes
Interferons	
IFN-α	Macrophages
IFN-β	Fibroblasts
IFN-γ	T lymphocytes and natural killer cells
Colony-Stimulating Factors	
Granulocyte CSF	Macrophages, T lymphocytes, fibroblasts, and endothelial cells
Macrophage CSF	Macrophages, T lymphocytes, fibroblasts, and endothelial cells
Granulocyte-macrophage CSF	Macrophages, T lymphocytes, fibroblasts, endothelial cells, and mesangial cells
Growth Factors	
TGF-β	Macrophages, T lymphocytes, and mesangial cells
EGF	Macrophages
FGF	Macrophages, endothelial cells, and platelets
PDGF	Macrophages, endothelial cells, platelets, and mesangial cells
ILGF-1	Macrophages and mesangial cells
Endothelins	
Endothelin 1	Endothelial, mesangial, and renal epithelial cells
Endothelin 2	Endothelial cells
Endothelin 3	Endothelial cells

by generating a variety of different cytokines, including interleukins IL-2 through IL-7, TNF-α/β, IFN-γ, all three of the colony-stimulating factors (GM-CSF, M-CSF, G-CSF), and TGF-β. These cytokines, which in themselves are non-antigen-specific, serve to expand and differentiate the cellular components necessary for executing a specific cell-mediated response.[4] T-lymphocyte-derived cytokines are also responsible for the recruitment and differentiation of antibody-producing B lymphocytes.

Endothelial Cell-Derived Cytokines

Endothelial cells not only line the entire vascular system but are actively involved in the cytokine network and host defense mechanisms. In addition, they are involved in wound repair and healing. Studies have shown that endothelial cells are also involved in angiogenesis, coagulation, antigen presentation to T lymphocytes, leukocyte homing, and inflammation. When activated, they become a source of cytokine production and have been shown to secrete IL-1, IL-6, IL-8, G-CSF, M-CSF, GM-CSF, FGF, PDGF, and all three isotypes of endothelin.

Fibroblast-Derived Cytokines

Apart from the mechanical stability fibroblasts impart to tissues and organs, they are active cells and play important roles in wound healing and the formation of collagen, fibronectin, and proteoglycans. However, like endothelial cells, fibroblasts can produce cytokines such as IL-1, IL-6, TNF-α, IFN-β, and all the CSFs.

INTERACTIONS BETWEEN CYTOKINES AND THE KIDNEY

Many cytokines can act as stimuli or mitogens for glomerular cells by interacting with high-affinity receptors on cell membranes. The major interactions appear to be with mesangial cells and vascular endothelium, although endothelins have been shown to modulate certain aspects of renal physiology (Fig. 19-1).

Interactions with the Mesangium

There is growing evidence that mesangial cells are tissue-resident macrophages and can perform accessory cell functions. It has also been shown that mesangial cells can respond to extracellular cytokine stimulation in a manner similar to that of other macrophages. Both IL-1 and TNF-α have been shown to affect the glomerulus by inducing mesangial cells to produce a series of reactive molecules such as prostanglandin E_2 (PGE_2) and platelet-activating factor.[5] Studies on mesangial cell cultures demonstrated that IL-1 and TNF-α could induce mRNA expression for IL-1, IL-6, IL-8, TNF-α, GM-CSF, and M-CSF. Assays performed on supernatants from cytokine-activated mesangial cell cultures demonstrated that IL-8 was actively produced and that it caused human monocytes to become chemotactic.[6] Mesangial cells have also been shown to exhibit enhanced expression of the intercellular adhesion molecule ICAM-1 following stimulation with IFN-γ, TNF-α, and IL-1.[7]

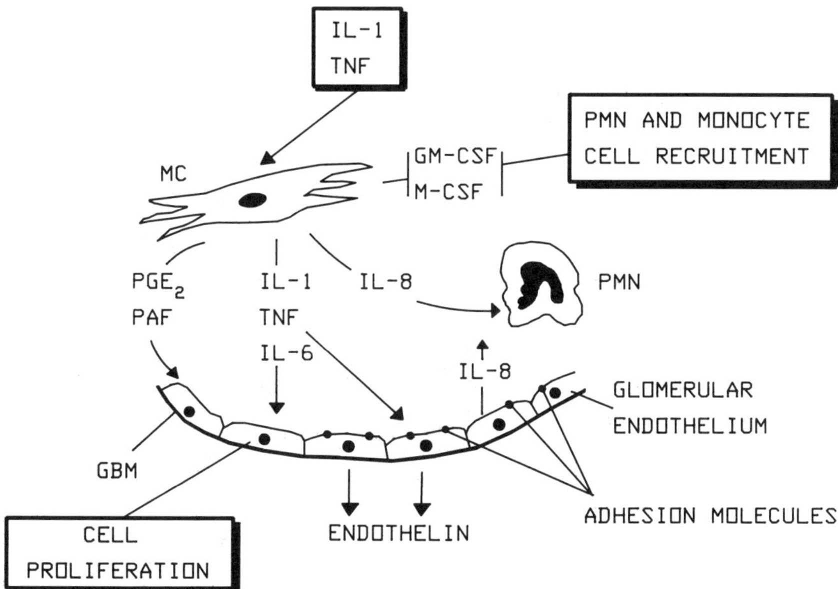

Fig. 19-1. The interactions between cytokines and the kidney glomerulus. Following stimulation by interleukin-1 (IL-1) and tumor necrosis factor (TNF), mesangial cells (MC) secrete prostaglandin E_2 (PGE_2), platelet activation factor (PAF), interleukins (IL-1, IL-6, IL-8), TNF, and colony-stimulating factors (GM-CSF, M-CSF). These cytokines induce the glomerular endothelium to proliferate, express adhesion molecules, and release IL-8, which in turn aids in the adhesion of polymorphonuclear cells (PMN) to the endothelial lining of the glomerular basement membrane (GBM) and their migration through the membrane. Activated endothelial cells also release endothelin into the circulation.

Interactions with Glomerular Endothelium

The vascular endothelium controls the migratory activity of polymorphonuclear cells through the expression of adhesion molecules. Stimulation of capillary endothelial cells by IL-1 and TNF-α lead to increased adhesion between endothelial cells and leukocytes by inducing enhanced expression of the endothelial leukocyte adhesion molecule (ELAM)-1 and the intercellular adhesion molecule (ICAM)-1.[8] Stimulation by IL-1 and TNF-α can also induce endothelial cells to produce IL-8, a cytokine that regulates the transmigrational activity of neutrophils through vessel walls.[9] IL-1, IL-6, and TNF-α can cause endothelial cell proliferation and cytokine secretion, and stimulation by these cytokines can induce superoxide and oxygen free radical release from cultured endothelial cells.[10]

Cytokine Regulation of Renal Physiology

During events such as hypoxia/anoxia, drug toxicity, or inflammation, endothelial cells become activated to synthesize and release the cytokine endothelin, which has been shown to have an important role in renal physiology and possibly also a role in the pathophysiology of renal disease. A number of activities have been ascribed to this cytokine, including vasoconstriction, modulation of ion transport, regulation of eicosanoid synthesis, and neurotransmitter function. In the kidney it has been shown to be a potent vasoconstrictor and glomerular filtration rate depressant, increasing both afferent and efferent renal vascular resistance and producing contraction of the mesangial cells, which in turn produces a reduction in the glomerular ultrafiltration coefficient (K_f). In addition, endothelin has been shown to modulate renin and atrial natriuretic peptide release.[11,12] Although the role of endothelin in renal disease is still unclear, increased levels have been associated with postischemic renal failure, cyclosporin toxicity, and hypertension in renal disease patients.[12]

THE ROLE OF CYTOKINES IN RENAL DISEASE

Although the relationship of cytokines to the pathogenesis of renal disease is still unclear, there are two major areas in which cytokine activity is clearly important—localized inflammation, especially in glomerulonephritis,[13] and the formation of scar tissue during wound healing and repair.

Cytokines and Tissue Inflammation

During infections macrophage stimulation can induce the synthesis of cytokine mRNAs followed by the secretion of IL-1, IL-6, TNF-α, M-CSF, G-CSF, and GM-CSF, and it has been shown that many different cells contain small or minute amounts of cytokine mRNA, even in the absence of any form of stimulation.[14] This may represent a mechanism for rapid cytokine production in response to inflammatory stimuli. Activated macrophages produce more IL-1 and TNF-α than do their resting counterparts, which may reflect their exposure to greater concentrations of stimuli at the inflammation site. Other factors, such as complement and immune complexes, that are present at the inflammation site, stimulate cytokine production by their interactions with macrophages.[15] TNF-α and IL-1 directly induce the production of IL-1, TNF-α, IL-6, and the CSF family by macrophages, fibroblasts, and endothelial cells.[16] GM-CSF and IFN-γ enhance production of TNF-α and IL-1 as well as M-CSF and G-CSF, and TNF-α and IL-1 induce production of prostaglandins, particularly PGE_2, which inhibits their production and reduces the effects of IL-1 on T-cell activation. Excessive levels of IL-1 and TNF-α have the ability to regulate the expression of their own receptors. Cytokines, especially IL-1, TNF-α, and TGF-β, are involved in the recruitment and activation of phagocytic monocytes during inflammation. Both IL-1 and TNF-α can affect bone marrow release of myeloid cells, and injection of either of these agents in experimental conditions has been shown to induce the release of mature neutrophils into the circulation.[17] IL-1 and TNF-α

Table 19–2. The Role of Cytokines in Inflammation and Hypersensitivity

Cytokine	Event
IL-1	Alterations in vascular permeability
IL-1/TNF-α	Febrile response
IL-1/TNF-α	Enhanced leukocyte adherence to endothelium
IL-1/TNF-α	Induction of procoagulant state in endothelium
IL-1/TNF-α/IFN-γ	Induction of respiratory burst, free radical generation, and secretion of hydrolytic enzymes by neutrophils and monocytes; activation of natural killer cells
IL-1/TNF-α/IFN-γ	Granuloma formation
IL-2	Activation of cell-mediated immune responses
IL-3	Activation of mast cells and histamine release
IL-3	Recruitment of granulocytes and phagocytic monocytes from the bone marrow
IL-4/IL-5	Regulation of antibody production
IL-6	Release of acute-phase proteins
IL-8	Chemotactic stimuli for neutrophils and monocytes
CSFs	Recruitment of phagocytes from the bone marrow
Endothelin	Vascular constriction

can also induce both macrophages and neutrophils to increase superoxide generation, while TNF-α can increase granulocyte metabolism and affect specific neutrophil granules (Table 19-2).

Cytokines and Glomerulonephritis

The role of cytokines in the pathogenesis of human renal disease is evolving, and apart from the well documented roles of IL-1, IL-6, and TNF-α in localized and systemic inflammation,[18] there have been reports of cytokine production by mesangial cells in glomerulonephritis.[19,20] Other reports have shown that cultured mesangial cells can release oxygen free radicals following stimulation by IL-1 and TNF-α[21] and that the deposition of soluble immune complexes can stimulate human glomerular basement membrane to secrete IL-1 and TNF-α.[22] Patients with IgA nephropathy have been shown to possess increased levels of IL-2 and soluble IL-2 receptor, indicating a cell-mediated immune response,[23,24] while patients with nephrotic syndrome exhibit high levels of TNF-α.[25] In other studies patients with IgA mesangial proliferative glomerulonephritis demonstrated a selective increase in the production of IL-6.[26]

The Role of Cytokines in Renal Tissue Repair

There is evidence that cytokines are involved in tissue repair and remodeling of the injury site following inflammation or physical injury.[1] Studies have shown that macrophages can release several factors that are mitogenic to fibroblasts. IL-1, TNF-α, FGF, and TGF-β can promote fibroblast proliferation and collagen synthesis as well as the synthesis of proteases from fibro-

Table 19–3. Interactions between Cytokines and Fibroblasts in Wound Healing

Cytokine	Reaction
IL-1	Cell proliferation, secretion of PGE_2, secretion of collagen, secretion of proteoglycans, release of cytokines, expression of adhesion molecules
TNF-α	Cell proliferation, secretion of PGE_2, release of cytokines, secretion of collagenase
IFN-γ	Suppression of collagen secretion, HLA class II expression, expression of adhesion molecules
TGF-β	Cell proliferation, collagen secretion
FGF	Cell proliferation

blasts.[27] IL-1 and TNF-α induce the secretion of PGE_2 and under certain circumstances can induce secretion of collagenase. IFN-γ has been shown to stimulate fibroblasts to express HLA class II antigens and during inflammation to express the adhesion molecule ICAM-1, leading to lymphocyte adhesion to fibroblasts within the inflamed area. However, during the recovery phase, interferons act as mediators for the suppression of collagen synthesis[27] (Table 19-3).

DIALYSIS AND CYTOKINE ACTIVATION

Activation of cytokine production during hemodialysis can be caused by several different parameters, such as direct interaction with the dialyzer membrane, hypersensitivity to components within the membrane, complement activation, or the presence of endotoxins in the dialysis fluid or water supply[28,29] (Fig. 19-2). The effects of hemodialysis on cytokine production, especially IL-1, was first postulated by Henderson et al[30] who stated that adverse effects of dialysis were attributable to IL-1 production. This hypothesis has been supported by other workers, who have shown that IL-1 but not TNF-α is elevated during the initial hemodialysis treatment but that both cytokines are significantly elevated in long-term hemodialysis patients. These studies also demonstrated that IL-1 alone is elevated post-treatment, whereas TNF-α levels remain the same pre- and postdialysis.[31]

The role played by the dialysis membrane in polymorphonuclear neutrophil (PMN) and monocyte activation is still unclear. Reports on complement activation and its effects on PMN function have indicated that membranes composed of several different materials, especially cuprophane, are able to activate PMNs through complement activation within the membrane.[32] In such cases, generation of the anaphylatoxic complement component C5a can stimulate cytokine release by macrophages and histamine release by basophils and mast cells,[33] thus leading to inflammation and hypersensitivity reactions. Other workers have recently reported that hemodialysis patients in stable condition demonstrated no increases in IL-4, IL-6, TNF-α, or GM-CSF either during or after treatment with either new or reused

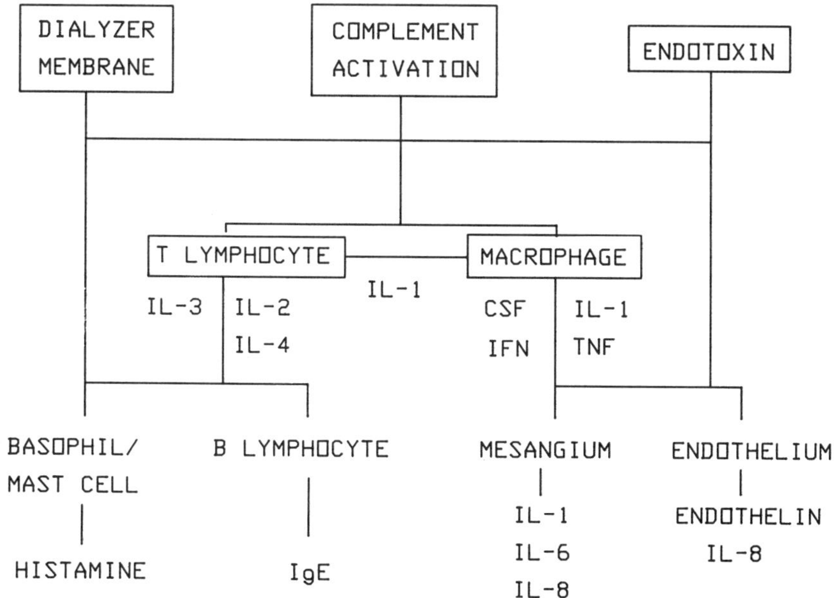

Fig. 19-2. Pathways leading to the production and secretion of cytokines during hemodialysis via theoretical interactions between dialyzer membranes, activated complement, endotoxin, and cytokine-producing cells.

polyacrylonitrile or cuprophane membranes. However, slight elevations in IL-1, IL-2, and IL-2 receptor were noted in 6 of 10 patients with renal disease when compared with normal subjects. In another study IL-2 was shown to be elevated in hemodialysis patients both pre- and post-treatment; in these patients IL-1 and IL-2 levels rose by approximately 50 percent following treatment. A similar situation was described in CAPD patients, where post-treatment samples demonstrated elevations of approximately 40 percent for IL-1 and 30 percent for IL-2. The IL-2 to IL-1 ratio was elevated in all patients with renal disease when compared with a control group[35] (Fig. 19-3).

In dialysis patients exhibiting allergic reactions, to components of either the membrane or dialysis fluid, elevations in IL-2, IL-3, IL-4, and IL-5 can be expected. IL-3 is the major cytokine responsible for promoting mast cell growth and differentiation, while IL-4 has been shown to induce B lymphocyte immunoglobulin switching to the secretion of IgE and enhances the expression of IgE Fc receptors.[36] IL-5 is an important factor for the growth and differentiation of eosinophils.[36]

During dialysis, patients often undergo imbalances in certain micronutrients such as zinc, copper and magnesium. All of these minerals can effect immunologic activity, including cytokine production. Zinc is perhaps the most important element and has been shown to be decreased in patients undergoing hemodialysis and continuous ambulatory peritoneal dialysis.[37]

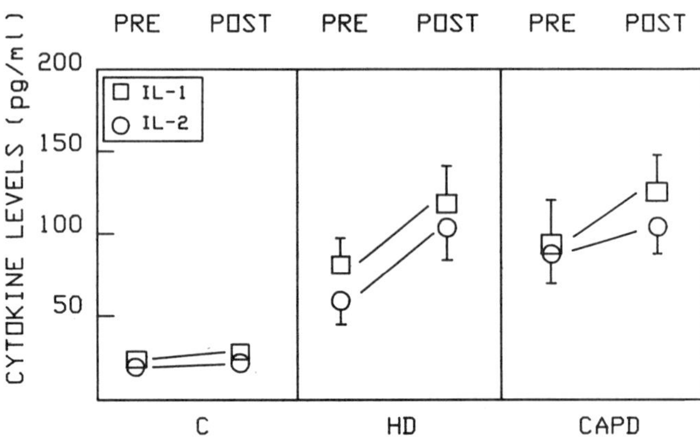

Fig. 19-3. Measurement of cytokine levels pre- and postdialysis. Comparison of results obtained from a group of hemodialysis (HD) and peritoneal dialysis (CAPD) patients following a single treatment session. Levels are compared with those of a control group (C) of healthy individuals.

Zinc concentrations can affect IL-1 production by macrophages in vitro, which suggests the potential importance of this element in immune or inflammatory regulation. Magnesium is another mineral that is lost during dialysis and treatment with diuretics. In experimental models hypomagnesemia has been shown to induce irritability associated with an allergic or proinflammatory state. Blood and urinary histamine levels were shown to be elevated in the magnesium-deficient animals, especially following an immunoglobulin E-eliciting antigenic challenge.[38] These findings suggest that magnesium deficiency can augment a hypersensitive state and enhance activation of IL-2, IL-3, IL-4, and IL-5.

REFERENCES

1. Whicher JT, Evans SW: Cytokines and disease. Clin Chem 36:1269, 1990
2. Whitacre CC: Immunology: a state of the art lecture. Ann N Y Acad Sci 594:1, 1990
3. Durum SK, Oppenheim JJ: Macrophage-derived mediators: interleukin 1, tumor necrosis factor, interleukin 6, interferon, and related cytokines. p. 639. In Paul WE (ed): Fundamental Immunology. Raven Press, New York, 1989
4. Gillis S: T-cell-derived lymphokines. p. 621. In Paul WE: Fundamental Immunology. Raven Press, New York, 1989
5. Topley N, Floege J, Wessel K et al: Prostaglandin E_2 production is synergistically increased in cultured human glomerular mesangial cells by combination of IL-1 and tumor necrosis factor. J Immunol 143:1989, 1989
6. Zoja C, Wang JM, Bettoni S et al: Interleukin-1 beta and tumor necrosis factor-alpha induce gene expression and production of leukocyte chemotactic factors, colony-stimulating factors, and interleukin-6 in human mesangial cells. Am J Pathol 138:991, 1991

7. Brannan DC, Jaynikar AH, Takai F et al: Mesangial cell accessory functions: mediation by intercellular adhesion molecules. Kidney Int 38:1038, 1990
8. Jutila MA, Berg EL, Kishimoto TK et al: Inflammation-induced endothelial cell adhesion to lymphocytes, neutrophils, and monocytes. Role of homing receptors and other adhesion molecules. Transplantation 48:727, 1989
9. Huber AR, Kunkel SL, Todd RF et al: Regulation of transendothelial neutrophil migration by endogenous interleukin-8. Science 254:99, 1991
10. Matsubara T, Ziff M: Increased superoxide anion release from human endothelial cells in response to cytokines. J Immunol 137:3295, 1986
11. Rubanyi GM, Parker Botelho LH: Endothelins. FASEB J 5:2713, 1991
12. Kon V, Badr KF: Biological actions and pathophysiologic significance of endothelin in the kidney. Kidney Int 40:1, 1991
13. Williams JD, Davies M: Eicosanoids and cytokines in glomerular injury. p. 123. In Pusey CD (ed): Immunology of Renal Diseases. Kluwer, Boston, 1991
14. Carlos TM, Harlan JM: Membrane proteins involved in phagocyte adherence to endothelium. Immunol Rev 114:5, 1990
15. Ramos BF, Qureshi R, Olsen KM, et al: The importance of mast cells for the neutrophil influx in immune complex-mediated peritonitis in mice. J Immunol 145:1868, 1990
16. Nathan CF: Secretory products of macrophages. J Clin Invest 79:319, 1987
17. Goldblum SE: The role of cytokines in injury. p. 191. In Kimball ES (ed): Cytokines and Inflammation. CRC Press, Boca Raton, Florida, 1991
18. Emery P, Salmon M: The immune response. 2. Systemic mediators of inflammation. Br J Hosp Med 45:164, 1991
19. Wardla EH: Cytokine growth factors and glomerulonephritis. Nephron 57:257, 1991
20. Weis JH, Yamashita W, Liu YJ et al: The biology of mesangial cells in glomerulonephritis. Proc Soc Exp Biol Med 195:150, 1990
21. Radaka HH, Maier B, Topley N et al: Interleukin 1-alpha and tumor necrosis factor-alpha induce oxygen radical production in mesangial cells. Kidney Int 37:767, 1990
22. Vissara MD, Fantana JD, Wiggins R et al: Glomerular basement membrane-containing immune complexes stimulate tumor necrosis factor and interleukin-1 production by human monocytes. Am J Pathol 134:1, 1989
23. Lai KN, Laung JD, Lai FM et al: T-lymphocyte activation in IgA nephropathy: serum-soluble interleukin-2 receptor levels, interleukin-2 production, and interleukin-2 receptor suppression by cultured lymphocytes. J Clin Immunol 9:485, 1989
24. Schana FP, Mastrolitti G, Jirillo E et al: Increased production of interleukin-2 and IL-2 receptor in primary IgA nephropathy. Kidney Int 35:875, 1989
25. Suranyi MG, Quiza C, Gausch A et al: Cytokine levels in patients with the nephrotic syndrome, abstracted. Kidney Int 37:445(A), 1990
26. Dohi K, Iwano M, Muraguchi A et al: The prognostic significance of urinary interleukin 6 in IgA nephropathy. Clin Nephrol 35:1, 1991
27. Piela TH, Korn JH: Lymphokines and cytokines in the reparative process. p. 255. In Cohen S (ed): Lymphokines and the Immune Response. CRC Press, Boca Raton, Florida, 1990
28. Bingle M, Lonnemann G, Koch KM et al: Plasma interleukin-1 activity during hemodialysis: the influence of dialysis membranes. Nephron 50:273, 1988
29. Lonnemann G, Bingle M, Floege J et al: Detection of endotoxin-like interleukin-1 inducing activity during in vitro hemodialysis. Kidney Int 33:29, 1988

30. Henderson LW, Koch KM, Dinarello CA et al: Hemodialysis hypotension: the interleukin hypothesis. Blood Purif 1:3, 1983
31. Descamps-Latscha B, Herblin A, Nguyen AT et al: Respective influence of uremia and hemodialysis on whole blood phagocyte oxidative metabolism, and circulating interleukin-1 and tumor necrosis factor. p. 183. In Horl WH, Schollmeyer PJ (eds): New Aspects of Human Polymorphonuclear Leukocytes. Plenum, New York, 1991
32. Bohler J, Donauer J, Schollmeyer P et al: Blood flow dependent granulocyte activation in membranes with and without complement activation. p. 215. In Horl WH, Schollmeyer PJ (eds): New Aspects of Human Polymorphonuclear Leukocytes. Plenum, New York, 1991
33. Lewis SL: C5a receptors on neutrophils and monocytes from chronic dialysis patients. p. 167. In Horl WH, Schollmeyer PJ (eds): New Aspects of Human Polymorphonuclear Leukocytes. Plenum, New York, 1991
34. Vaziri ND, Kaupke CJ, Yousefi S et al: Cytokine levels during dialysis. ASAIO Trans 37:M389, 1991
35. Kimmel PL, Phillips TM, Phillips EA et al: Effect of renal replacement therapy on cellular cytokine production in patients with renal disease. Kidney Int 38:129, 1990
36. Herrod HG: Interleukins in immunology and allergic diseases. Ann Allergy 63:269, 1989
37. Kimmel PL, Phillips TM, Lew SQ et al: Zinc and peritoneal macrophage function. p. 191. In La Greca G, Ronco C, Feriani M et al (eds): Peritoneal Dialysis. Wichtig Editore, Milan, 1991
38. Wei W, Frantz KB: A synergism of antigen challenge and severe magnesium deficiency on blood and urinary histamine levels in rats. J Am Coll Nutr 9:616, 1990

Index

Page numbers followed by f *indicate figures; those followed by* t *indicate tables*